T0263231

Human Milk for Preterm Infants

Editors

FRANCIS B. MIMOUNI
BERTHOLD KOLETZKO

CLINICS IN PERINATOLOGY

www.perinatology.theclinics.com

Consulting Editor
LUCKY JAIN

March 2017 • Volume 44 • Number 1

ELSEVIER

1600 John F. Kennedy Boulevard • Suite 1800 • Philadelphia, Pennsylvania, 19103-2899

http://www.theclinics.com

CLINICS IN PERINATOLOGY Volume 44, Number 1
March 2017 ISSN 0095-5108, ISBN-13: 978-0-323-50983-1

Editor: Kerry Holland
Developmental Editor: Casey Potter

Clinics in Perinatology (ISSN 0095-5108) is published quarterly by Elsevier Inc., 360 Park Avenue South, New York, NY 10010-1710. Months of issue are March, June, September, and December. Business and Editorial Offices: 1600 John F. Kennedy Blvd., Ste. 1800, Philadelphia, PA 19103-2899. Customer Service Office: 3251 Riverport Lane, Maryland Heights, MO 63043. Periodicals postage paid at New York, NY and additional mailing offices. Subscription prices are $299.00 per year (US individuals), $532.00 per year (US institutions), $350.00 per year (Canadian individuals), $651.00 per year (Canadian institutions), $433.00 per year (international individuals), $651.00 per year (international institutions), $100.00 per year (US students), and $195.00 per year (Canadian and international students). International air speed delivery is included in all Clinics subscription prices. All prices are subject to change without notice. **POSTMASTER:** Send address changes to *Clinics in Perinatology*, Elsevier Health Sciences Division, Subscription Customer Service, 3251 Riverport Lane, Maryland Heights, MO 63043. **Customer Service: Telephone: 1-800-654-2452** (U.S. and Canada); **1-314-447-8871** (outside U.S. and Canada). **Fax: 1-314-447-8029. E-mail: journalscustomerservice-usa@elsevier.com** (for print support); **journalsonlinesupport-usa@elsevier.com** (for online support).

Reprints. For copies of 100 or more, of articles in this publication, please contact the Commercial Reprints Department, Elsevier Inc., 360 Park Avenue South, New York, NY 10010-1710. Tel. 212-633-3874; Fax: 212-633-3820; E-mail: reprints@elsevier.com.

Clinics in Perinatology is also published in Spanish by McGraw-Hill Interamericana Editores S.A., P.O. Box 5-237, 06500 Mexico D.F., Mexico.

Clinics in Perinatology is covered in *MEDLINE/PubMed (Index Medicus) Current Contents, Excepta Medica, BIOSIS and ISI/BIOMED.*

Contributors

CONSULTING EDITOR

LUCKY JAIN, MD, MBA
Richard W. Blumberg Professor and Interim Chairman, Emory University School of Medicine, Department of Pediatrics, Executive Medical Director and Interim Chief Academic Officer, Children's Healthcare of Atlanta, Atlanta, Georgia

EDITORS

FRANCIS B. MIMOUNI, MD, FAAP
Chief, Department of Neonatology, Shaare Zedek Medical Center, Jerusalem, Israel; President, Israeli Board of Pediatrics; Secretary General, International Neonatology Association; Professor Emeritus, Sackler Faculty of Medicine, Tel Aviv Sourasky Medical Center, Tel Aviv University, Tel Aviv, Israel

BERTHOLD KOLETZKO, MD, PhD
Professor of Paediatrics, Division of Metabolism and Nutritional Medicine, Dr von Hauner Childrens Hospital, University of Munich Medical Center, Ludwig-Maximilians-Universität Munich, Munich, Germany

AUTHORS

LARS BODE, PhD
Associate Professor, Department of Pediatrics, University of California, San Diego; Director, Mother-Milk-Infant Center of Research Excellence, School of Medicine, University of California, San Diego, La Jolla, California

RACHEL BUFFIN, MD
Neonatal Unit, Hôpital de la Croix-Rousse; Rhone-Alpes Auvergneregional Human Milk Bank, Hôpital de la Croix-Rousse, Lyon, France

NICOLE THERESA CACHO, DO, MPH
Assistant Professor, Division of Neonatology, Department of Pediatrics, University of Florida, Gainesville, Florida

HANS DEMMELMAIR, PhD
Professor, Division of Metabolism and Nutritional Medicine, Dr von Hauner Childrens Hospital, University of Munich Medical Center, Ludwig-Maximilians-Universität Munich, Munich, Germany

CATHERINE J. FIELD, RD, PhD
Department of Agricultural, Food and Nutritional Science, University of Alberta, Edmonton, Alberta, Canada

CHRISTOPH FUSCH, MD, PhD, FRCPC
Professor of Pediatrics, Division of Neonatology, McMaster University, Hamilton, Ontario, Canada; Department of Pediatrics, Paracelsus Medical School, General Hospital of Nuremberg, Nuremberg, Germany

GERHARD FUSCH, PhD
Division of Neonatology, Department of Pediatrics, McMaster University, Hamilton, Ontario, Canada

RANGMAR GOELZ, MD
Department of Neonatology, University Children's Hospital, Tuebingen, Germany

KLAUS HAMPRECHT, MD, PhD
Professor, Institute of Medical Virology, University Hospital of Tuebingen, Tuebingen, Germany

BEN T. HARTMANN, PhD
Perron Rotary Express Mothers' Milk Bank, Neonatology Clinical Care Unit, King Edward Memorial Hospital, Subiaco, Western Australia, Australia; Centre for Neonatal Research and Education, The University of Western Australia, Perth, Western Australia, Australia

TRICIA J. JOHNSON, PhD
Professor, Health Systems Management, Rush University Medical Center, Chicago, Illinois

BERTHOLD KOLETZKO, MD, PhD
Professor of Paediatrics, Division of Metabolism and Nutritional Medicine, Dr von Hauner Childrens Hospital, University of Munich Medical Center, Ludwig-Maximilians-Universität Munich, Munich, Germany

GYNTER KOTRRI, BHSc
Division of Neonatology, Department of Pediatrics, McMaster University, Hamilton, Ontario, Canada

CELIA KWAN, BHSc
Division of Neonatology, Department of Pediatrics, McMaster University, Hamilton, Ontario, Canada

BO LÖNNERDAL, PhD
Distinguished Professor Emeritus of Nutrition and Internal Medicine, Department of Nutrition, University of California, Davis, California

BODIL M. LARSEN, RD, PhD
Department of Agricultural, Food and Nutritional Science; Department of Pediatrics, Nutrition Services, Alberta Health Services, University of Alberta, Edmonton, Alberta, Canada

BEATRICE E. LECHNER, MD
Assistant Professor, Department of Pediatrics, Women and Infants Hospital of Rhode Island; Department of Pediatrics, Alpert School of Medicine, Brown University, Providence, Rhode Island

ERIN D. LEWIS, PhD
Department of Agricultural, Food and Nutritional Science, University of Alberta, Edmonton, Alberta, Canada

RONIT LUBETZKY, MD
Sackler Faculty of Medicine, Tel Aviv University; Department of Pediatrics, Dana Dwek Children's Hospital, Tel Aviv Sourasky Medical Center, Tel Aviv, Israel

DROR MANDEL, MD
Sackler Faculty of Medicine, Tel Aviv University; Department of Neonatology, Dana Dwek Children's Hospital, Tel Aviv Sourasky Medical Center, Tel Aviv, Israel

PAULA P. MEIER, PhD, RN
Director, Clinical Research and Lactation, Neonatal Intensive Care Unit, Professor, Women, Children, and Family Nursing, Rush University Medical Center, Rush University; Professor, Pediatrics, Rush Medical College, Chicago, Illinois

FRANCIS B. MIMOUNI, MD, FAAP
Chief, Department of Neonatology, Shaare Zedek Medical Center, Jerusalem, Israel; President, Israeli Board of Pediatrics; Secretary General, International Neonatology Association; Professor Emeritus, Sackler Faculty of Medicine, Tel Aviv Sourasky Medical Center, Tel Aviv University, Tel Aviv, Israel

SARA MOUKARZEL, PhD
Postdoctoral Fellow, Department of Pediatrics, University of California, San Diego; Executive Director, Mother-Milk-Infant Center of Research Excellence, School of Medicine, University of California, San Diego, La Jolla, California

NATALIE NATHAN, BSc
Sackler Faculty of Medicine, Tel Aviv University; Department of Pediatrics, Dana Dwek Children's Hospital, Tel Aviv Sourasky Medical Center, Tel Aviv, Israel

JOSEF NEU, MD
Professor, Division of Neonatology, Department of Pediatrics, University of Florida, Gainesville, Florida

LESLIE A. PARKER, PhD, ARNP
Clinical Associate Professor, Biobehavioral Nursing Science, College of Nursing, University of Florida, Gainesville, Florida

ALOKA L. PATEL, MD
Associate Professor, Department of Pediatrics-Neonatology, Rush University Medical Center; Department of Women, Children, and Family Nursing, Rush University College of Nursing, Rush University, Chicago, Illinois

JEAN-CHARLES PICAUD, MD, PhD
President of French Human Milk Bank Association (ADLF) and European Milk Bank Association (EMBA), Neonatal Unit; Rhone-Alpes Auvergneregional Human Milk Bank, Hôpital de la Croix-Rousse, Lyon, France; Lyon Sud Charles Merieux School of Medicine, Université Claude Bernard Lyon 1; Rhone-Alpes Human Nutrition Research Center, Hôpital Lyon Sud, Pierre-Bénite, France; European Milk Bank Association (EMBA), Milano, Italy

CAROLINE RICHARD, RD, PhD
Department of Agricultural, Food and Nutritional Science, University of Alberta, Edmonton, Alberta, Canada

BEVERLY ROSSMAN, PhD, RN
Assistant Professor, Department of Women, Children, and Family Nursing, Rush University College of Nursing, Rush University, Chicago, Illinois

BETTY R. VOHR, MD
Professor, Department of Pediatrics, Women and Infants Hospital of Rhode Island; Department of Pediatrics, Alpert School of Medicine, Brown University, Providence, Rhode Island

SIVAN YOCHPAZ, MD
Department of Pediatrics, Dana Dwek Children's Hospital, Tel Aviv Sourasky Medical Center, Tel Aviv, Israel

EKHARD E. ZIEGLER, MD
Department of Pediatrics, University of Iowa, Iowa City, Iowa

Contents

Best practices translating the evidence for high-dose human milk (HM) feeding for preterm infants during neonatal intensive care unit (NICU) hospitalization have been described, but their implementation has been compromised. Although the rates of any HM feeding have increased over the last decade, efforts to help mothers maintain HM provision through to NICU discharge have remained problematic. Special emphasis should be placed on prioritizing the early lactation period of coming to volume so that mothers have sufficient HM volume to achieve their personal HM feeding goals. Donor HM does not provide the same risk reduction as own mother's HM.

The immune system of preterm infants is immature, placing them at increased risk for serious immune-related complications. Human milk provides a variety of immune protective and immune maturation factors that are beneficial to the preterm infant's poorly developed immune system. The most studied immune components in human milk include antimicrobial proteins, maternal leukocytes, immunoglobulins, cytokines and chemokines, oligosaccharides, gangliosides, nucleotides, and long-chain polyunsaturated fatty acids. There is growing evidence that these components contribute to the lower incidence of immune-related conditions in the preterm infant. Therefore, provision of these components in human milk, donor milk, or formula may provide immunologic benefits.

This article summarizes evidence regarding whether a donor human milk (DHM) and/or an exclusively human milk (EHM) diet decreases the incidence of necrotizing enterocolitis (NEC) and the dose of human milk (HM) necessary to reduce the risk of NEC in premature infants. Additional research regarding protection afforded by DHM and EHM is necessary as well as research elucidating the exact dose of HM necessary for NEC risk reduction. Research is also needed to determine whether there is a

raw breast milk (BM). Actual data support negative influence on long-term cognitive development. Concerning prevention, only heat inactivation eliminates virus infectivity, and short-term heat inactivation is most preservative; this can be applied effectively under routine conditions. Short-term heat inactivation for 5 minutes at 62°C maintains the benefits of feeding BM without the disadvantages of CMV transmission.

The provision of donor human milk avoids the risks associated with early infant formula feeding only when maternal milk is unavailable. Donor human milk-banking services (DHMBS) should provide an effective clinical service that causes no harm to donors or recipients. This article aims to begin the process of defining the minimum acceptable standard required for safe donor human milk banking in the neonatal unit. An assessment process is established to consider the potential risks and benefits of milk banking to both recipients and donors. These risks and benefits define the clinical responsibility of DHMBS and their social responsibility.

Animal studies show that the lactation period contributes to metabolic programming of the offspring and that oral leptin and insulin show bioactivity. Stage of lactation, duration of gestation, maternal body composition, and maternal diet seem to influence the concentrations of small molecules in human milk. Variability of small molecule concentrations seems higher in preterm milk than in term milk. Insulin in human milk shows concentrations similar to plasma. Leptin concentration is lower in milk than in plasma and reflects maternal body mass index. Early in lactation, leptin could contribute to mediating the association between maternal and infant body composition.

This study is a systematic review of the macronutrient and energy composition of preterm human milk to enable the practicing neonatologist to make informed nutritional decisions in preterm infants. Meta-analyses were conducted in all the studies that reported total energy, true protein, fat, and lactose. Protein content decreased massively (by one-half) and significantly from day 1 to 3 at week 10 to 12. There was a significant linear increase in fat, lactose, and energy content during the same timeframe. Theoretic calculations on energy and macronutrient intake of preterm infants must be made according to a lactation time-specific manner.

There is evidence that multinutrient fortification of human milk increases in-hospital growth of preterm infants, but fortification has not been shown to improve long-term growth and neurodevelopmental outcome. We aimed to ascertain whether randomized controlled trials have determined the effect of early versus late introduction of fortifiers on growth and/or other outcomes, and have compared the efficacy/adverse effects of human milk–based versus cow milk–based fortifiers. We conclude that there is little evidence that early introduction of human milk fortification affects important outcomes, and limited evidence that a bovine fortifier places the infant at a higher risk of NEC.

Human milk contains many bioactive proteins that are likely to be involved in the better outcomes of breast-fed infants compared with those fed infant formula. Bovine milk proteins or protein fractions may be able to provide some of these benefits and may, therefore, be used for preterm infants. Recombinant human milk proteins are likely to exert bioactivities similar to those of the native human milk proteins, but considerable research is needed before they can be used in routine care of preterm infants.

Human milk oligosaccharides (HMOs) are a group of approximately 200 different unconjugated sugar structures in human milk proposed to support infant growth and development. Data from several preclinical animal studies and human cohort studies suggest HMOs reduce preterm infant mortality and morbidity by shaping the gut microbiome and protecting against necrotizing enterocolitis, candidiasis, and several other immune-related diseases. Current feeding practices and clinical algorithms do not consider infant HMO intake when assessing dietary adequacy or disease risk. Advancements in HMO analytical methodologies and HMO synthesis facilitate cohort and intervention studies to investigate which particular HMOs are most relevant in supporting preterm infants.

Human milk analyzers can measure macronutrient content in native breast milk to tailor adequate supplementation with fortifiers. This article reviews all studies using milk analyzers, including (i) evaluation of devices, (ii) the impact of different conditions on the macronutrient analysis of human milk, and (iii) clinical trials to improve growth. Results lack consistency, potentially due to systematic errors in the validation of the device, or pre-analytical sample preparation errors like homogenization. It is crucial to introduce good laboratory and clinical practice when using these devices, otherwise a non-validated clinical usage can severely affect growth outcomes of infants.

PROGRAM OBJECTIVE

The goal of *Clinics in Perinatology* is to keep practicing perinatologists, neonatologists, obstetricians, practicing physicians and residents up to date with current clinical practice in perinatology by providing timely articles reviewing the state of the art in patient care.

TARGET AUDIENCE

Perinatologists, neonatologists, obstetricians, practicing physicians, residents and healthcare professionals who provide patient care utilizing findings from *Clinics in Perinatology*.

LEARNING OBJECTIVES

Upon completion of this activity, participants will be able to:
1. Review the macronutrient and hormonal components of human milk.
2. Discuss developmental outcomes of infants fed human milk.
3. Recognize the importance of human milk for preterm infants.

ACCREDITATION

The Elsevier Office of Continuing Medical Education (EOCME) is accredited by the Accreditation Council for Continuing Medical Education (ACCME) to provide continuing medical education for physicians.

The EOCME designates this enduring material for a maximum of 15 *AMA PRA Category 1 Credit*(s)™. Physicians should claim only the credit commensurate with the extent of their participation in the activity.

All other health care professionals requesting continuing education credit for this enduring material will be issued a certificate of participation.

DISCLOSURE OF CONFLICTS OF INTEREST

The EOCME assesses conflict of interest with its instructors, faculty, planners, and other individuals who are in a position to control the content of CME activities. All relevant conflicts of interest that are identified are thoroughly vetted by EOCME for fair balance, scientific objectivity, and patient care recommendations. EOCME is committed to providing its learners with CME activities that promote improvements or quality in healthcare and not a specific proprietary business or a commercial interest.

The planning committee, staff, authors and editors listed below have identified no financial relationships or relationships to products or devices they or their spouse/life partner have with commercial interest related to the content of this CME activity:
Lars Bode, PhD; Rachel Buffin, MD; Nicole Theresa Cacho, DO, MPH; Hans Demmelmair, PhD; Catherine J. Field, RD, PhD; Anjali Fortna; Christoph Fusch, MD, PhD, FRCPC; Gerhard Fusch, PhD; Rangmar Goelz, MD; Klaus Hamprecht, MD, PhD; Ben T. Hartmann, PhD; Kerry Holland; Lucky Jain, MD, MBA; Tricia J. Johnson, PhD; Berthold Koletzko, MD, PhD; Gynter Kotrri, BHSc; Celia Kwan, BHSc; Bodil M. Larsen, RD, PhD; Beatrice E. Lechter, MD; Erin D. Lewis, PhD; Ronit Lubetzky, MD; Dror Mandel, MD; Paula P. Meier, PhD, RN; Francis B. Mimouni, MD, FAAP; Sara Moukarzel, PhD; Palani Murugesan; Natalie Nathan, BSc; Josef Neu, MD; Leslie A. Parker, PhD, ARNP; Aloka L. Patel, MD; Jean-Charles Picaud, MD, PhD; Caroline Richard, RD, PhD; Beverly Rossman, PhD, RN; Betty R. Vohr, MD; Sivan Yochpaz, MD; Ekhard E. Ziegler, MD.

The planning committee, staff, authors and editors listed below have identified financial relationships or relationships to products or devices they or their spouse/life partner have with commercial interest related to the content of this CME activity:
Bo Lönnerdal, PhD is on the speakers' bureau for Mead Johnson & Company, LLC, is a consultant/advisor for Arla Foods; Semper; Hero; Albion Laboratories, Inc; Biostine; and HiPP, has research support from Mead Johnson & Company, LLC and Arla Foods, and receives royalties/patents from Hero.

UNAPPROVED/OFF-LABEL USE DISCLOSURE

The EOCME requires CME faculty to disclose to the participants:
1. When products or procedures being discussed are off-label, unlabelled, experimental, and/or investigational (not US Food and Drug Administration [FDA] approved); and
2. Any limitations on the information presented, such as data that are preliminary or that represent ongoing research, interim analyses, and/or unsupported opinions. Faculty may discuss information about pharmaceutical agents that is outside of FDA-approved labelling. This information is intended solely for CME and is not intended to promote off-label use of these medications. If you have any questions, contact the medical affairs department of the manufacturer for the most recent prescribing information.

TO ENROLL

To enroll in the *Clinics in Perinatology* Continuing Medical Education program, call customer service at 1-800-654-2452 or sign up online at http://www.theclinics.com/home/cme. The CME program is available to subscribers for an additional annual fee of $235 USD.

METHOD OF PARTICIPATION

In order to claim credit, participants must complete the following:

1. Complete enrolment as indicated above.
2. Read the activity.
3. Complete the CME Test and Evaluation. Participants must achieve a score of 70% on the test. All CME Tests and Evaluations must be completed online.

CME INQUIRIES/SPECIAL NEEDS

For all CME inquiries or special needs, please contact elsevierCME@elsevier.com.

CLINICS IN PERINATOLOGY

THE CLINICS ARE AVAILABLE ONLINE!
Access your subscription at:
www.theclinics.com

Foreword

Dairy Cows, Famines, and What Neonatologists Can Learn from Them

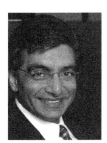

Lucky Jain, MD, MBA
Consulting Editor

Newborn calves deprived of their mother's milk early in life seldom survive, even if they are fed a perfectly balanced artificial formula. They die of overwhelming infections because cows rely on their colostrum to transfer a vast array of antibodies to their calves in the first few hours of life. Days after birth, this cycle continues, with cows gaining important colonization information about their babies by licking them and then transferring antibodies specific to those pathogens in their milk. Pretty remarkable adaptation to a situation where transplacental transfer of antibodies is limited. Farmers who raise cattle know this biologic secret well and make sure that newborn calves receive plenty of mother's milk, even in regions where milk is a scarce commodity.

While the impact of mother's milk deprivation is not as striking in humans, a respectable body of literature confirms significant advantages attached to breast milk. These benefits vary from lower mortality (in breast-fed babies born in nations with poor alternatives to mother's milk) to softer cognitive and immune benefits in resource-rich nations with safe hygienic conditions and optimally balanced formulas. How mother's milk achieves these remarkable biologic effects was poorly understood for a long time, with benefits limited to associations seen mostly through epidemiologic data. Recent studies provide strong biologic models for how these effects are achieved. Extracellular vesicles in milk, for example, harbor a variety of compounds, including lipids, proteins, noncoding RNAs, and messenger RNAs that have the capability of mediating subtle but important changes in the newborn.[1] Exosomes are particularly important because they carry a tightly regulated message and play an essential role in cell-to-cell communication. Encapsulation in exosomes confers protection against enzymatic and nonenzymatic degradation of biologic messengers and provides a pathway for their cellular uptake by endocytosis of exosomes. Evidence suggests

Clin Perinatol 44 (2017) xv–xvii
http://dx.doi.org/10.1016/j.clp.2016.12.002
0095-5108/17/© 2016 Published by Elsevier Inc.

> **Box 1**
> **Suggested benefits of human-milk feeding for preterm infants**
>
> - Dose-related decreases in NICU length of stay and lower morbidity including risk of the following:
>   - Sepsis
>   - Necrotizing enterocolitis
>   - Urinary tract infection
> - Benefits persist beyond NICU stay
> - Improved gastrointestinal function and integrity via the following:
>   - Decreased gastric pH
>   - Increased gastrointestinal motility
>   - Accelerated mucosal immunity
>   - Improved gut microflora
>   - Decreased mucosal permeability leading to reduced bacterial translocation
> - Improvement in indexes of neurodevelopment that persists into adolescence
>
> *Adapted from* Raiten DJ, Steiber AL, Hand RK. Executive summary: evaluation of the evidence to support practice guidelines for nutritional care of preterm infants-the Pre-B Project. Am J Clin Nutr 2016;103(2):604S.

that exosomes in milk are transported by a variety of cells and are delivered to peripheral tissues to mediate distal tissue effects. Low concentrations of dietary microRNAs may alter gene expression. Such biologic pathways could then begin to explain the observed advantages in breastfed infants such as higher Mental Developmental Index, Psychomotor Development Index, and Preschool Language Scale-3 than in those fed nutritionally equivalent formulas.

The biologic pathways that decrease the risk of necrotizing enterocolitis are also well described. Human milk is believed to compensate for the immature systems by lowering gastric pH, enhancing intestinal motility, decreasing epithelial permeability, and altering the composition of bacterial flora.[2]

These and other benefits of breast milk are summarized in **Box 1**.[3] Yet, large swaths of communities have moved away from breastfeeding, and the rigorous requirements of today's workforce make it harder for young mothers to keep up with round-the-clock demands on a breastfeeding mother's time. Societies and the medical community will need to come up with new strategies to promote and sustain a strong breastfeeding culture.[4]

This issue of *Clinics in Perinatology* focuses entirely on human milk feeding in preterm infants. Drs Mimouni and Koletzko are to be congratulated for bringing together a superb set of state-of-the-art articles on this topic. As always, I am grateful to the editors, authors, and the publishing team at Elsevier (Kerry Holland and Casey Potter) for their superb assistance.

Lucky Jain, MD, MBA
Emory University School of Medicine
Department of Pediatrics
Children's Healthcare of Atlanta
2015 Uppergate Drive
Atlanta, GA 30322, USA

E-mail address:
ljain@emory.edu

REFERENCES

1. Zempleni J, Aguilar-Lozano A, Sadri M, et al. Biological activities of extracellular vesicles and their cargos from bovine and human milk in humans and implications for infants. J Nutr 2016. [Epub ahead of print].
2. Maffei D, Schanler RJ. Human milk is the feeding strategy to prevent necrotizing enterocolitis! Semin Perinatol 2016. [Epub ahead of print].
3. Raiten DJ, Steiber AL, Hand RK. Executive summary: evaluation of the evidence to support practice guidelines for nutritional care of preterm infants-the Pre-B Project. Am J Clin Nutr 2016;103(2):599S–605S.
4. Rollins NC, Bhandari N, Hajeebhoy N, et al. Lancet Breastfeeding Series Group. Why invest, and what it will take to improve breastfeeding practices? Lancet 2016;387:491–504.

Preface

Human Milk for Preterm Infants

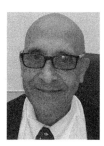
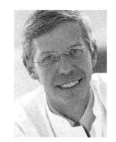

Francis B. Mimouni, MD, FAAP   Berthold Koletzko, MD, PhD
Editors

In a groundbreaking article, Lucas and colleagues[1] in 1990 reported the results of a prospective multicenter study on 926 preterm infants. The infants received either formula, their own mother's human milk, a combination of both, or donor human milk. Necrotizing enterocolitis (NEC) developed in 5.5% of infants and bore a mortality of 26%. Confirmed disease was 6 to 10 times more common in exclusively formula-fed babies than in those fed breast milk alone, and 3 times more common than in those who received both formula and breast milk. Pasteurized donor milk seemed to be as protective as raw maternal milk. Among babies born at more than 30 weeks' gestation, confirmed NEC was rare in those whose diet included breast milk, and it occurred 20 times more often in those fed formula only. Lucas and colleagues estimated that in British neonatal units, exclusive formula feeding could account for 500 extra cases of NEC each year, of which about 100 infants would die. By the time Lucas' article was published, it became also obvious that unfortified human milk could not provide for the unique nutritional needs of the preterm infant, in particular, very low-birth-weight infants, and would leave such an infant with significant nutritional deficiencies when reaching term age, in particular in terms of inadequate protein-to-energy and mineral-to-energy density ratios, ultimately leading to undermineralized bones and suboptimal lean body mass and length growth. Consequently, major efforts were done to develop human milk fortifiers and to find ways to improve their bioavailability.[2]

In the current issue of *Clinics in Perinatology*, world experts from several continents review the current evidence on the use of human milk in preterm infants. In particular, we are systematically reviewing the many studies that have described the unique macronutrient composition of preterm human milk: a systematic review of the use of "bedside" human milk analysis in the neonatal intensive care unit is presented by Professor Christoph Fusch and colleagues, from the McMaster University. Together with Professor Ekhard Ziegler from the University of Iowa, a Tel Aviv team presents a systematic review on human milk fortification. The Munich, Germany team led by Professor Koletzko presents the evidence about the need for women providing milk to their

Clin Perinatol 44 (2017) xix–xx
http://dx.doi.org/10.1016/j.clp.2016.12.001
0095-5108/17/© 2016 Published by Elsevier Inc.

preterm infants to take DHA supplements. Professor Bo Lönnerdal, from the University of California, Davis, gives an extensive review of recently identified bioactive proteins in human milk and their potential benefits for preterm infants. Dr Hans Demmelmair, from Munich, and Berthold Koletzko provide us with new insights into variation of metabolite and hormone contents in human milk. Professor Cathy Field, from Edmonton Alberta, Canada, and colleagues present us with the immune properties of human milk in relation to preterm infant feeding. Professor Jean-Charles Picaud, from the University of Lyon, France, and Rachel Buffin present us with state-of-the-art considerations about human milk treatment and quality of banked human milk. Professor Benjamin Hartmann, from Perth, reviews the issues of the use of donor milk, its collection, storage, and ensuring safety. Professor Klaus Hamprecht, from Tübingen, Germany, and Rangmar Goelz review the postnatal CMV infection through human milk in preterm infants, its transmission, clinical presentation, and methods of prevention; Professor Joseph Neu, from Gainesville, Florida, and colleagues present a systematic review about NEC and human milk feeding. Professor Betty Vohr, from Providence, and Beatrice Lechner offer us an expert review of the neurodevelopmental outcomes of preterm infants fed human milk. Finally Professor Paula Meier, from the Rush University in Chicago, and colleagues present the evidence-based methods that may promote human milk feeding of preterm infants.

We believe this issue will be of particular interest to neonatologists, neonatal nurse practitioners, neonatal nurses, as well as lactation consultants and pediatric dieticians.

Francis B. Mimouni, MD, FAAP
Shaare Zedek Medical Center
Tel Aviv University
12 Shmuel Bait Street
Jerusalem 913102, Israel

Berthold Koletzko, MD, PhD
Ludwig-Maximilians-Universität München
Dr von Hauner Children's Hospital
Lindwurmstrasse 4
D-80337 München, Germany

E-mail addresses:
fbmimouni@gmail.com (F.B. Mimouni)
office.koletzko@med.lmu.de (B. Koletzko)

REFERENCES

1. Lucas A, Cole TJ. Breast milk and neonatal necrotising enterocolitis. Lancet 1990; 336(8730):1519–23.
2. Tönz O, Schubiger G. Feeding of very-low-birth-weight infants with breast-milk enriched by energy, nitrogen and minerals: FM85. Helv Paediatr Acta 1985;40(4): 235–47.

Evidence-Based Methods That Promote Human Milk Feeding of Preterm Infants

An Expert Review

Paula P. Meier, PhD, RN*, Tricia J. Johnson, PhD, Aloka L. Patel, MD, Beverly Rossman, PhD, RN

KEYWORDS

- Human milk • Neonatal intensive care unit • Breast pump • Preterm infants
- Lactation initiation and maintenance

KEY POINTS

- The evidence for the use of human milk (HM) feedings during the neonatal intensive care unit (NICU) hospitalization for preterm infants has been slowly adopted into clinical best practices.
- In multiple instances, these best practices have been identified and tested, but are not adopted because of economical and ideological constraints.
- The early postbirth periods of maternal secretory activation and coming to volume appear to comprise a critical window for the protection of maternal HM provision through to NICU discharge.
- Lactation technologies that improve the use of HM during the NICU hospitalization have been detailed in the scientific literature, but not widely implemented.
- Donor HM feeding infrastructure costs can compete with costs for the acquisition of mother's own HM in the NICU, with implications for cost-effective prioritization of limited resources.

Human milk (HM, milk from the infant's own mother) feedings during the neonatal intensive care unit (NICU) hospitalization represent a cost-effective strategy to reduce disease burden and associated costs in preterm infants.[1–7] However, this evidence must be translated into NICU best practices that target barriers to high-dose HM feedings if preterm infants and their mothers are to receive the benefits of this knowledge. Although multiple studies have revealed effective interventions for modifying barriers to maternal lactation and HM feeding in this population, economic and ideological

Disclosure Statement: The authors have nothing to disclose.
Rush University Medical Center, 1653 West Congress Parkway, Chicago, IL 60612, USA
* Corresponding author.
E-mail address: Paula_Meier@rush.edu

concerns have limited their wide-scale adaptation.[8] As a result, many mothers of pre-term infants fail to achieve their HM feeding goals, and infants receive either donor HM or formula, neither of which achieves similar reduction in disease burden and cost.[9] This article

- Reviews data on the initiation and maintenance of lactation for mothers of preterm infants
- Summarizes best practices for protecting maternal HM volume during the NICU hospitalization
- Delineates predictable, preventable problems in the feeding of HM
- Details quality indicators that measure the effectiveness of NICU HM feeding programs

METHODOLOGY

The literature used to create this review spans multiple specialties, including preterm infants, nutrition, HM science, lactation physiology, breast pump dependency, NICU lactation support, and the economics of HM feeding for very low birthweight (VLBW, <1500 g birthweight) infants. These citations were accumulated over several years by the authors, who are primary researchers in this field. Thus, this expert review reflects current evidence, controversies, and implications for research and practice.

INITIATION AND MAINTENANCE OF LACTATION IN MOTHERS OF PRETERM INFANTS
Initiation of Lactation

The past decade is characterized by an increasing proportion of mothers who initiate lactation (begin providing HM) for their preterm infants,[3,10,11] many because they change the decision from formula to HM because of information they received from NICU health care providers.[12–14] Studies have confirmed that NICU messaging about the superiority of HM does not make mothers feel guilty or coerced, but instead is interpreted as needed information to make the best feeding decision for their infants.[12,13] Although black and/or low-income mothers have been especially likely to change from formula to HM after speaking with their infant's care providers,[12–14] black preterm infants in the United States remain less likely than their Caucasian counterparts to receive any HM, especially if their mothers have low income.[5,15–17] Specific talking points for sharing the science of HM with families of preterm infants have been published, and can standardize evidence-based messaging about providing HM within the NICU.[8,18,19]

Maintenance of Lactation

The maintenance of lactation, usually measured by whether the infant is still receiving partial or exclusive HM at the time of NICU discharge, (HM continuation through NICU discharge), remains a global problem, with only a handful of best practices demon-strated to be effective.[20–27] In a prospective cohort study, Hoban and colleagues re-ported that mothers of VLBW infants changed their HM feeding goals over the course of the NICU hospitalization, and became increasingly unlikely to achieve their goals for exclusive or partial HM as the hospitalization progressed.[14] It has been proposed that the profound dislike and inconvenience of long-term HM expression, maternal stress and fatigue, insufficient encouragement and assistance from family and friends, and inconsistent advice in the NICU all play a role in mothers' discontinuation of HM pro-vision prior to NICU discharge.[25–28] Furthermore, it is likely that some mothers, espe-cially those whose initial prebirth intent was to formula feed, revert back to their prebirth feeding goals, especially as the infant's condition improves and the mother perceives that "HM has done its job" of protecting from acquired morbidities.[8,14]

Maintenance of lactation is related to maternal human milk volume

The failure to maintain HM provision through to NICU discharge is related to insufficient pumped HM to meet the infant's nutritional requirements. However, it is not clear whether insufficient HM volume precedes less-intensive HM expression efforts or vice versa. For example, does the mother see that despite her best efforts, her pumped HM volume decreases, and she becomes discouraged and pumps less frequently, eventually discontinuing HM provision? Or, is the primary catalyst the dislike and inconvenience of pumping, such that the mother pumps less frequently, notes decreased HM volume and then decides that her growing preterm infant is doing well with partial supplements of formula or donor milk, ceasing HM provision altogether?[8,14,26] These distinctions are important, because they require different interventions to prevent early cessation of HM provision.

Successful initiatives to improve the maintenance of lactation

A handful of multi-institutional quality initiatives have demonstrated higher rates of HM provision at NICU discharge by adopting multidisciplinary infant nutrition and lactation teams that incorporate clear protocols for premature infants.[24] Other initiatives have focused on developing a NICU nursing lactation team, increasing availability of hospital-grade breast pumps, and implementing lactation rounds.[23] Larger statewide initiatives that report increased rates of HM feedings at NICU discharge have included multidisciplinary teams to provide education and advocacy for HM provision, to support establishing and maintaining HM supply, and to provide a consistent and comprehensive nutritional monitoring program.[22] Many of the evidence-based interventions to maintain lactation in this population such as timely access to effective and efficient breast pumps, freezer storage space, and proactive NICU-specific lactation care, have not been adopted due to the upstart economic investments that would be required (**Table 1**). In many instances, it is easier to acquire institutional approval for donor HM infrastructure than for programs that facilitate mothers' providing their own HM, despite the fact that own mothers' HM is more economical to provide and acquire and provides greater protection from acquired morbidities.[9,29,30]

Research Priorities to Improve the Initiation and Maintenance of Lactation in Mothers of Preterm Infants

Most previous studies addressing barriers to the initiation and maintenance of lactation in mothers of preterm infants have focused primarily on motivational and behavioral interventions such as skin-to-skin care, patterns of breast pump use, and models of support.[23–27,31–33] However, many breast pump-dependent mothers of preterm infants have chronic health problems or pregnancy and birth complications that impact lactation outcomes and that may be unresponsive to current behavioral and motivational interventions.[8,18,34] These complications, which include prepregnancy body mass index (BMI) greater than 25, preterm birth, Cesarean delivery and preeclampsia, as well as prolonged bedrest and medications to treat these complications, impact the hormonal processes that regulate secretory differentiation and early lactation.[35–41] However, because preterm infants require so little HM volume in the early postbirth period, these maternal HM volume problems can easily go unrecognized for days or weeks, making the problems more difficult to diagnose and manage. Thus, a research priority is understanding the role of maternal health complications that impact lactation outcomes for breast pump-dependent mothers of preterm infants, who are often ill themselves.

Table 1
Economic barriers to the initiation and maintenance of lactation: estimated average cost of required services per infant

	Barrier	Cost per Infant	Low	High	Assumptions
1	Provision of professionally produced, evidence-based materials targeting the importance of HM for preterm infants + monitoring of HM volume and goals for HM feeding	Brochure + education sheets = $10 Mother's Milk Volumes (MMV) record = $5.50 Maternal Goals record = $0.10	$15.60	$15.60	1 set of materials per infant
2	Hospital-grade electric breast pump rental for 3 mo (through term-corrected age)	$40 to $70 per month	$120.00	$210.00	3 mo rental; low estimate assumes $40 per month, wholesale cost; high estimate assumes $70/mo retail cost
3	Provision of pump kit	$32.91 cost per kit	$32.91	$32.91	1 kit per infant
4	Access to custom-fitted breast shields for effective, efficient and comfortable HM removal	$7 retail cost	$7.00	$7.00	1 set per infant
5	Provision of sufficient numbers of hospital-grade HM storage containers for pumped HM	$0.21 cost per container (Jegier 2013)	$89.46	$134.19	Low estimate assumes 6 containers/d (350 mL/120 × 1.2 rounded to next multiple of 3); high estimate assumes 9 containers/d (700 mL/120 × 1.2 rounded to next multiple of 3); for 71-d NICU stay
6	Access to NICU-specific lactation support from NICU-based certified breastfeeding peer counselors (BPCs) during coming to volume, weekly group forums, and on an individual basis, as needed	$18/h + 26% fringe benefits	$417.11	$539.79	71-d NICU stay; $18/h + 26% fringe benefits; low estimate assumes 2 BPCs for 44 infants per day; high estimate assumes 2 BPC for 33 infants per day

7	Availability of NICU freezers for safe storage of all pumped HM (eg, not telling mothers to store HM in the home and bring it in as needed)	$8000 cost per freezer	$6.92	$10.37	Storage for 15 infants per freezer; low estimate assumes 15 y life; high estimate assumes 10 y life; for 71 d length of NICU stay
8	Use of HM waterless warmers to avoid HM contamination with waterborne pathogens	$773 cost per warmer	$30.07	$50.12	1 warmer per infant for 71 d NICU stay; low estimate assumes 5 y life; high estimate assumes 3 y life
9	Use of liners for waterless warmer	$3.25 cost per liner	$230.75	$230.75	1 liner/d for 71 d NICU stay
10	Basic creamatocrit and/or other HM analysis technology to individualize HM feedings and HM collection strategies	$1500 per creamatocrit	$0.38	$0.63	1 creamatocrit per NICU; assumes 800 NICU admissions per year; low estimate assumes 5 y life; high estimate assumes 3 y life
11	Availability of infant scales for measuring HM intake during breastfeeding	$1500 per scale	$3.89	$6.48	1 scale per 15 infants for NICU stay; low estimate assumes 5 y life; high estimate assumes 3 y life
Total			$954.08	$1237.84	

Costs reported in 2015 US dollars.
Based on Average length of NICU stay for VLBW infants of 71 days from RUMC data.
Abbreviation: RUMC, Rush University Medical Center.

Another research priority is addressing the mothers' consistent reports about the dislike and inconvenience of breast pump use. Mothers of preterm infants are completely breast pump dependent, meaning that the breast pump regulates the lactation processes of HM removal and mammary gland stimulation, which are critical to continued HM production.[34] Despite the reality that breast pump dependency will continue for weeks or months, surprisingly few rigorous studies have examined features of breast pumps, breast pump suction patterns, breast shield sizing, and other product-related considerations such as the ability to warm breast shields.[34,42,43] Whereas it is known that breast pump evaluations in this population should include objective outcomes that include effectiveness, efficiency, comfort and convenience of the breast pump, the primary outcome measures in most studies continue to be pumped HM volume and maternal "preferences," both of which lack rigor and are affected by multiple extraneous variables.[34] Thus, a critical research priority for the maintenance of lactation in mothers of preterm infants is the improvement in the design of breast pumps and breast pump supplies so that they optimize efficiency and convenience, consistent with mothers' concerns.[34,44] Unfortunately, ideological barriers to breast pump research affect the study and dissemination of findings from industry-funded trials as well as the selection of breast pumps for clinical NICU use based on data versus compliance with World Health Organization (WHO) code marketing interpretation and other ideologic initiatives.[44,45]

PROTECTING MATERNAL HUMAN MILK VOLUME IN BREAST PUMP-DEPENDENT MOTHERS OF PRETERM INFANTS

Breast pump-dependent mothers of preterm infants have specific, predictable barriers to the initiation and maintenance of lactation, which do not affect mothers of healthy term infants. These lactation processes and barriers have been delineated in 2 recent review papers,[8,34] and are summarized in **Table 2** according to the stage of lactation: initiation, coming to volume, and the maintenance of established lactation. Of particular concern are initiation and coming to volume, because the first 2 weeks after-birth are critical for transition of the mammary gland from secretory differentiation to secretory activation, and little is known about these processes in breast pump-dependent mothers of preterm infants.[37,40,42,46] Furthermore, several studies indicate that daily pumped HM volume at either week 1 or week 2 after birth in this population predicts HM continuation at NICU discharge (Aloka L. Patel, MD, personal communication, 2016).[34,47,48] In 1 recently completed study, mothers of VLBW infants who successfully experienced coming to volume (eg, achieving HM volume ≥500 mL/d by day 14 after birth) were over 3 times more likely to provide HM at NICU discharge than mothers who did not achieve this threshold (Aloka L. Patel, MD, personal communication, 2016).

Early Lactation: Initiation and Coming to Volume

The early postbirth lactation stages of initiation and coming to volume warrant further detail, because they pose predictable problems for breast pump-dependent mothers of preterm infants and should be monitored and addressed proactively.[34] The initiation of lactation coincides with the closure of tight junctions in the mammary epithelium,[37,46] a process that is disrupted and/or delayed by preterm and/or complicated birth,[40] lack of exposure to human infant-specific sucking patterns,[42] delayed breast pump use,[49,50] early hormonal contraception,[51] and prolonged hand expression in the absence of breast pump use.[52]

Table 2
Critical periods for protecting maternal milk volume in breast pump dependent mothers of preterm infants

Critical Period	Problem	Impact	Best Practice(s)	References
Initiation	• Lack of understanding about the mechanisms that trigger secretory differentiation and regulate lactation • Multiple risk factors for delayed or impaired initiation of lactation • Use of ideology vs evidence about method and timing of milk removal/mammary gland stimulation • Early administration of hormonal contraceptives • Economic barriers for access to equipment and NICU-specific lactation care	• Interference with rapid post-birth decline in progesterone • Lack of timely mammary gland stimulation to complete secretory activation (lactogenesis II) • Impaired or delayed secretory activation segues into permanent low milk volume	• Assure that mothers are taught about the potential impact of hormonal contraception during the maternity hospitalization on the initiation of lactation so they can make an informed decision about its timing • Screen mothers for risk factors for delayed or impaired onset of lactation (eg, hypertension, obesity, Cesarean delivery) and share this information (and a plan for monitoring) with them • Do not use exclusive hand expression in the absence of breast pump stimulation • Initiate pumping within the first hour after birth • Use a breast pump suction pattern that mimics the human infant during the initiation of lactation and has been shown to increase HM volume compared with standard breast pump suction patterns • Assure mothers have access to NICU lactation care providers with expertise in breast pump dependency	34,40–42,44,49–52,79–84

(continued on next page)

Table 2
(continued)

Critical Period	Problem	Impact	Best Practice(s)	References
Coming to volume	• Lack of understanding about change from endocrine to autocrine regulation of lactation • Unclear messaging for mothers about necessity of frequent and complete HM removal to effect this transition • Lack of proactive lactation care strategies that prevent and/or detect early problems with HM volume	• Mothers who fail to come to volume by 14 d after birth are statistically unlikely to provide sufficient HM through to NICU discharge • Overlooking common pitfalls during coming to volume can translate into long-term HM volume problems	• Educate mothers about the critical nature of coming to volume, emphasizing that most HM volume problems present during this time, and must be managed quickly and correctly • Share HM targets ($\geq$500 mL/d) for postbirth day 14 or before • Explain and use Coming to Volume Assessment tool to detect and manage modifiable HM volume problems • Explain and use My Mom Pumps for Me! maternal HM volume log • Assess pumping technique by watching mothers use the pump daily during coming to volume ○ Check for correct breast shield sizing, pumping pressures, and thorough breast emptying	18,34,79

| Maintenance of established lactation | • Lack of proactive strategies to monitor changes in mothers' personal goals for providing HM through to NICU discharge
• Inadequate proactive counseling/teaching about common problems/scenarios that reduce HM volume during the later NICU hospitalization
• Lack of support for long-term pumping | • As the duration of the NICU hospitalization increases, mothers do not achieve their personal HM feeding goals
• Infants do not receive the highest possible NICU dose of HM, reducing protection from potentially preventable morbidities | • Meet with each mother weekly to review and update personal HM feeding goals (Use "My Feeding Plans" tool)
• Proactively review common scenarios that reduce HM volume during the late NICU hospitalization
  ○ Substituting a feeding at breast for breast pump use (Need to pump after breastfeeding)
  ○ Returning to employment and reducing total daily pumping time or using less effective (portable) breast pump
• Incorporate NICU-based breastfeeding peer counselors and mother-to-mother support for long-term pumping | 14,26,27,32,75,79,85 |

Coming to volume refers to the lactation stage between the onset of lactogenesis II and the establishment of a threshold HM volume, typically $\geq$500 mL/d.[34] This transition heralds the autocrine control of lactation,[53] via the suckling-induced prolactin surge[54] and feedback inhibition of lactation.[55] Coming to volume in a breast pump-dependent mother with a NICU infant is impaired by easily overlooked conditions that lead to HM stasis, thereby triggering feedback inhibition of lactation. These conditions include using an ineffective breast pump that does not empty the breasts thoroughly, improperly fitted breast shields that obstruct the outflow of HM from the ducts, inappropriate breast pump suction pressures, short pumping sessions, and long intervals between breast pump use.[34] Furthermore, several lines of evidence suggest that the early postbirth stages of initiation and coming to volume are critical periods for the programming of lactation structures and functions, making it difficult or impossible for mothers with low HM volume to catch up after these critical periods have passed.[34,42,52]

Clinical Tools to Monitor Coming to Volume and Maternal Human Milk Feeding Goals

All available evidence indicates that the NICU staff should prioritize the first 14 days after birth using proactive interventions to achieve maternal HM volume measures that are $\geq$500 mL/d.[18,34] A NICU toolkit for managing these early lactation phases has been described and includes a user-friendly pumping diary (My Mom Pumps for Me!), the Coming to Volume Assessment Tool, and a weekly maternal feeding goals interview tool (My Plans for Feeding my Baby at NICU discharge) that assures mothers' individual HM feeding goals are monitored and supported.[18] Whereas the costs for these interventions are often assumed to be unaffordable, in reality they are economical (see **Table 1**), especially considering that the cost savings afforded to each additional fed milliliter of HM during the first 14 days after birth is valued at $534 toward reduction in NICU costs of care, exclusive of costs specifically attributed to necrotizing enterocolitis.[2]

IMPROVING THE USE OF HUMAN MILK FOR PRETERM INFANTS

Considerable global variation exists in the storage, handling, fortification, and feeding of HM in the NICU, as detailed in 2 recent review papers.[3,8] Barriers to the integration of evidence-based practices to improve the use of HM for preterm infants include lack of HM/lactation specialists with NICU expertise, cost of investment in resources, and ideologic objections to the use of technology that makes breastfeeding unnatural.

Safe Handling of Pumped Human Milk in the Neonatal Intensive Care Unit

When HM is pumped, transferred among containers, stored, warmed, fortified, and fed via gavage infusion, there are multiple avenues for compromising the nutritional and bioactive components that actually reach the infant.[3,8] Furthermore, HM is easily contaminated during these processes and can serve as an excellent medium for bacterial growth, especially if HM has been previously frozen. These concerns are the most comprehensively addressed by feeding freshly pumped HM that has not been either refrigerated or frozen (eg, directly from mother to infant), and this strategy should be prioritized to the greatest possible extent.[3,8] **Table 3** summarizes best practices for safe handling of pumped HM in the NICU.

New data about changes in the integrity of HM with storage have significant clinical implications for conserving pumped HM.[56–58] Slutzah and colleagues reported that freshly pumped, unfortified HM is safely fed after refrigeration for 96 hours.[56] Separate

Table 3
Safe handling of pumped human milk for preterm infant feeding in the neonatal intensive care unit

Objective	Best Practices

A. Maximize nutritive and bioactive components	• Feed freshly pumped, never-frozen, HM to greatest possible extent
	  ○ Freshly pumped, unfortified HM can be refrigerated for up to 96 h
	• Do not pasteurize mother's own HM
	• Implement mechanism for identifying pumped colostrum and transitional HM so it can be fed in the order it is pumped during advancement of enteral feedings
	  ○ Alternate colostrum and transitional HM with freshly pumped HM after 72 h postfeed initiation if colostrum and transitional HM collections have been previously frozen
	• Minimize number of temperature changes (eg, serial refrigeration + warming)

B. Optimize nutrient delivery and utilization	• Feed freshly pumped, never-frozen, HM to greatest possible extent • Use strategies to minimize the impact of exogenous additives on the delivery and utilization of HM components • Feed HM by intermittent rather than continuous gavage infusion to prevent lipid entrapment in infusion tubing and resultant loss of nutritional lipid and energy • Invert syringe (bevel upward) if intermittent feedings are placed on an infusion pump to assure HM lipid is delivered to infant • Flush HM remaining in infusion tubing after feeding with 1-2 mL air so that infant receives as much of trapped lipid as possible
C. Minimize bacterial contaminants and bacterial growth	• Feed freshly pumped, never-frozen, HM to greatest possible extent • Standardize protocols for collection, storage and transport of HM that are user-friendly and easily understood by NICU families • Assure all HM specimens are collected and stored in sterile receptacles • Store all pumped HM in industrial NICU refrigerators and freezers that are tamper proof and routinely monitored for appropriate temperature maintenance • Do not implement a routine culturing surveillance program for pumped HM, as this approach has been shown ineffective in minimizing bacteria • Use waterless warming and thawing techniques to prevent HM contamination • Feed previously frozen HM within 24 h of thawing
D. Eliminate errors in HM fed to the wrong infant	• Implement an HM management system that minimizes the risk of HM being fed to the wrong infant • Engage parents in the importance of accurate labeling of HM receptacles and other activities (such as checking that all pumped HM is moved from 1 NICU room to another with the infant) per individual NICU protocol

Data from Meier PP, Patel AL, Bigger HR, et al. Human milk feedings in the neonatal intensive care unit. In: Rajendram R, Preedy VR, Patel VB, editors. Diet and nutrition in critical care. New York: Springer-Verlag; 2015. p. 807–22; and Meier PP, Rossman B, Patel AL, et al. Human milk in the neonatal intensive care unit. In: A state-of-the-art view about human milk and lactation. Stuttgart (Germany): Thieme, in press.

studies suggest that pumped HM can be thawed and refrozen at least 1 time[59] (allowing transfer of HM from large containers into smaller ones for smaller-volume feeds), and that HM from serial pumpings can be safely added to previously pumped HM over a 24-hour period.[60]

There is no evidence to inform whether HM storage and preparation should be centralized within a milk bank area or prepared at the bedside by the NICU nurse. A centralized service is potentially safer with respect to misallocation of HM (eg, infant receiving another mother's HM), although this assumption has not been tested. Centralized preparation may also be more efficient and convenient, especially if donor HM is used to supplement mothers' own HM. In contrast, HM preparation at the bedside by a NICU nurse enables more individualization of the feeding that potentially impacts infant outcome. For example, the NICU nurse can prioritize fresh versus frozen HM, colostrum versus mature HM and other strategies that are impossible when a centralized service has already prepared 12 or 24 hours of HM feedings in advance. The pros and cons of each practice have been reviewed recently.[8] One single-center study has demonstrated a reduction in the rate of HM misallocation in the NICU with the adoption of an electronic HM tracking/scanning system, while others have implemented nonelectronic measures to reduce errors.[61,62]

Within- and Between-Mother Variability in Pumped Human Milk and Impact on Infant Growth

The within- and between-mother variability in pumped HM fed in the NICU has been documented for decades.[3,8] Of all HM components, lipid, which contributes 50% to 60% of HM calories, is the most variable, with 1 study of pumped HM specimens provided by NICU mothers revealing minimum and maximum values for caloric density of 604 kCal/L and 1098 kCal/L, respectively.[63] Multiple modifiable factors contribute to lipid variability, which can be quickly identified and managed using the creamatocrit or other more costly HM analysis technologies.[3,63] **Table 4** summarizes common NICU scenarios that result in low-lipid, high-lactose HM being fed, with resultant slow infant weight gain and potential feed intolerance. Recent review papers on this topic provide extensive clinical examples of the impact of low-lipid HM on infant growth and feed intolerance.[3,8] Although the adequacy of protein impacts infant growth, HM protein varies little after the first month of lactation, during which time protective and growth proteins (eg, secretory immunoglobulin A [IgA], lactoferrin, epidermal growth factor) are more concentrated that nutritive protein.[64,65]

FEEDING AT BREAST IN THE NEONATAL INTENSIVE CARE UNIT

Feeding at breast for preterm infants can be conceptualized as a series of steps, including: breast pump use at the infant's bedside, skin-to-skin holding, tasting HM (suckling after breast pump use to remove all or some of the HM), and finally consuming full feedings at the breast.[18,66–69] There are no data to indicate that infants must attain a threshold weight or gestational age to begin tasting HM, and several studies reveal that preterm infants remain more physiologically stable during breast than bottle feeding.[8] However, a myriad of international studies suggest that preterm infants are prone to underconsumption of HM during exclusive at-breast feeding until they reach approximately term, corrected age despite the fact that the mother has more than enough HM and can remove it effectively with a breast pump.[3,8]

Table 4
Factors influencing the human milk lipid received by the preterm infant

Factor	Impact	Best Practices
Pumping		
• Long intervals between pumpings yield a low-lipid, high lactose HM	• Longer intervals between pumpings (such as during sleep or return to employment) result in low-lipid HM in the first pumping after the longer interval, whereas • Shorter intervals (such as every 2 h pumpings during a visit to the NICU) result in a high-lipid HM in the first pumping after the interval	• If sufficient HM volume, freeze low-lipid HM for use after NICU discharge, and • Feed HM collected after shorter interpump intervals • HM can be pooled over a 24 h period in the same storage container to decrease this within-mother variability
• Not emptying breasts thoroughly yields a low-lipid, high-lactose HM	• HM that flows from the first few minutes of a pumping is low-lipid (foremilk), whereas • Following milk ejection and through to thorough breast emptying, the HM lipid increases significantly	• Do not teach mothers to use a standard time to complete pumping such as 10 or 15 min • Emphasize that time to complete breast emptying is individual • Teach mothers the concept of foremilk and hindmilk so that they understand the importance of complete breast emptying
• Inadvertently separating foremilk and hindmilk with small pumping/storage receptacles	• Container filled from the earlier part of the pumping will be low-lipid HM, whereas • Container filled from the later part of the pumping will be high-lipid HM, and • These differences may translate into calories that are 3 times higher in the last vs first pumped receptacle	• Avoid the use of these products for mothers whose pumped HM volume exceeds the capacity of the receptacle • Teach all mothers the importance of not separating HM during pumping (unless used as a strategy to concentrate hindmilk lipid)
Storage		
• HM is not homogenized, so lipid separates and rises to the top of the storage container • Freezing disrupts the HM fat globule membrane	• Mothers may think there is something wrong with the pumped HM if not informed about separation of lipid • Lipid becomes difficult to thoroughly mix	• Teach mothers that lipid rises to the top of the storage container and that it is a different color from the rest of the HM • Develop and implement protocols that assure the HM is thoroughly mixed • Recognize that this process takes extra time for the bedside RN

(continued on next page)

Table 4
(continued)

Factor	Impact	Best Practices
Handling		
• Lipid adheres to crevices of storage containers or lids and is not transferred to feeding receptacles	• Lipid is not delivered to the infant • This is a commonly overlooked contribution to slow weight gain	• Assure that HM feeding protocols include guidelines for transferring as much HM lipid as possible by thorough checking and mixing • Do not use HM storage bags in the NICU because lipid is very difficult to remove from corner crevices
Feeding		
• Lipid is poorly delivered with slow-infusion gavage feedings	• Lipid is trapped in infusion tubings • The slowest infusion rates yield the greatest lipid trapping (loss)	• Avoid continuous infusions of HM • Use intermittent, gravity gavage feedings when possible • If intermittent gavage feedings are administered by infusion pump, use the most rapid rate that is safe • Use creamatocrit or HM analysis to diagnose/ manage the degree of lipid trapping if continuous infusions must be used
• Lipid rises to the top of HM infusion instruments and is poorly delivered in a horizontal position	• Significant lipid loss can occur over a 24 h period • Infant receives equivalent of defatted HM with a greater proportion of calories from lactose • This problem is a significant source of caloric loss	• Place the infusion syringe so that the bevel is pointing up so as much lipid as possible is moved from the syringe into the infusion tubing
• Lipid is trapped in infusion tubing if not flushed post-feed with air	• Even when intermittent gavage feedings are administered by infusion pump, lipid is trapped in the infusion tubing • This is worsened when the nurse adds extra HM to the prescribed feed volume, knowing that a final 2 mLs will remain in the tubing at the end of the feeding (which is discarded) • The infant does not receive the trapped lipid	• Do not add extra HM to compensate for the volume remaining in the tubing at the end of the infusion; instead • Flush the remaining HM from the infusion tubing using a slow air purge

(continued on next page)

Table 4
(continued)

Factor	Impact	Best Practices
• During breastfeeds the preterm infant may not consume sufficient volume to remove lipid-rich hindmilk	• Mothers often have more HM in the breast than the preterm infant can consume • Infants can consume sufficient HM volume (as measured by test weights) and still gain weight slowly if the intake reflects low-lipid foremilk that flows at the beginning of the feeding • Failure to remove hindmilk at the end of the feeding also impacts the feedback inhibitor of lactation with resultant downregulation of HM volume	• Until the preterm infant is able to effectively and efficiently consume all of the HM from a single breast, bottle supplements of pumped HM can consist of fractionated hindmilk, as needed • Recognize that slow weight gain when consuming an adequate volume of HM from the breast does not mean that the infant needs extra fortification or formula products • This scenario is easily diagnosed and managed using a combination of creamatocrits with pumped HM and test weights
• Frequent switching the infant between breasts potentiates low-lipid foremilk intake	• Due to weak suction pressures, the preterm infant may not consume an adequate HM volume at the breast • Consuming an adequate HM volume is facilitated when maternal HM flow is rapid, such as with postmilk ejection • The common strategy of switching breasts after 5 min of sucking is meant to facilitate intake at breast, but • It potentiates low-lipid, high-volume feedings • In extreme circumstances infant may demonstrate symptoms of lactose intolerance, including explosive stools and slow weight gain	• Do not recommend this approach with recently discharged preterm infants • It is preferable to provide some pumped HM (as hindmilk as necessary) to provide sufficient HM intake until the infant is capable of exclusive at-breast feeding

Data from Meier PP, Patel AL, Bigger HR, et al. Human milk feedings in the neonatal intensive care unit. In: Rajendram R, Preedy VR, Patel VB, editors. Diet and nutrition in critical care. New York: Springer-Verlag; 2015. p. 807–22; and Meier PP, Rossman B, Patel AL, et al. Human milk in the neonatal intensive care unit. In: A state-of-the-art view about human milk and lactation. Stuttgart (Germany): Thieme, in press.

Human Milk Transfer During Breastfeeding Requires Mature Infant Suction Pressures

This ineffective and inefficient HM removal by preterm infants is caused by weak intraoral suction pressures that are critical to breastfeeding but not bottle feeding. Suction pressures strengthen as the infant matures, as does the ability to stay awake and alert during the feeding and not slip off the breast repeatedly.[8] **Fig. 1** depicts HM intake by breast and bottle during the first 4 weeks after discharge in VLBW infants whose mothers had adequate HM for their requirements.[70] As demonstrated in **Fig. 1**, mothers have adequate volumes of HM and can remove it with a breast pump, but the infant cannot remove the available HM during exclusive breastfeeding. **Fig. 1** can be used to help families understand that NICU discharge does not mean that breastfeeding will magically work, because the mother and infant are no longer separated. In fact, the breast continues to synthesize HM only because additional breast pump use removes HM effectively and efficiently. Early discontinuation of breast pump use during this transition to exclusive at-breast feedings predisposes to low HM volume and inadequate infant intake.[8]

Use of Evidence-Based Lactation Technologies to Facilitate Breastfeeding

The first month after discharge can be extremely difficult for breastfeeding mothers with preterm infants, in part because lactation technologies that can guide this transition are not commonly employed. First, test weights performed during the last week or two in the NICU using accurate scales can help individualize breastfeeding strategies for use in the home.[8] For example, if serial test weights reveal that the infant consumes only 5 to 10 mL at breast, more bottle supplement of HM is required than if the infant consumes 80% of the prescribed volume. Multiple studies of test weights to measure HM intake during breastfeeding reveal that they are accurate, acceptable by mothers, and cannot be replaced by clinical indices such as counting swallows or checking for milk in the infant's mouth.[44,71,72] One randomized study revealed that mothers of preterm infants can use test-weights in the home after NICU discharge to manage supplements and complements of their pumped HM until infants can consume exclusive breastfeeds.[73]

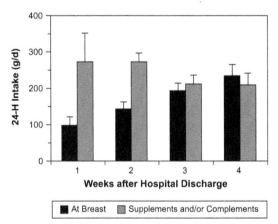

Fig. 1. Volume of milk consumed at the breast and as extra milk (supplements and complements of pumped mothers' milk) during the first 4 weeks at home in premature infants discharged from the neonatal intensive care unit. (*Courtesy of* N. Hurst, PhD, Houston, TX; P. Meier, PhD, Chicago, IL; and J. Engstrom, PhD, Chicago, IL.)

A second lactation aid that can be useful during this transition is the ultrathin silicone nipple shield, which partially compensates for weak suction pressures by creating and maintaining a nipple shape for the infant to latch onto.[8,70,74] Although not originally designed as a milk transfer device, evidence indicates that use of the nipple shield increases HM transfer during breastfeeding in preterm infants for whom maintaining sufficient suction pressure to extract HM is suboptimal or impossible.[8] Multiple ideological objections to nipple shield use in this population abound, including that it decreases HM transfer, decreases maternal HM volume, looks like a bottle nipple, and is addictive. In contrast, data indicate that the nipple shield can serve as a short-term lactation aid in this population until suction pressures mature sufficiently to allow effective and efficient transfer of HM during exclusive breastfeeding.[8,70,74]

EVIDENCE-BASED QUALITY INDICATORS THAT TARGET HIGH-DOSE HUMAN MILK FEEDINGS

Given the link between high-dose HM feedings and improved short- and long-term health and cost outcomes, many NICUs and have established quality improvement initiatives for the use of HM. The most commonly used metrics are the proportion of preterm infants who ever receive HM and the proportion who are still receiving any or exclusive HM at the time of NICU discharge. However, Bigger and colleagues, using data from a prospective cohort study, revealed that significant proportions of VLBW infants who were discharged as no HM had received very high-dose HM feedings through the first 14 and 28 days of life.[75] These data, which emphasize collecting measures of dose (in mL/kg/d or as a proportion of total enteral feeding), in addition to the ever received and still receiving HM quality indicators, are consistent with findings that link early high-dose HM to the reduction in the risk of necrotizing enterocolitis and sepsis and associated increased costs.[75]

Another concern in developing quality improvement initiatives for the use of HM is the increasing tendency to combine own mother's HM and donor HM into the same metric, which is often called human milk-fed or breast milk-fed.[9] The distinction between own mother's HM and donor HM is critical when measuring quality outcomes, because donor HM does not provide similar risk reduction from sepsis, bronchopulmonary dysplasia (BPD), and neurodevelopmental problems when compared to mother's own HM.[9,76] Many of the bioactive components in HM are mother-specific elements, such as probiotic bacteria (HM microbiome) and accompanying prebiotic oligosaccharides,[77,78] and multiple other HM components are reduced or eradicated due to longitudinal changes in lactation (eg, early HM vs later HM), preterm versus term HM, storage, freeze–thaw cycle and pasteurization, all of which impact donor HM.[9] Furthermore, the processes involved in achieving high rates of mother's own HM feedings in the NICU are completely different from acquiring donor HM, and scarce funds are often invested into establishing a donor HM infrastructure rather than in acquiring HM from the infant's own mother.[9]

SUMMARY

Although the evidence for high-dose HM feeding for preterm infants during NICU hospitalization is widely accepted, best practices that translate and implement this evidence into daily clinical NICU care have been slow to follow. These best practices have been delineated, and model programs for improving the use of HM during NICU hospitalization have been described. However, increasing the rates of high-dose HM feedings for this population requires an economic investment in personnel, equipment, and supplies, as well as a commitment to select best practices based on evidence rather than ideology. Special emphasis should be placed on prioritizing the early lactation period of coming to volume, so that mothers have sufficient HM volume to achieve their personal HM feeding goals. Finally, it is important to recognize that donor HM does not provide the same risk reduction as own mother's HM for multiple morbidities in preterm infants, providing evidence for the channeling of limited resources into NICU programs that promote the use of mother's own HM.

REFERENCES

1. Patel A, Johnson T, Engstrom J, et al. Impact of early human milk on sepsis and health care costs in very low birthweight infants. J Perinatol 2013;33(7):514–9.
2. Johnson TJ, Patel AL, Bigger HR, et al. Cost savings of human milk as a strategy to reduce the incidence of necrotizing enterocolitis in very low birth weight infants. Neonatology 2015;107(4):271–6.
3. Meier PP, Patel AL, Bigger HR, et al. Human milk feedings in the neonatal intensive care unit. In: Rajendram R, Preedy VR, Patel VB, editors. Diet and nutrition in critical care. New York: Springer-Verlag; 2015. p. 807–22.
4. Patel AL, Johnson TJ, Robin B, et al. Influence of own mother's milk on bronchopulmonary dysplasia and costs. Arch Dis Child Fetal Neonatal Ed 2016. [Epub ahead of print].
5. Vohr BR, Poindexter BB, Dusick AM, et al. Beneficial effects of breast milk in the neonatal intensive care unit on the developmental outcome of extremely low birth weight infants at 18 months of age. Pediatrics 2006;118(1):e115–23.
6. Vohr BR, Poindexter BB, Dusick AM, et al. Persistent beneficial effects of breast milk ingested in the neonatal intensive care unit on outcomes of extremely low birth weight infants at 30 months of age. Pediatrics 2007;120(4):e953–9.
7. Belfort MB, Anderson PJ, Nowak VA, et al. Breast milk feeding, brain development, and neurocognitive outcomes: a 7-year longitudinal study in infants born at less than 30 weeks' gestation. J Pediatr 2016;177:133–9.e1.
8. Meier PP, Rossman B, Patel AL, et al. Human milk in the neonatal intensive care unit. In: A state-of-the-art view about human milk and lactation. Stuttgart (Germany): Thieme, in press.
9. Meier PP, Patel AL, Esquerra-Zwiers A. Donor human milk update 2016: evidence, mechanisms and priorities for research and practice. J Pediatr 2016. [Epub ahead of print].
10. Colaizy TT, Morriss FH. Positive effect of NICU admission on breastfeeding of preterm US infants in 2000 to 2003. J Perinatol 2008;28(7):505–10.
11. Colaizy TT, Saftlas AF, Morriss FH Jr. Maternal intention to breast-feed and breastfeeding outcomes in term and preterm infants: pregnancy risk assessment monitoring system (PRAMS), 2000-2003. Public Health Nutr 2012;15(4):702–10.
12. Sisk PM, Lovelady CA, Dillard RG. Effect of education and lactation support on maternal decision to provide human milk for very-low-birth-weight infants. Adv Exp Med Biol 2004;554:307–11.
13. Miracle DJ, Meier PP, Bennett PA. Mothers' decisions to change from formula to mothers' milk for very-low-birth-weight infants. J Obstet Gynecol Neonatal Nurs 2004;33(6):692–703.
14. Hoban R, Bigger H, Patel AL, et al. Goals for human milk feeding in mothers of very low birth weight infants: how do goals change and are they achieved during the NICU hospitalization? Breastfeed Med 2015;10(6):305–11.

15. Lee HC, Gould JB. Factors influencing breast milk versus formula feeding at discharge for very low birth weight infants in California. J Pediatr 2009;155(5): 657–62.e1-2.
16. Sisk PM, Lovelady CA, Dillard RG, et al. Maternal and infant characteristics associated with human milk feeding in very low birth weight infants. J Hum Lact 2009; 25(4):412–9.
17. Pineda RG. Predictors of breastfeeding and breastmilk feeding among very low birth weight infants. Breastfeed Med 2011;6(1):15–9.
18. Meier PP, Patel AL, Bigger HR, et al. Supporting breastfeeding in the neonatal intensive care unit: rush mother's milk club as a case study of evidence-based care. Pediatr Clin North Am 2013;60(1):209–26.
19. Rodriguez NA, Miracle DJ, Meier PP. Sharing the science on human milk feedings with mothers of very-low-birth-weight infants. J Obstet Gynecol Neonatal Nurs 2005;34(1):109–19.
20. Davanzo R, Monasta L, Ronfani L, et al. Breastfeeding in neonatal intensive care unit study group. breastfeeding at NICU discharge: a multicenter Italian study. J Hum Lact 2013;29(3):374–80.
21. Riley B, Schoeny M, Rogers L, et al. Barriers to human milk feeding at discharge of very low-birthweight infants: evaluation of neighborhood structural factors. Breastfeed Med 2016;11:335–42.
22. Lee HC, Kurtin PS, Wight NE, et al. A quality improvement project to increase breast milk use in very low birth weight infants. Pediatrics 2012;130(6):e1679–87.
23. Bixby C, Baker-Fox C, Deming C, et al. A multidisciplinary quality improvement approach increases breastmilk availability at discharge from the neonatal intensive care unit for the very-low-birth-weight infant. Breastfeed Med 2016;11:75–9.
24. University of California San Diego Health. Supporting Premature Infant Nutrition (SPIN) Web site. 2016. Available at: https://health.ucsd.edu/specialties/obgyn/maternity/newborn/nicu/spin/about/Pages/default.aspx. Accessed May 10, 2016.
25. Hurst N, Engebretson J, Mahoney JS. Providing mother's own milk in the context of the NICU: a paradoxical experience. J Hum Lact 2013;29(3):366–73.
26. Rossman B, Kratovil AL, Greene MM, et al. "I have faith in my milk": the meaning of milk for mothers of very low birth weight infants hospitalized in the neonatal intensive care unit. J Hum Lact 2013;29(3):359–65.
27. Rossman B, Engstrom JL, Meier PP, et al. "They've walked in my shoes": mothers of very low birth weight infants and their experiences with breastfeeding peer counselors in the neonatal intensive care unit. J Hum Lact 2011;27(1):14–24.
28. Fleurant E, Schoeny M, Hoban R, et al. Barriers to human milk feeding at discharge of VLBW infants: maternal goal setting as a key social factor. Breastfeed Med 2016;12(1).
29. Jegier BJ, Johnson TJ, Engstrom JL, et al. The institutional cost of acquiring 100 mL of human milk for very low birth weight infants in the neonatal intensive care unit. J Hum Lact 2013;29(3):390–9.
30. Jegier BJ, Meier P, Engstrom JL, et al. The initial maternal cost of providing 100 mL of human milk for very low birth weight infants in the neonatal intensive care unit. Breastfeed Med 2010;5(2):71–7.
31. Rossman B, Engstrom JL, Meier PP. Healthcare providers' perceptions of breastfeeding peer counselors in the neonatal intensive care unit. Res Nurs Health 2012;35(5):460–74.
32. Rossman B, Greene MM, Meier PP. The role of peer support in the development of maternal identity for "NICU moms". J Obstet Gynecol Neonatal Nurs 2015; 44(1):3–16.

33. Strand H, Blomqvist YT, Gradin M, et al. Kangaroo mother care in the neonatal intensive care unit: staff attitudes and beliefs and opportunities for parents. Acta Paediatr 2014;103(4):373–8.
34. Meier PP, Patel AL, Hoban R, et al. Which breast pump for which mother: an evidence-based approach to individualizing breast pump technology. J Perinatol 2016;36(7):493–9.
35. Hernandez LL, Grayson BE, Yadav E, et al. High fat diet alters lactation outcomes: possible involvement of inflammatory and serotonergic pathways. PLoS One 2012;7(3):e32598.
36. Neville MC, Webb P, Ramanathan P, et al. The insulin receptor plays an important role in secretory differentiation in the mammary gland. Am J Physiol Endocrinol Metab 2013;305(9):E1103–14.
37. Neville MC. Introduction: tight junctions and secretory activation in the mammary gland. J Mammary Gland Biol Neoplasia 2009;14(3):269–70.
38. Hurst NM. Recognizing and treating delayed or failed lactogenesis II. J Midwifery Womens Health 2007;52(6):588–94.
39. Rasmussen KM. Association of maternal obesity before conception with poor lactation performance. Annu Rev Nutr 2007;27:103–21.
40. Cregan MD, De Mello TR, Kershaw D, et al. Initiation of lactation in women after preterm delivery. Acta Obstet Gynecol Scand 2002;81(9):870–7.
41. Hartmann PE, Cregan MD, Ramsay DT, et al. Physiology of lactation in preterm mothers: initiation and maintenance. Pediatr Ann 2003;32(5):351–5.
42. Meier PP, Engstrom JL, Janes JE, et al. Breast pump suction patterns that mimic the human infant during breastfeeding: greater milk output in less time spent pumping for breast pump-dependent mothers with premature infants. J Perinatol 2012;32(2):103–10.
43. Meier PP, Engstrom JL, Hurst NM, et al. A comparison of the efficiency, efficacy, comfort, and convenience of two hospital-grade electric breast pumps for mothers of very low birthweight infants. Breastfeed Med 2008;3(3):141–50.
44. Meier PP, Engstrom JL, Patel AL, et al. Improving the use of human milk during and after the NICU stay. Clin Perinatol 2010;37(1):217–45.
45. Meier PP. Concerns regarding industry-funded trials: letter to the editor. J Hum Lact 2005;21(2):121–3.
46. Pang WW, Hartmann PE. Initiation of human lactation: secretory differentiation and secretory activation. J Mammary Gland Biol Neoplasia 2007;12(4):211–21.
47. Hill PD, Aldag JC, Chatterton RT, et al. Comparison of milk output between mothers of preterm and term infants: the first 6 weeks after birth. J Hum Lact 2005;21(1):22–30.
48. Wilson E, Christensson K, Brandt L, et al. Early provision of mother's own milk and other predictors of successful breast milk feeding after very preterm birth: a regional observational study. J Hum Lact 2015;31(3):393–400.
49. Parker LA, Sullivan S, Krueger C, et al. Association of timing of initiation of breast-milk expression on milk volume and timing of lactogenesis stage II among mothers of very low-birth-weight infants. Breastfeed Med 2015;10(2):84–91.
50. Parker LA, Sullivan S, Krueger C, et al. Effect of early breast milk expression on milk volume and timing of lactogenesis stage II among mothers of very low birth weight infants: a pilot study. J Perinatol 2012;32(3):205–9.
51. Berens P, Labbok M. Academy of Breastfeeding Medicine. ABM clinical protocol #13: contraception during breastfeeding, revised 2015. Breastfeed Med 2015;10:3–12.
52. Lussier MM, Brownell EA, Proulx TA, et al. Daily breastmilk volume in mothers of very low birth weight neonates: a repeated-measures randomized trial of hand

expression versus electric breast pump expression. Breastfeed Med 2015;10: 312–7.

53. Knight CH, Peaker M, Wilde CJ. Local control of mammary development and function. Rev Reprod 1998;3(2):104–12.

54. Glasier A, McNeilly AS, Howie PW. The prolactin response to suckling. Clin Endocrinol (Oxf) 1984;21(2):109–16.

55. Blatchford DR, Hendry KA, Wilde CJ. Autocrine regulation of protein secretion in mouse mammary epithelial cells. Biochem Biophys Res Commun 1998;248(3): 761–6.

56. Slutzah M, Codipilly CN, Potak D, et al. Refrigerator storage of expressed human milk in the neonatal intensive care unit. J Hum Lact 2010;26(3):233–4.

57. Schanler RJ, Fraley JK, Lau C, et al. Breastmilk cultures and infection in extremely premature infants. J Perinatol 2011;31(5):335–8.

58. Handa D, Ahrabi AF, Codipilly CN, et al. Do thawing and warming affect the integrity of human milk? J Perinatol 2014;34(11):863–6.

59. Rechtman DJ, Lee ML, Berg H. Effect of environmental conditions on unpasteurized donor human milk. Breastfeed Med 2006;1(1):24–6.

60. Stellwagen LM, Vaucher YE, Chan CS, et al. Pooling expressed breastmilk to provide a consistent feeding composition for premature infants. Breastfeed Med 2013;8:205–9.

61. Dougherty D, Nash A. Bar coding from breast to baby: a comprehensive breast milk management system for the NICU. Neonatal Netw 2009;28(5):321–8.

62. Drenckpohl D, Bowers L, Cooper H. Use of the six sigma methodology to reduce incidence of breast milk administration errors in the NICU. Neonatal Netw 2007; 26(3):161–6.

63. Meier PP, Engstrom JL, Zuleger JL, et al. Accuracy of a user-friendly centrifuge for measuring creamatocrits on mothers' milk in the clinical setting. Breastfeed Med 2006;1(2):79–87.

64. Lonnerdal B. Bioactive proteins in human milk: mechanisms of action. J Pediatr 2010;156(2 Suppl):S26–30.

65. Molinari CE, Casadio YS, Hartmann BT, et al. Proteome mapping of human skim milk proteins in term and preterm milk. J Proteome Res 2012;11(3):1696–714.

66. Nyqvist KH, Anderson GC, Bergman N, et al. State of the art and recommendations. kangaroo mother care: application in a high-tech environment. Breastfeed Rev 2010;18(3):21–8.

67. Spatz DL. Ten steps for promoting and protecting breastfeeding for vulnerable infants. J Perinat Neonatal Nurs 2004;18(4):385–96.

68. Hurst NM, Valentine CJ, Renfro L, et al. Skin-to-skin holding in the neonatal intensive care unit influences maternal milk volume. J Perinatol 1997;17:213–7.

69. Davanzo R, Brovedani P, Travan L, et al. Intermittent kangaroo mother care: a NICU protocol. J Hum Lact 2013;29(3):332–8.

70. Meier P, Patel AL, Wright K, et al. Management of breastfeeding during and after the maternity hospitalization for late preterm infants. Clin Perinatol 2013;40(4): 689–705.

71. Meier PP, Engstrom JL. Test weighing for term and premature infants is an accurate procedure. Arch Dis Child Fetal Neonatal Ed 2007;92(2):F155–6.

72. Haase B, Barreira J, Murphy PK, et al. The development of an accurate test weighing technique for preterm and high-risk hospitalized infants. Breastfeed Med 2009;4(3):151–6.

73. Hurst NM, Meier PP, Engstrom JL, et al. Mothers performing in-home measurement of milk intake during breastfeeding of their preterm infants: maternal reactions and feeding outcomes. J Hum Lact 2004;20(2):178–87.
74. Meier PP, Brown LP, Hurst NM, et al. Nipple shields for preterm infants: effect on milk transfer and duration of breastfeeding. J Hum Lact 2000;16(2):106–14.
75. Bigger HR, Fogg LJ, Patel A, et al. Quality indicators for human milk use in very low-birthweight infants: are we measuring what we should be measuring? J Perinatol 2014;34(4):287–91.
76. Quigley M, McGuire W. Formula versus donor breast milk for feeding preterm or low birth weight infants. Cochrane Database Syst Rev 2014;(4):CD002971.
77. Collado MC, Cernada M, Neu J, et al. Factors influencing gastrointestinal tract and microbiota immune interaction in preterm infants. Pediatr Res 2015;77(6): 726–31.
78. Underwood MA, Gaerlan S, De Leoz ML, et al. Human milk oligosaccharides in premature infants: absorption, excretion, and influence on the intestinal microbiota. Pediatr Res 2015;78(6):670–7.
79. Meier PP, Engstrom JL, Rossman B. Breastfeeding peer counselors as direct lactation care providers in the neonatal intensive care unit. J Hum Lact 2013; 29(3):313–22.
80. Lopez LM, Grey TW, Stuebe AM, et al. Combined hormonal versus nonhormonal versus progestin-only contraception in lactation. Cochrane Database Syst Rev 2015;(3):CD003988.
81. Cregan MD, de Mello TR, Hartmann PE. Pre-term delivery and breast expression: consequences for initiating lactation. Adv Exp Med Biol 2000;478:427–8.
82. Hartmann P, Cregan M. Lactogenesis and the effects of insulin-dependent diabetes mellitus and prematurity. J Nutr 2001;131(11):3016S–20S.
83. Mulready-Ward C, Sackoff J. Outcomes and factors associated with breastfeeding for <8 weeks among preterm infants: findings from 6 states and NYC, 2004-2007. Matern Child Health J 2013;17(9):1648–57.
84. Dewey KG. Maternal and fetal stress are associated with impaired lactogenesis in humans. J Nutr 2001;131(11):3012S–5S.
85. Esquerra-Zwiers A, Rossman B, Meier P, et al. "It's somebody else's milk": unraveling the tension in mothers of preterm infants who provide consent for pasteurized donor human milk. J Hum Lact 2016;32(1):95–102.

The Importance of Human Milk for Immunity in Preterm Infants

Erin D. Lewis, PhD[a], Caroline Richard, RD, PhD[a],
Bodil M. Larsen, RD, PhD[a,b], Catherine J. Field, RD, PhD[a,*]

KEYWORDS

- Leukocytes • Inflammation • Maturation • Peptides • Gangliosides
- Immunoglobulins • Long-chain polyunsaturated fatty acids

KEY POINTS

- Preterm infants have a lower number of immune cells, lower functional capacity, and dysregulated inflammatory response compared with term infants.
- Human milk provides a variety of immune protective and immune maturation factors that are predicted to be important for immune development in the preterm infant.
- The most studied immune components in human milk include antimicrobial proteins, maternal leukocytes, immunoglobulins, cytokines and chemokines, oligosaccharides, gangliosides, nucleotides, and long-chain polyunsaturated fatty acids.
- Provision of these components in human milk, donor milk, or formula may provide immunologic benefits to the preterm infant.

INTRODUCTION

The immune system of preterm infants is immature, placing them at increased risk for serious immune-related complications. Human milk contains immunologic components that have the potential to provide immune benefits to the preterm infants.

IMMUNE SYSTEM DEVELOPMENT AND THE PRETERM INFANT

The infant, particularly the preterm infant, is born with an immune system that is distinct from an adult's. Maturation occurs in the early postnatal period and is influenced by the infant's diet (breast milk and foods) and environment (pathogens,

Disclosure Statement: The authors have nothing to disclose.
[a] Department of Agricultural, Food and Nutritional Science, University of Alberta, 8602 112 Street, Edmonton, Alberta T6G 2E1, Canada; [b] Department of Pediatrics, Nutrition Services, Alberta Health Services, University of Alberta, 8440 112 Street, Edmonton, Alberta T6G 2B7, Canada
* Corresponding author. 4-126A Li Ka Shing Centre for Health Research Innovation, University of Alberta, Edmonton, Alberta T6G2E1, Canada.
E-mail address: catherine.field@ualberta.ca

Clin Perinatol 44 (2017) 23–47
http://dx.doi.org/10.1016/j.clp.2016.11.008
0095-5108/17/© 2016 Elsevier Inc. All rights reserved.

allergens, microflora) (reviewed in Ref.[1]). The acquired/adaptive immune system, consisting of T and B lymphocytes, recognizes foreign pathogens and antigens after presentation by antigen-presenting cells (APCs). However, because of low antigen exposure in utero, the infant acquired immune system is naïve at birth, lacking the immunologic memory and functionality of the adult (reviewed in Ref.[2]). Because of this, the innate immune system (which includes mast cells, neutrophils, natural killer [NK] cells, monocytes/macrophages, dendritic cells [DCs], basophils, and eosinophils) serves as the primary immune defense for the infant. Although the infant relies on their innate immune system, it is reported to produce fewer cytokines than the adult, in response to various challenges.[3]

OVERVIEW OF THE IMMUNE IMMATURITY OF THE PRETERM INFANT

Preterm infants have increased risk of infections compared with term infants, partly attributed to immune immaturity. Further, preterm infants are reported to have poorer immunosurveillance and a hyperregulated or dysregulated inflammatory response compared with term infants.

The major differences are as follows:

1. Lower concentration of circulating T cells, a higher proportion of naïve T cells, and a smaller bone marrow neutrophil storage pool.
2. Lower functional capacity of most immune cells (macrophages, neutrophils, DCs, NK cells, T and B cells).
3. Lower production of immunoactive proteins (complement and cytokines, immunoglobulin) when challenged.

Details of the differences and perturbations that characterize the preterm immune system have been comprehensively reviewed by others[4–10] and are summarized in **Table 1**.

CLINICAL BENEFITS OF HUMAN MILK TO THE IMMUNE HEALTH OF PRETERM INFANTS

Provision of human milk, has been demonstrated to reduce the risk of many immune-related conditions in preterm infants.

Necrotizing Enterocolitis

Necrotizing enterocolitis (NEC) is the most frequent and serious cause of gastrointestinal-related morbidity and mortality in preterm infants (reviewed in Ref.[11]). The inability to appropriately defend against microbes, and regulate inflammation and wound healing, contribute to the high systemic concentrations of inflammatory mediators (interleukin [IL]-1, IL-6, IL-8, and tumor necrosis factor [TNF]-α) characteristic of NEC (reviewed in Ref.[11]). Studies have demonstrated that preterm infants, including very preterm infants (<32 weeks), fed mother's milk[12,13] or donor milk[14] have lower incidence of NEC than those not exposed to human milk (Cochrane review by Quigley and colleagues[14]). This suggests that components in milk modulate this condition, possibly through their immune properties.

Allergies and Other Atopic Diseases

Allergies and other atopic diseases (asthma, allergic rhinitis, and atopic dermatitis) are more commonly observed in a preterm infant and believed to result from a failure to develop tolerance to an antigen.[15,16] Tolerance is a state of local and systemic immune unresponsiveness to antigens that occurs early in life.[17] At birth, the immune system is characterized by a predominant type 2 T-helper (Th2) cytokine response

Table 1
Components of the immune system in preterm infants

Components of the Immune System	Role and Function	In Preterm Infant	Ref
Physical Barrier			
Skin	Prevent penetration of pathogens.	The epidermal barrier function fully develops at approximately the 32nd to 34th week of gestation. The skin of very PT infants is immature and more susceptible to rupture.	4
Mucous membranes	Mucous and secretory components in the respiratory and gastrointestinal tracts protect against the entry of pathogens.	The gastrointestinal tract is not fully mature in PT infants with lower gastric acidity. ↓ amounts of MHC receptors and secretory components are detectable until 29th week of gestation. ↓ number of B cells that produce antibodies before the first postnatal week.	120–123
Innate immune system			
Complement system proteins	On activation, the complement system (≈ 20 proteins) generates different molecules (C3a, C3) that release inflammatory mediators, and stimulate chemotaxis and phagocytosis and microbial lysis.	↓ amounts of proteins (C1, C4, and factor B) of the complement system before the third trimester of pregnancy. ↓ pathogen-killing abilities and deficiency in the pattern-recognition receptor mannose-binding lectin in PT vs term infants. ↑ with gestational age.	6,8,124,125

(continued on next page)

Table 1
(continued)

Components of the Immune System	Role and Function	In Preterm Infant	Ref
Monocytes and macrophages	Phagocytize microorganisms and intracellular destruction with toxic substances (superoxide anions, hydroxyl radicals, nitric oxide, lysozyme). They are APCs expressing MHC classes I and II that can induce T-cell proliferation through the secretion of cytokines. Leukocytes	↓ capacity at processing/presenting antigens and cytokines production in infants vs adults. ↓ cytokine production (IFN-γ and TNF-α) from monocytes in PT vs term infants.	5,9,18,126–128
Neutrophils	(neutrophils, macrophages and lymphocytes) can also release APPs that bind and destroy microorganisms.	↑ in cytokines and APPs production with gestational age. ↓ neutrophils storage pool before 32nd week of gestation. ↓ amounts of molecules involved in the recruitment of neutrophils to the site of infection (P-selectin, L-selectin, E-selectin, CR3) in PT vs term infants. ↓ capacity of neutrophils to deal with pathogens (ex: ↓ respiratory activity) in PT vs term infants. ↑ with gestational age.	7,129–133
DCs		Similar number of DCs and level of TLR9 in PT and term infants vs adults. ↓ lower capacity to produce IFN-α on TLR9 challenge in PT vs term infants.	134
NK cells	Ability to lyse infected cells (tumor and virus-infected cells) but also bacteria, parasites, and fungi.	Similar (or slightly higher) number of NK cells in term infants vs adult. ↓ NK cytotoxic activity (less efficient) in term infants vs adult. ↓ number of NK cells and NK activity in PT vs term infants.	135,136

Adaptive immune system

T cells	Need to be stimulated by APC to get activated and then regulate immune responses by producing cytokines (Th1 and Th2). Also play a role in activating NK cells, monocytes, and B cells.	↓ T cells proliferative response (IL-2), production of Th1 cytokines (IFN-γ), and cytolytic activity in infants vs adults. ↓ absolute number of T cells and proliferative capacity in PT vs term infants.	5,137,138
B cells	Activated by T cells. Main producer of Ig antibodies for the specific humoral immunity. Igs are involved in OT.	↓ production of Ig antibodies in term infants vs adults. ↓ expression of CD40, CD40L, and TNF family receptors needed for B-cell activation and effective antibody response in PT vs term infants.	125,139
Passive immune system	Maternal IgG transfer to the fetus through the placenta to compensate for the lack of antibodies produced.	Transfer for IgG starts at approximately the 32nd to 34th week of gestation. ↑ with gestational age.	10,140

Abbreviations: ↑, higher; ↓, lower; APC, antigen-presenting cell; APP, antimicrobial proteins and peptide; DC, dendritic cell; IFN-γ, interferon gamma; Ig, immunoglobulin; IL, interleukin; MHC, major histocompatibility complex; NK, natural killer; OT, oral tolerance; PT, preterm; TLR, toll-like receptor; TNF-α, tumor necrosis factor-alpha.

From Blumer N, Pfefferle PI, Renz H. Development of mucosal immune function in the intrauterine and early postnatal environment. Curr Opin Gastroenterol 2007;23(6):655–60; with permission.

and maturation during infancy is associated with an improved Th1 response.[18] It is hypothesized that maintenance of an exaggerated Th2 response (production of IL-4, IL-5, IL-6, and IL-13) over a Th1 response (ie, IL-2, interferon [IFN]-γ, and TNF-α) increases the risk for allergies and other atopic diseases.[19] Feeding human milk has been demonstrated to promote the development of tolerance in the infant[20] and is associated with a lower risk for allergies, including food allergy,[20] asthma (systematic review and meta-analysis by Dogaru and colleagues[21]), and atopic dermatitis (reviewed in Ref.[15]).

Bronchopulmonary Dysplasia

Bronchopulmonary dysplasia (BPD) occurs in approximately 16% to 23% of preterm infants.[22] The development of BPD is commonly attributed to the impairment of innate immune responses, a predominant Th2 response, and dysregulation of inflammation (reviewed in Ref.[23]). Exclusive breastfeeding is associated with a lower incidence of BPD,[24] and providing donor human milk reduces the incidence of BPD among preterm infants.[25]

Retinopathy of Prematurity

Retinopathy of prematurity (ROP) is a major cause of blindness, and preterm infants are at increased risk. It is hypothesized that poor long-chain polyunsaturated fatty acid (LCPUFA) status[26] in conjunction with an exaggerated and poorly regulated inflammatory response[27] are involved in ROP pathogenesis. Recently, a systematic review concluded that any exposure to human milk protected the preterm infants from ROP,[28] suggesting a role for n-3 LCPUFAs and the factors that regulate inflammation present in human milk.

IMMUNE COMPONENTS IN HUMAN MILK

There are many components of human milk that may contribute to the immune-related clinical benefits of human milk to the preterm infant. These components (**Table 2**) can be grouped into 2 roles: immune protection and immune development/maturation. Key components are discussed as follows.

Protective Factors

- Help maintain immune barrier functions and protect gastrointestinal epithelium by preventing colonization of pathogenic bacteria and dysbiosis of microbiome.
- Provide direct (passive) immunity to the infant protecting the infant from microbial challenges.
- Exert anti-inflammatory (immune regulatory) effects.

Development/Maturation Factors

- Promote maturation, differentiation, and development of infant's gut-associated lymphoid tissue (GALT), and systemic immune system.
- Promote the development of tolerance to environmental and dietary antigens and the microbiome.

Immune components in human milk (see **Table 2**) have immune protective and/or immune maturation roles that are particularly beneficial to the preterm infant's poorly developed immune system (see **Table 1**). The functions of some key immune components found in human milk, and how the components play or may play a role in immune protection or maturation of preterm infants will follow. There is evidence that there are differences in composition of immune factors in preterm and term milk (summarized in

Table 2 Immune protective and developmental factors in human milk		
Protective	**Developmental**	**Both**
Lactoferrin	G-CSF	Leukocytes
Lysozyme	IGF-1 and IGF-2	Immunoglobulins
Lactadherin	Cytokines	Cytokines
Lactoperoxidase	CXC Chemokines	CXC Chemokines
α-lactoglobulin	Bifidus factor	MCP-1
κ-casein	TGF-β and TGF-α	EGF
Defensins	Nucleotides	Oligosaccharides
Haptocorrin		Gangliosides
Cytokines		Glycoaminoglycans
CXCL-9 (MIP)		Bifidus factor
IP-10		LCPUFA (AA, DHA)
sCD14		miRNAs
TNF-RI		
Mucins		

Abbreviations: AA, arachidonic acid; DHA, docosahexaenoic acid; EGF, epidermal growth factor; G-CSF, granulocyte-macrophage colony-stimulating factor; IGF, insulinlike growth factor; IP, interferon gamma (IFN)-γ-inducible protein; LCPUFA, long-chain polyunsaturated fatty acid; MCP, monocyte-chemotactic protein 1; MIP, monokine induced by IFN-γ; miRNA, microRNA; TGF, transforming growth factor; TNF, tumor necrosis factor.

Adapted from Hosea Blewett HJ, Cicalo MC, Holland CD, et al. The immunological components of human milk. Adv Food Nutr Res 2008;54:49.

Table 3); however, the implications for the preterm infant are not yet known, so human milk will refer to both.

Antimicrobial Proteins and Peptides

Many of the proteins and peptides present in human milk have antimicrobial properties beneficial to the preterm infant. A more detailed description is covered in Bo Lönnerdal's article, "Bioactive Proteins in Human Milk – Potential Benefits for Preterm Infants," in this issue.

Lactoferrin

Lactoferrin is one of the most abundant antimicrobial proteins in human milk and can directly protect the infant from enteric pathogens and promote the development of GALT and the infant's systemic immune system (reviewed in Ref.[29]). In support of this, a recent Cochrane review concluded that lactoferrin supplementation decreased the risk of NEC and late-onset sepsis in preterm infants.[30]

Lysozyme

Lysozyme is an antimicrobial protein in human milk that functions with lactoferrin (reviewed in Ref.[31]). Intestinal tissue from infants with NEC were found to have very few lysozyme-producing intestinal cells compared with infants without NEC,[32] suggesting that exogenous lysozymes in milk may be a critical factor for NEC protection. This hypothesis was confirmed in a study using a pig model, in which sows were genetically modified to produce human lysozyme in milk[33] and the nursing piglets from these sows had a better ability to inhibit *Escherichia coli* growth in the duodenum.[33]

Lactadherin

Lactadherin is a milk fat globule membrane protein that has been shown to prevent rotavirus infection, which is common in preterm infants and in human intestinal cells.[34]

Table 3
Immune components in human milk and the implications for preterm infant's immunity

Component	Function for Infant	VPT[2] Compared with Term Milk	PT Compared with Term Milk
Proteins			
Lactoferrin	Antimicrobial, iron carrier	Lower in VPT[36,141]	No difference[38,142,143]
Lysozyme	Antimicrobial	Higher in VPT[38,144] No difference[141,142,145]	
Lactadherin	Antimicrobial	Lower in VPT[36]	
Defensins	Antimicrobial		Higher in PT (only defensin-α)[38,39]
MicroRNAs	Lymphocyte development, inflammatory mediator		Unknown
Cellular			
Macrophages	Phagocytosis, pathogen defense, lymphocyte activation	Higher in VPT colostrum[146,147]	No difference[114]
Neutrophils	Unknown		Higher in PT[114,146]
Lymphocytes	Lymphocyte development, inflammatory mediator		No difference[114]
Immunoglobulins			
sIgA/IgA	Antimicrobial, pathogen binding inhibition	Higher in VPT[65,141]	Higher in PT[148] No difference[38,142]
IgG	Antimicrobial, antibody-mediated cytotoxicity		No difference[148]
IgM	Antimicrobial, antibody-mediated cytotoxicity		No difference[148]
Cytokines			
IL-1β	Inflammatory mediatory, intestinal and immune system trophic factor	No difference[63]	No difference[113]
IL-2	Modulates T-cell development		Higher in PT (colostrum only)[113]
IL-6	Intestinal trophic factor, inflammatory mediator, B-cell activation		Lower in PT[113]
IL-8	Intestinal trophic factor, recruitment of maternal leukocytes	Lower in VPT[63,65]	No difference[113,149]

(continued on next page)

Table 3
(continued)

Component	Function for Infant	VPT[2] Compared with Term Milk	PT Compared with Term Milk
IL-10	Intestinal trophic factor, anti-inflammatory cytokine, promote tolerance	Higher in VPT[63]	
IFN-γ	Stimulates Th1 inflammatory response, suppresses Th2 allergic response		No difference[38]
TNF-α	Proinflammatory cytokine	Lower in VPT[65]	No difference[38]
Chemokines and other soluble factors			
CXCR-1	Cytokine receptor		Higher in PT[149]
CXCR-2	Cytokine receptor		No difference[149]
CXCL-9 (MIP)	Antimicrobial, NK and T-cell chemoattractant		No difference[115]
IP-10	Antimicrobial, NK and T-cell chemoattractant		No difference[115]
sCD14	Inflammatory mediator, promote differentiation and activation of lymphocytes		Higher in PT[38]
TNF-RI	Reduces TNF-α activity, mediates inflammation	Lower in VPT[150]	
G-CSF	Stimulates neutrophil growth and differentiation, intestinal trophic factor		Lower in PT[71]
MCP-1	T-cell chemoattractant		Lower in PT (mature milk)[151]
Growth factors			
TGF-β and TGF-α	Intestinal trophic factor, promote tolerance	Higher in VPT[65]	Higher in PT[79] No difference[38]
EGF	Intestinal trophic factor, promote tolerance	Higher in VPT[65]	Higher in PT[79]
IGF-1 and IGF-2	Promote development and maturation of gastrointestinal cells		No difference[152]

(continued on next page)

Table 3
(continued)

Component	Function for Infant	VPT[2] Compared with Term Milk	PT Compared with Term Milk
Oligosaccharides			
HMO	Promote colonization of commensal bacteria, pathogen binding		Higher in PT[89,153]
Gangliosides	Prebiotic, suppress inflammation		GM3 lower and GD3 higher in PT[98]
Other immune factors			
LCPUFAs	Promote tolerance and Th1 response		Higher in PT[154]
Nucleotides	Intestinal trophic factor, promote differentiation and activation of lymphocytes		AMP lower in PT, hypoxan lower in PT[155]
Food antigens	Promote tolerance		Unknown

Abbreviations: EGF, epidermal growth factor; G-CSF, granulocyte-macrophage colony-stimulating factor; HMO, human milk oligosaccharides; IFN-γ, interferon gamma; Ig, immunoglobulin; IGF, insulinlike growth factor; IL, interleukin; IP, interferon gamma (IFN)-γ-inducible protein; LCPUFA, long-chain polyunsaturated fatty acid; MCP, monocyte-chemotactic protein 1; MIP, monokine induced by IFN-γ; PT, preterm; TGF, transforming growth factor; TNF-α, tumor necrosis factor-alpha; VPT, very preterm (<32 weeks).

From Blumer N, Pfefferle PI, Renz H. Development of mucosal immune function in the intrauterine and early postnatal environment. Curr Opin Gastroenterol 2007;23(6):655–60; with permission.

In support of this observation, lactadherin concentrations in human milk were inversely associated with symptoms of infection in rotavirus-infected newborns.[35] Interestingly, lactadherin concentrations are approximately 1.5-fold lower in preterm milk compared with term milk,[36] which may partly explain why complications of rotavirus infection are more severe in preterm infants.

Defensins
Defensins (α and β) are antimicrobial peptides secreted by Paneth cells. Preterm infants are reported to have a reduced ability to secrete these peptides (reviewed in Ref.[37]), therefore human milk provides defensins to the preterm infant. Defensin-α concentrations are reported to be higher in both preterm colostrum[38] and mature milk,[39] compared with term colostrum and mature milk. Human milk–derived defensin-β inhibited the growth of 2 common bacterial strains associated with NEC (*Salmonella* and *E coli*),[40] suggesting a role in reducing the risk of NEC.

MicroRNAs
MicroRNAs (miRNAs) are abundant in human milk, and have a wide array of immunologic functions including effects on immune development and maturation, cell signaling, and inflammatory responses (reviewed in Ref.[41]). Expression of 4 miRNAs was different in peripheral blood of preterm infants with BPD compared with control infants[42] and the miRNA profile (21 different miRNAs) in intestinal tissues from preterm infants with NEC differed from surgical control subjects.[43] Although these studies

suggest that aberrant expression of miRNA may be related to the pathogenesis of immune-related conditions in preterm infants, studies are needed to demonstrate that miRNA in human milk could be beneficial for the immune system of the preterm infant.

Maternal Leukocytes

Maternal leukocytes in human milk are present in an activated phenotype and are hypothesized to play a key role in bridging the gap between the naïve immune system of the infant and the immune system of the child (reviewed in Refs.[44,45]). The major maternal leukocytes are briefly discussed.

Macrophages

Macrophages found in human milk express activation markers, have phagocytic abilities, secrete immunoregulatory factors, and have been found to contain engulfed secretory immunoglobulin A (sIgA), suggesting that they may modulate lymphocyte functions and aid in bacterial defense in the gut (reviewed in Ref.[46]). The percentage of macrophages was found to be lower in milk from mothers with infants diagnosed with cow's milk allergy or atopic dermatitis,[47] suggesting a role for maternal macrophages in development of tolerance. Moreover, in infants who develop infections, the concentration of macrophages in human milk was found to increase,[48] suggesting that the presence of macrophages has a role in regulating infections in the infant.

Neutrophils

Neutrophils are also found in human milk expressing activation markers (reviewed in Ref.[46]). However, ex vivo studies have demonstrated that neutrophils have decreased polarity, motility, and adherence once secreted into milk, suggesting lower functional capacity. It is believed that neutrophils confer maternal immunologic protection (reviewed in Ref.[46]); however, reduced neutrophil functional capacity has been linked to NEC risk,[49] warranting further research on the role of milk-derived neutrophils.

Lymphocytes

Lymphocytes, mainly memory T (expressing CD45RO+) and B (expressing immunoglobulin [Ig]D-CD27+) are found in human milk (reviewed in Ref.[45]). Additionally, human milk lymphocytes are found to express markers of activation and mucosal homing markers, suggesting these cells are derived from the maternal mucosal immune system (reviewed in Ref.[45]). Memory and activated lymphocytes found in human milk could compensate for the naivety of the infant immune system, and promote infant T-cell development and maturation (reviewed in Ref.[46]). Several studies have demonstrated that when the infant has infections, including measles, gastrointestinal, respiratory, or influenza, the number of leukocytes in human milk increases. This suggests an important role for maternal milk leukocytes in infant immunosurveillance (reviewed in Ref.[44]). Although animal models have demonstrated activated, maternal leukocytes from breast milk are transferred to the infant gastrointestinal tract and circulation (reviewed in Ref.[50]), direct clinical evidence is lacking.

Immunoglobulins

Immunoglobulins are transferred systemically via the placenta from the mother to infant late in the third trimester, placing the preterm infant at an immunologic disadvantage. IgA/sIgA is the most abundant antibody in human milk and provides critical antimicrobial defenses to the immature infant gut by preventing pathogens from attaching to mucosal surfaces, neutralizing microbial toxins while providing passive immunity to the infant (reviewed in Ref.[51]). IgG and IgM are less abundant than IgA in milk, but have also been demonstrated to have immunosurveillance properties for the infant (reviewed in Ref.[52]). Several studies have demonstrated that sIgA concentrations in human milk are inversely associated with risk of atopy in infants.[53] In contrast, a recent Cochrane review concluded that the oral administration of a combination of bovine IgG/IgA did not reduce the incidence of NEC in preterm infants.[54] This suggests that bovine immunoglobulins are not the same as human, or that immunoglobulins may function in conjunction with other components in milk. A Cochrane review concluded that intravenous administration of IgG results in a 3% reduction in sepsis, but did not affect the incidence of NEC or BPD.[55] Two clinical trials demonstrated that intravenous administration of IgM-enriched immunoglobulin did not significantly reduce mortality rate from sepsis in preterm infants (reviewed in Ref.[56]). Collectively, these studies suggest that immunoglobulins have limited antimicrobial function on their own, or it is the specific type of immunoglobulin found in maternal milk that confers immune benefits. This may have implications on the role of immunoglobulins in donor milk.

Cytokines

Cytokines are signaling molecules that confer a variety of immunologic functions, including immune protection and immune function/development/maturation. Human milk contains an array of cytokines, including IL-1β, IL-2, IL-4, IL-5, IL-6, IL-8, IL-10, IFN-γ, and TNF-α (reviewed in Ref.[45]). Neonates have limited ability to produce many cytokines found in human milk (reviewed in Ref.[57]); therefore, human milk may serve as an important source. Previous research has demonstrated that some milk cytokines are protected from degradation and have activity in the infant intestine[58] (reviewed in Ref.[59]). Although the in vivo effects of milk-derived cytokines on the infant have not been established, it is hypothesized, based on their known functions, that cytokines present in human milk influence the development and maturation of the preterm infant's immune system. Cytokines may also be involved in reducing the risk of certain immune-related conditions in preterm infants. Some proposed effects of cytokines on the infant's immune system are:

1. Promote the development of a Th1 response. IFN-γ in particular is involved in the Th1 inflammatory response, suppression of a Th2 allergic response, and increases antigen presentation by APCs (reviewed in Ref.[60]). IL-2, IL-6, and TNF-α may also have a role in promoting a Th1 response in the preterm infant.
2. Aid in maturation of neonatal leukocytes. IL-1β has a role in cell differentiation and proliferation and IL-2 is a proliferative cytokine that stimulates T cells (reviewed in Ref.[60]). IL-2 in human milk may aid in the development of the immature T-lymphocyte population in the preterm infant.[61]
3. Regulation of inflammation. IL-1β and IL-6 are inflammatory mediators involved in activation of the acute phase of the immune response, which may assist in the regulation of inflammation in the preterm infant (reviewed in Ref.[60]). TNF-α is a proinflammatory cytokine involved in the regulation of inflammation (reviewed in Ref.[60]) and it is possible that human milk TNF-α may also compensate for the lower production by neonatal monocytes/macrophages (see **Table 1**). TNF-receptor 1 (TNF-R1) has been demonstrated ex vivo to reduce TNF-α activity by binding to TNF-α,[62] and may be useful in blocking endogenously produced TNF-α by the infant intestine and mediating the anti-inflammatory effects of human milk. IL-10 also acts as an anti-inflammatory cytokine. Very preterm milk contains 84% higher concentrations of IL-10 compared with term milk,[63] which may be important for mediating the excessive inflammatory response in the preterm infant.

4. Enhanced immunoglobulin production. IL-6 has been demonstrated in vitro to stimulate B-cell immunoglobulin production,[64] which is reduced in infants compared with adults (see **Table 1**). IL-10 is a primary regulator of the inflammatory response and contributes to the differentiation and development of infant IgA-producing cells (reviewed in Ref.[60]). It is believed that IL-10 may be involved in the prevention of allergy, but experimental support is mixed.

5. Maturation of the infant gastrointestinal system. IL-8 facilitates the maturation of the infant intestine and acts as a chemoattractant for neutrophils, thus having an important role in innate immunity (reviewed in Ref.[60]). Interestingly, very preterm colostrum[65] and very preterm mature milk[63] are reported to have less IL-8 compared with both preterm and term milk, yet implications of this have not been investigated.

Chemokines and Other Soluble Immune Components

CXC chemokines

CXC chemokines, including IFN-γ-inducible protein (IP-10) and monokine induced by IFN-γ (MIP), are involved in chemotaxis, neutrophil trafficking, Th1 response, and development of lymphoid tissues to aid in defense against bacterial infection (reviewed in Ref.[66]). CXC chemokine receptors (CXCR) including *CXCR-1* and *CXCR-2* are expressed on immune cells of the innate immune system and act as receptors for cytokines, including IL-8 (reviewed in Ref.[66]). In vitro, IP-10 and MIP have been shown to protect against *E coli* and *Listeria monocytogenes* in peripheral blood mononuclear cells.[67] The presence of these antimicrobial CXC chemokines in milk may provide some immune protection to the preterm infant; however, in vivo evidence is lacking.

Monocyte-chemotactic protein 1 and CC chemokines

Monocyte-chemotactic protein 1 (MCP-1) and CC chemokines promote homing of leukocytes to lymphoid tissue, including Th2 cell recruitment and macrophage and NK cell migration (reviewed in Ref.[60]). The implications for the preterm infant are unknown; however, the presence of MCP-1 in human milk has the potential to assist in recruitment of maternal leukocytes to sites of infection and aid in host defenses.

Soluble CD14

Soluble CD14 (sCD14) is a soluble receptor that acts as an acute-phase protein to mediate inflammation and promote a Th1 response (reviewed in Ref.[60]). In vitro, sCD14 has been demonstrated to stimulate B-cell growth and differentiation, and assist in the activation of neonatal B cells, which would help with antibody production.[68] Lower concentrations of sCD14 in human milk are inversely associated with atopy or eczema[69] and asthma[70] in infants. Thus, the high levels of sCD14 in human milk may contribute to the benefits of feeding human milk on incidence of allergy and atopic disease. However, specific studies in preterm infants, who are at greater risk of allergy and atopic diseases, are lacking.

Granulocyte-colony stimulating factor

Granulocyte-colony stimulating factor (G-CSF) is important for neutrophil growth and differentiation. G-CSF receptors are present in the intestine, suggesting that G-CSF may also assist in the maturation of GALT.[71] In a randomized control trial, oral G-CSF treatment reduced the risk of NEC in preterm infants.[72] Furthermore, a clinical trial found that administration of G-CSF improved survival in preterm infants with sepsis-induced neutropenia. However, G-CSF is reported to be 50% lower in preterm milk,[71] which may be disadvantageous to the immature gastrointestinal immune system and lower neutrophil function observed in preterm infants.

Growth Factors

Growth factors in human milk are present in high concentrations, which are advantageous to the preterm infant for maturation and protection of the intestine. Additionally, growth factors interact with IL-10 and play a key role in the promotion of immunologic tolerance (reviewed in Ref.[46]).

Transforming growth factor-β

Transforming growth factor-β (TGF-β), along with other regulatory cytokines and growth factors, is believed to play a role in the maturation and promotion of infant immune responses and promote development of the gastrointestinal system and tolerance (reviewed in Ref.[73]). TGF-β concentrations in human milk were inversely associated with risk of atopy[74] and wheeze[75] in infants. A systematic review concluded that TGF-β concentrations in human milk were negatively associated with infant outcomes of allergy, including serum levels of β-lactoglobulin and casein-specific IgA and IgG antibodies,[76] suggesting TGF-β in human milk may be important in reducing risk of infant allergy. In vitro, TGF-β was shown to reduce endotoxin-induced inflammatory cytokine responses by intestinal macrophages.[77] Further, in a model of transgenic mice pups deficient in TGF-β, NEC-like intestinal injury was induced and orally supplemented TGF-β was protective to the pup.[77] Collectively, these studies suggest that TGF-β plays a role in reducing the risk of NEC and atopic diseases in the preterm infant; however, clinical trials are required to confirm this hypothesis.

Epidermal growth factor

Epidermal growth factor (EGF) plays an important role in cellular proliferation and maturation and acts in conjunction with other immune factors to assist in development of GALT (reviewed in Ref.[78]). Very preterm milk contains 60% to 80% higher concentrations of EGF compared with preterm and term,[79] which may be a compensatory mechanism to account for the lack of placental transfer of EGF. There is increasing evidence that EGF in human milk may be protective against NEC (reviewed in Ref.[80]). In animal models, EGF-supplemented formula in rodents reduced the incidence of NEC,[81] downregulated proinflammatory cytokines, and upregulated anti-inflammatory cytokines,[82] and maintained intestinal barrier function.[83]

Insulinlike growth factors

Insulinlike growth factors (IGF) promote cell growth, which may aid in the development and maturation of the infant's gastrointestinal tract (reviewed in Ref.[84]). Intraperitoneal IGF-1 was protective in a rodent model of NEC,[85] suggesting its presence in human milk may confer similar benefits to preterm infants.

Oligosaccharides

Oligosaccharides, including gangliosides and glycans, are abundant in human milk, with concentrations 100-fold to 1000-fold higher than bovine milk (reviewed in Ref.[86]). The immunologic functions are discussed briefly and is detailed elsewhere in this issue (see Sara Moukarzel and Lars Bode's article, "Human Milk Oligosaccharides and the Preterm Infant: A Journey in Sickness and in Health," in this issue).

Human milk oligosaccharides

Human milk oligosaccharides (HMOs) are prebiotic agents that promote the colonization of beneficial bacteria in the colon, prevent pathogen adhesion to intestinal surfaces, and alter responses in GALT (reviewed in Ref.[86]). HMO-supplemented formula reduced the pathology score in a rodent model of NEC.[87] HMO diversity is thought to be beneficial, as individual oligosaccharides bind differently to specific pathogens. Preterm milk is reported to have a lower HMO diversity,[88,89] which may increase susceptibility/risk of the preterm infant. In vitro, cord blood mononuclear cells incubated with HMOs increase the IFN-γ, IL-4, and IL-13–producing T cells, and T-cell activation markers,[90] suggesting that HMOs may influence maturation of lymphocytes. Despite this, 2 recent reviews concluded that there is insufficient evidence to provide HMOs to preterm infants to reduce the risk of NEC.[91,92]

Ganglioside

Ganglioside composition in human milk is unique, with higher concentrations of GD3 and GM3 compared with bovine milk or infant formula. There is considerable evidence that gangliosides have roles in pathogen inhibition, development and maturation of the infant's GALT, and oral tolerance (reviewed in Ref.[93]). In animals, ganglioside-supplemented formulas (mixtures of GM3, GD3, and GD1) altered the inflammatory response (increased anti-inflammatory IL-10 and decreased proinflammatory TNF-α and IL-6), decreased the incidence and pathology of NEC,[94] and increased the number of Th1 and Th2 cytokine-secreting lymphocytes[95] and IgA-secreting cells in GALT. In humans, ganglioside-supplemented formula decreased E coli and increased bifidobacterial in feces of infants, suggesting a modulation of the gut microbiome.[96] Furthermore, ex vivo ganglioside exposure (GD3, GM1, GM3) of infant intestinal sections treated with E coli lipopolysaccharide reduced the production of proinflammatory cytokines (IL-1 β, IL-6, and IL-8).[97] It is unknown if the lower concentrations (approximately 65%) of GM3[98] in preterm milk compared with term milk have implications for the preterm infant.

Food Antigens

The exposure to food-specific antigens present in human milk, including ovalbumin (egg), β-lactoglobulin (milk), Ara h1/Ara h2 (peanuts), and gliadin (wheat), may modulate immune responses and contribute to the development of tolerance in the infant (reviewed in Ref.[16]). The induction of oral tolerance by dietary antigens in human milk may be dependent on the presence of other regulatory factors (TGF-β, cytokines, and probiotics)[99] and n-3 LCPUFA.[100] Administering food-specific antigens in maternal milk of rodents induced oral tolerance to egg[101] and peanuts,[102] possibly by promoting a Th1 response.[103] Similarly, the Ara h1/Ara h2-specific antibodies from human milk were shown to bind IgE and desensitize cells involved in an allergic response in mice.[104] However, the potential protective effect of dietary antigens is still controversial, as a recent Cochrane review of human trials concluded that avoidance of dietary antigens (eg, cow's milk, eggs) during lactation by women at high risk of having a child with an allergy might reduce the risk of atopic eczema in infants.[105] Clearly, better-designed trials are needed to confirm or refute the role of food antigens in human milk.

Nucleotides

Nucleotides and nucleic acids comprise approximately 20% of nonprotein nitrogen content in human milk and have a variety of immune-related functions, including modulation of intestinal lymphocytes, cytokines, and immunoglobulins; maturation of the gastrointestinal tract; and pathogen defense (reviewed in Ref.[106]). Most recently, a neonatal pig model of intrauterine growth restriction demonstrated that nucleotide-supplemented formula increased plasma concentrations of IgA and IL-1β and leukocyte number compared with unsupplemented formula.[107] A systematic review and meta-analysis concluded that nucleotide-supplemented infant formula, compared with breast milk or control formula, improved antibody response to several immunizations (influenza, polio, diphtheria) and reduced the number of diarrheal episodes,[108] suggesting a role not only in pathogen protection but also in immune maturation.

Long-Chain Polyunsaturated Fatty Acids

Concentrations of LCPUFAs arachidonic (AA) and docosahexaenoic (DHA) acid in human milk vary considerably based on diet and geographic location.[109] Although they constitute less than 1% of total fatty acids in human milk, there is evidence that these 2 LCPUFAs have a beneficial effect on immune system development and the establishment of tolerance in infants (reviewed in Refs.[46,110]). Epidemiologic studies suggest an inverse association between human milk DHA content and the development of atopic disease in children with family history of atopic disease (reviewed in Ref.[110]). Human and rodent[100] studies suggest that supplementing the maternal diet with DHA during lactation, thereby increasing the human milk DHA content, alters infants' immune function and promotes the establishment of oral tolerance in the first year of life (reviewed in Ref.[110]). Furthermore, preterm infants fed formula supplemented with AA and DHA had a higher proportion of memory T cells and better cytokine response to immune challenge, consistent with human milk feeding, compared with unsupplemented formula.[111] A meta-analysis concluded that supplementation with n-3 PUFA (DHA alone, or a mixture from fish oil or algae) reduced the risk of BPD and NEC, with no effect on risk of ROP, in very preterm infants.[112] Overall, providing additional LCPUFA to preterm infants, through breast milk or infant formula, appears to confer important immunologic benefits.

CONCLUSIONS AND CONSIDERATIONS FOR FUTURE RESEARCH

Overall, there is evidence that immune components present in human milk play a role in reducing the incidence of a variety of immune-related conditions (NEC, ROP, BPD, and allergies) in the preterm infant. Immune components present in human milk, including antimicrobial proteins, leukocytes, cytokines and chemokines, immunoglobulin, growth factors, oligosaccharides, LCPUFAs, and nucleotides, play important roles in both protection and maturation of the infant's naïve immune system. There are several considerations for future research that will aid in further understanding of how these immune components confer immunologic benefit, including the following:

1. Identifying specific immune needs of the preterm infant. Few studies have looked specifically at preterm immune development. The studies that have examined this population typically group all infants born at less than 37 weeks together.
2. Identifying the concentrations of immune factors in human milk and the effect of maternal diet, health, physiology, and environmental exposures. For example, composition of immune components in milk has been demonstrated to be greatly affected by lactation stage,[38,113–116] and therefore stage of lactation should be considered when feeding a preterm infant.
3. Standardizing and clarifying reporting of composition of human milk (volume, methods, maternal factors, gestational age).
4. Using clinical trials to identify the importance of immune components in milk on immune health in preterm infants. There are many components that have not been studied and function has only been hypothesized and most studies that have examined components in vivo have been in term infants or animal models of term infants. Additionally, most clinical trials have explored these by adding singularly to infant formula, and it is known that the immune system develops differently

in both term[117] and preterm[111] fed formula compared with human milk. The ideal study needs to alter these in mother's milk, ideally by changing her diet or physiologic state, and determining the outcome in the infant.

5. Ensuring that human milk provides the appropriate concentration of immune-benefiting compounds for the preterm infant. This includes determining if a preterm mother's milk is sufficient to meet the special immune needs of the infant and optimization of immune components in pasteurized donor milk that have been shown to change with pasteurization[118] (reviewed in Ref.[119]).

Best Practices

What is the current practice?

Preterm infants

Best Practice/Guideline/Care Path Objective(s)
1. Provide mother's own milk when possible + fortifiers to meet requirements of preterm infant for optimal growth.
2. Provide donor milk when not enough milk is produced + fortifiers to meet requirements of preterm infant for optimal growth.
3. If it is not possible to provide sufficient human milk (mothers or donor) consider supplementing with a preterm infant formula that has additional compounds added in which there is evidence from clinical trials (lactoferrin, G-CSF, gangliosides, nucleotides, and AA + DHA) that there is some benefit to the preterm infant's immune system.

What changes in current practice are likely to improve outcomes?

Adapt donor milk to consider infant gestational age or lactation stage so as to ensure the immunologic benefits to the preterm infant. Alternative pasteurization methods may preserve more immunologic components in human milk.

Summary Statement

Immune components (including antimicrobial proteins, leukocytes, cytokines and chemokines, immunoglobulins, growth factors, oligosaccharides, nucleotides, and LCPUFAs) present in human milk are critical for protection against immune-related conditions and maturation and development of the immune system in the preterm infant.

ACKNOWLEDGMENTS

The authors thank Laura VanderSluis for critically reviewing this article. Research was supported by a Natural Sciences and Engineering Research Council (NSERC) Discovery Grant (RES0008127) to C.J. Field. E.D. Lewis is recipient of an NSERC Doctoral Scholarship and Izaak Walton Killam Memorial Scholarship. C. Richard is recipient of postdoctoral fellowships from the Canadian Institutes of Health Research and Izaak Walton Killam Memorial Fellowship.

REFERENCES

1. Blumer N, Pfefferle PI, Renz H. Development of mucosal immune function in the intrauterine and early postnatal environment. Curr Opin Gastroenterol 2007; 23(6):655–60.
2. Perez-Cano FJ, Franch A, Castellote C, et al. The suckling rat as a model for immunonutrition studies in early life. Clin Dev Immunol 2012;2012:537310.
3. Marodi L. Innate cellular immune responses in newborns. Clin Immunol 2006; 118(2–3):137–44.

4. Cartlidge P. The epidermal barrier. Semin Neonatol 2000;5(4):273–80.
5. Garcia AM, Fadel SA, Cao S, et al. T cell immunity in neonates. Immunol Res 2000;22(2–3):177–90.
6. McGreal EP, Hearne K, Spiller OB. Off to a slow start: under-development of the complement system in term newborns is more substantial following premature birth. Immunobiology 2012;217(2):176–86.
7. Nussbaum C, Sperandio M. Innate immune cell recruitment in the fetus and neonate. J Reprod Immunol 2011;90(1):74–81.
8. Sharma AA, Jen R, Butler A, et al. The developing human preterm neonatal immune system: a case for more research in this area. Clin Immunol 2012;145(1): 61–8.
9. Strunk T, Currie A, Richmond P, et al. Innate immunity in human newborn infants: prematurity means more than immaturity. J Matern Fetal Neonatal Med 2011; 24(1):25–31.
10. van den Berg JP, Westerbeek EA, van der Klis FR, et al. Transplacental transport of IgG antibodies to preterm infants: a review of the literature. Early Hum Dev 2011;87(2):67–72.
11. Hunter CJ, Upperman JS, Ford HR, et al. Understanding the susceptibility of the premature infant to necrotizing enterocolitis (NEC). Pediatr Res 2008;63(2): 117–23.
12. Herrmann K, Carroll K. An exclusively human milk diet reduces necrotizing enterocolitis. Breastfeed Med 2014;9(4):184–90.
13. Sullivan S, Schanler RJ, Kim JH, et al. An exclusively human milk-based diet is associated with a lower rate of necrotizing enterocolitis than a diet of human milk and bovine milk-based products. J Pediatr 2010;156(4):562–7.e1.
14. Quigley MA, Henderson G, Anthony MY, et al. Formula milk versus donor breast milk for feeding preterm or low birth weight infants. Cochrane Database Syst Rev 2007;(4):CD002971.
15. Iyengar SR, Walker WA. Immune factors in breast milk and the development of atopic disease. J Pediatr Gastroenterol Nutr 2012;55(6):641–7.
16. Tawia S. Development of oral tolerance to allergens via breastmilk. Breastfeed Rev 2015;23(3):35–9.
17. Pabst O, Mowat AM. Oral tolerance to food protein. Mucosal Immunol 2012;5(3): 232–9.
18. Hartel C, Adam N, Strunk T, et al. Cytokine responses correlate differentially with age in infancy and early childhood. Clin Exp Immunol 2005;142(3):446–53.
19. Prescott SL. Early origins of allergic disease: a review of processes and influences during early immune development. Curr Opin Allergy Clin Immunol 2003;3(2):125–32.
20. van Odijk J, Kull I, Borres MP, et al. Breastfeeding and allergic disease: a multidisciplinary review of the literature (1966-2001) on the mode of early feeding in infancy and its impact on later atopic manifestations. Allergy 2003;58(9): 833–43.
21. Dogaru CM, Nyffenegger D, Pescatore AM, et al. Breastfeeding and childhood asthma: systematic review and meta-analysis. Am J Epidemiol 2014;179(10): 1153–67.
22. Fanaroff AA, Stoll BJ, Wright LL, et al. Trends in neonatal morbidity and mortality for very low birthweight infants. Am J Obstet Gynecol 2007;196(2):147.e1-8.
23. Madurga A, Mizikova I, Ruiz-Camp J, et al. Recent advances in late lung development and the pathogenesis of bronchopulmonary dysplasia. Am J Physiol Lung Cell Mol Physiol 2013;305(12):L893–905.

24. Spiegler J, Preuss M, Gebauer C, et al. Does breastmilk influence the development of bronchopulmonary dysplasia? J Pediatr 2016;169:76–80.e4.

25. Schanler RJ, Lau C, Hurst NM, et al. Randomized trial of donor human milk versus preterm formula as substitutes for mothers' own milk in the feeding of extremely premature infants. Pediatrics 2005;116(2):400–6.

26. Harris WS, Baack ML. Beyond building better brains: bridging the docosahexaenoic acid (DHA) gap of prematurity. J Perinatol 2015;35(1):1–7.

27. Sood BG, Madan A, Saha S, et al. Perinatal systemic inflammatory response syndrome and retinopathy of prematurity. Pediatr Res 2010;67(4):394–400.

28. Bharwani SK, Green BF, Pezzullo JC, et al. Systematic review and meta-analysis of human milk intake and retinopathy of prematurity: a significant update. J Perinatol 2016;36(11):913–20.

29. Donovan SM. The role of lactoferrin in gastrointestinal and immune development and function: a preclinical perspective. J Pediatr 2016;173(Suppl):S16–28.

30. Pammi M, Abrams SA. Oral lactoferrin for the prevention of sepsis and necrotizing enterocolitis in preterm infants. Cochrane Database Syst Rev 2015;(2):CD007137.

31. Lonnerdal B. Bioactive proteins in human milk: health, nutrition, and implications for infant formulas. J Pediatr 2016;173(Suppl):S4–9.

32. Coutinho HB, da Mota HC, Coutinho VB, et al. Absence of lysozyme (muramidase) in the intestinal Paneth cells of newborn infants with necrotising enterocolitis. J Clin Pathol 1998;51(7):512–4.

33. Lu D, Li Q, Wu Z, et al. High-level recombinant human lysozyme expressed in milk of transgenic pigs can inhibit the growth of *Escherichia coli* in the duodenum and influence intestinal morphology of sucking pigs. PLoS One 2014; 9(2):e89130.

34. Kvistgaard AS, Pallesen LT, Arias CF, et al. Inhibitory effects of human and bovine milk constituents on rotavirus infections. J Dairy Sci 2004;87(12): 4088–96.

35. Newburg DS, Peterson JA, Ruiz-Palacios GM, et al. Role of human-milk lactadherin in protection against symptomatic rotavirus infection. Lancet 1998; 351(9110):1160–4.

36. Molinari CE, Casadio YS, Hartmann BT, et al. Proteome mapping of human skim milk proteins in term and preterm milk. J Proteome Res 2012;11(3):1696–714.

37. Salzman NH, Underwood MA, Bevins CL. Paneth cells, defensins, and the commensal microbiota: a hypothesis on intimate interplay at the intestinal mucosa. Semin Immunol 2007;19(2):70–83.

38. Trend S, Strunk T, Lloyd ML, et al. Levels of innate immune factors in preterm and term mothers' breast milk during the 1st month postpartum. Br J Nutr 2016;115(7):1178–93.

39. Wang XF, Cao RM, Li J, et al. Identification of sociodemographic and clinical factors associated with the levels of human beta-defensin-1 and human beta-defensin-2 in the human milk of Han Chinese. Br J Nutr 2014;111(5):867–74.

40. Baricelli J, Rocafull MA, Vazquez D, et al. Beta-defensin-2 in breast milk displays a broad antimicrobial activity against pathogenic bacteria. J Pediatr (Rio J) 2015;91(1):36–43.

41. Alsaweed M, Hepworth AR, Lefevre C, et al. Human milk microRNA and total RNA differ depending on milk fractionation. J Cell Biochem 2015;116(10): 2397–407.

42. Wu YT, Chen WJ, Hsieh WS, et al. MicroRNA expression aberration associated with bronchopulmonary dysplasia in preterm infants: a preliminary study. Respir Care 2013;58(9):1527–35.

43. Ng PC, Chan KY, Leung KT, et al. Comparative miRNA expressional profiles and molecular networks in human small bowel tissues of necrotizing enterocolitis and spontaneous intestinal perforation. PLoS One 2015;10(8):e0135737.

44. Hassiotou F, Geddes DT. Immune cell-mediated protection of the mammary gland and the infant during breastfeeding. Adv Nutr 2015;6(3):267–75.

45. Hosea Blewett HJ, Cicalo MC, Holland CD, et al. The immunological components of human milk. Adv Food Nutr Res 2008;54:45–80.

46. Field CJ. The immunological components of human milk and their effect on immune development in infants. J Nutr 2005;135(1):1–4.

47. Jarvinen KM, Suomalainen H. Leucocytes in human milk and lymphocyte subsets in cow's milk-allergic infants. Pediatr Allergy Immunol 2002;13(4):243–54.

48. Riskin A, Almog M, Peri R, et al. Changes in immunomodulatory constituents of human milk in response to active infection in the nursing infant. Pediatr Res 2012;71(2):220–5.

49. Lam HS, Cheung HM, Poon TC, et al. Neutrophil CD64 for daily surveillance of systemic infection and necrotizing enterocolitis in preterm infants. Clin Chem 2013;59(12):1753–60.

50. Zhou L, Yoshimura Y, Huang Y, et al. Two independent pathways of maternal cell transmission to offspring: through placenta during pregnancy and by breastfeeding after birth. Immunology 2000;101(4):570–80.

51. Corthesy B. Multi-faceted functions of secretory IgA at mucosal surfaces. Front Immunol 2013;4:185.

52. Hurley WL, Theil PK. Perspectives on immunoglobulins in colostrum and milk. Nutrients 2011;3(4):442–74.

53. Orivuori L, Loss G, Roduit C, et al. Soluble immunoglobulin A in breast milk is inversely associated with atopic dermatitis at early age: the PASTURE cohort study. Clin Exp Allergy 2014;44(1):102–12.

54. Foster JP, Seth R, Cole MJ. Oral immunoglobulin for preventing necrotizing enterocolitis in preterm and low birth weight neonates. Cochrane Database Syst Rev 2016;(4):CD001816.

55. Ohlsson A, Lacy JB. Intravenous immunoglobulin for preventing infection in preterm and/or low birth weight infants. Cochrane Database Syst Rev 2013;(7):CD000361.

56. Tarnow-Mordi W, Isaacs D, Dutta S. Adjunctive immunologic interventions in neonatal sepsis. Clin Perinatol 2010;37(2):481–99.

57. Field CJ, Clandinin MT, Van Aerde JE. Polyunsaturated fatty acids and T-cell function: implications for the neonate. Lipids 2001;36(9):1025–32.

58. Calhoun DA, Lunoe M, Du Y, et al. Concentrations of granulocyte colony-stimulating factor in human milk after in vitro simulations of digestion. Pediatr Res 1999;46(6):767–71.

59. Garofalo R. Cytokines in human milk. J Pediatr 2010;156(2 Suppl):S36–40.

60. Agarwal S, Karmaus W, Davis S, et al. Immune markers in breast milk and fetal and maternal body fluids: a systematic review of perinatal concentrations. J Hum Lact 2011;27(2):171–86.

61. Bryan DL, Forsyth KD, Gibson RA, et al. Interleukin-2 in human milk: a potential modulator of lymphocyte development in the breastfed infant. Cytokine 2006; 33(5):289–93.

62. Buescher ES, McWilliams-Koeppen P. Soluble tumor necrosis factor-alpha (TNF-alpha) receptors in human colostrum and milk bind to TNF-alpha and neutralize TNF-alpha bioactivity. Pediatr Res 1998;44(1):37–42.
63. Mehta R, Petrova A. Very preterm gestation and breastmilk cytokine content during the first month of lactation. Breastfeed Med 2011;6(1):21–4.
64. Dienz O, Eaton SM, Bond JP, et al. The induction of antibody production by IL-6 is indirectly mediated by IL-21 produced by CD4+ T cells. J Exp Med 2009; 206(1):69–78.
65. Castellote C, Casillas R, Ramirez-Santana C, et al. Premature delivery influences the immunological composition of colostrum and transitional and mature human milk. J Nutr 2011;141(6):1181–7.
66. Palomino DC, Marti LC. Chemokines and immunity. Einstein (Sao Paulo) 2015; 13(3):469–73.
67. Cole AM, Ganz T, Liese AM, et al. Cutting edge: IFN-inducible ELR- CXC chemokines display defensin-like antimicrobial activity. J Immunol 2001;167(2): 623–7.
68. Filipp D, Alizadeh-Khiavi K, Richardson C, et al. Soluble CD14 enriched in colostrum and milk induces B cell growth and differentiation. Proc Natl Acad Sci U S A 2001;98(2):603–8.
69. Jones CA, Holloway JA, Popplewell EJ, et al. Reduced soluble CD14 levels in amniotic fluid and breast milk are associated with the subsequent development of atopy, eczema, or both. J Allergy Clin Immunol 2002;109(5):858–66.
70. Rothenbacher D, Weyermann M, Beermann C, et al. Breastfeeding, soluble CD14 concentration in breast milk and risk of atopic dermatitis and asthma in early childhood: birth cohort study. Clin Exp Allergy 2005;35(8):1014–21.
71. Calhoun DA, Lunoe M, Du Y, et al. Granulocyte colony-stimulating factor is present in human milk and its receptor is present in human fetal intestine. Pediatrics 2000;105(1):e7.
72. El-Ganzoury MM, Awad HA, El-Farrash RA, et al. Enteral granulocyte-colony stimulating factor and erythropoietin early in life improves feeding tolerance in preterm infants: a randomized controlled trial. J Pediatr 2014;165(6):1140–5.e1.
73. Penttila IA. Milk-derived transforming growth factor-beta and the infant immune response. J Pediatr 2010;156(2 Suppl):S21–5.
74. Kalliomaki M, Ouwehand A, Arvilommi H, et al. Transforming growth factor-beta in breast milk: a potential regulator of atopic disease at an early age. J Allergy Clin Immunol 1999;104(6):1251–7.
75. Oddy WH, Halonen M, Martinez FD, et al. TGF-beta in human milk is associated with wheeze in infancy. J Allergy Clin Immunol 2003;112(4):723–8.
76. Oddy WH, Rosales F. A systematic review of the importance of milk TGF-beta on immunological outcomes in the infant and young child. Pediatr Allergy Immunol 2010;21(1 Pt 1):47–59.
77. Maheshwari A, Kelly DR, Nicola T, et al. TGF-beta2 suppresses macrophage cytokine production and mucosal inflammatory responses in the developing intestine. Gastroenterology 2011;140(1):242–53.
78. Tang X, Liu H, Yang S, et al. Epidermal growth factor and intestinal barrier function. Mediators Inflamm 2016;2016:1927348.
79. Dvorak B, Fituch CC, Williams CS, et al. Increased epidermal growth factor levels in human milk of mothers with extremely premature infants. Pediatr Res 2003;54(1):15–9.
80. Coursodon CF, Dvorak B. Epidermal growth factor and necrotizing enterocolitis. Curr Opin Pediatr 2012;24(2):160–4.

81. Dvorak B, Halpern MD, Holubec H, et al. Epidermal growth factor reduces the development of necrotizing enterocolitis in a neonatal rat model. Am J Physiol Gastrointest Liver Physiol 2002;282(1):G156–64.

82. Halpern MD, Dominguez JA, Dvorakova K, et al. Ileal cytokine dysregulation in experimental necrotizing enterocolitis is reduced by epidermal growth factor. J Pediatr Gastroenterol Nutr 2003;36(1):126–33.

83. Clark JA, Doelle SM, Halpern MD, et al. Intestinal barrier failure during experimental necrotizing enterocolitis: protective effect of EGF treatment. Am J Physiol Gastrointest Liver Physiol 2006;291(5):G938–49.

84. Howarth GS. Insulin-like growth factor-I and the gastrointestinal system: therapeutic indications and safety implications. J Nutr 2003;133(7):2109–12.

85. Ozen S, Akisu M, Baka M, et al. Insulin-like growth factor attenuates apoptosis and mucosal damage in hypoxia/reoxygenation-induced intestinal injury. Biol Neonate 2005;87(2):91–6.

86. Bode L. The functional biology of human milk oligosaccharides. Early Hum Dev 2015;91(11):619–22.

87. Autran CA, Schoterman MH, Jantscher-Krenn E, et al. Sialylated galacto-oligosaccharides and 2'-fucosyllactose reduce necrotising enterocolitis in neonatal rats. Br J Nutr 2016;116(2):294–9.

88. De Leoz ML, Wu S, Strum JS, et al. A quantitative and comprehensive method to analyze human milk oligosaccharide structures in the urine and feces of infants. Anal Bioanal Chem 2013;405(12):4089–105.

89. Gabrielli O, Zampini L, Galeazzi T, et al. Preterm milk oligosaccharides during the first month of lactation. Pediatrics 2011;128(6):e1520–31.

90. Eiwegger T, Stahl B, Schmitt J, et al. Human milk–derived oligosaccharides and plant-derived oligosaccharides stimulate cytokine production of cord blood T-cells in vitro. Pediatr Res 2004;56(4):536–40.

91. Vandenplas Y, Zakharova I, Dmitrieva Y. Oligosaccharides in infant formula: more evidence to validate the role of prebiotics. Br J Nutr 2015;113(9):1339–44.

92. Mugambi MN, Musekiwa A, Lombard M, et al. Probiotics, prebiotics infant formula use in preterm or low birth weight infants: a systematic review. Nutr J 2012;11:58.

93. Rueda R. The role of dietary gangliosides on immunity and the prevention of infection. Br J Nutr 2007;98(Suppl 1):S68–73.

94. Xu J, Anderson V, Schwarz SM. Dietary GD3 ganglioside reduces the incidence and severity of necrotizing enterocolitis by sustaining regulatory immune responses. J Pediatr Gastroenterol Nutr 2013;57(5):550–6.

95. Vazquez E, Gil A, Rueda R. Dietary gangliosides positively modulate the percentages of Th1 and Th2 lymphocyte subsets in small intestine of mice at weaning. Biofactors 2001;15(1):1–9.

96. Rueda R, Sabatel JL, Maldonado J, et al. Addition of gangliosides to an adapted milk formula modifies levels of fecal *Escherichia coli* in preterm newborn infants. J Pediatr 1998;133(1):90–4.

97. Schnabl KL, Larsen B, Van Aerde JE, et al. Gangliosides protect bowel in an infant model of necrotizing enterocolitis by suppressing proinflammatory signals. J Pediatr Gastroenterol Nutr 2009;49(4):382–92.

98. Rueda R, Garcia-Salmeron JL, Maldonado J, et al. Changes during lactation in ganglioside distribution in human milk from mothers delivering preterm and term infants. Biol Chem 1996;377(9):599–601.

99. Verhasselt V, Milcent V, Cazareth J, et al. Breast milk-mediated transfer of an antigen induces tolerance and protection from allergic asthma. Nat Med 2008; 14(2):170–5.
100. Richard C, Lewis ED, Goruk S, et al. Feeding a diet enriched in docosahexaenoic acid to lactating dams improves the tolerance response to egg protein in suckled pups. Nutrients 2016;8(2):103.
101. Yamamoto T, Tsubota Y, Kodama T, et al. Oral tolerance induced by transfer of food antigens via breast milk of allergic mothers prevents offspring from developing allergic symptoms in a mouse food allergy model. Clin Dev Immunol 2012;2012:721085.
102. Lopez-Exposito I, Song Y, Jarvinen KM, et al. Maternal peanut exposure during pregnancy and lactation reduces peanut allergy risk in offspring. J Allergy Clin Immunol 2009;124(5):1039–46.
103. Verhasselt V. Is infant immunization by breastfeeding possible? Philos Trans R Soc Lond B Biol Sci 2015;370(1671):1–6.
104. Bernard H, Ah-Leung S, Drumare MF, et al. Peanut allergens are rapidly transferred in human breast milk and can prevent sensitization in mice. Allergy 2014; 69(7):888–97.
105. Kramer MS, Kakuma R. Cochrane in context: maternal dietary antigen avoidance during pregnancy or lactation, or both, for preventing or treating atopic disease in the child. Evid Based Child Health 2014;9(2):484–5.
106. Sauer N, Mosenthin R, Bauer E. The role of dietary nucleotides in single-stomached animals. Nutr Res Rev 2011;24(1):46–59.
107. Che L, Hu L, Liu Y, et al. Dietary nucleotides supplementation improves the intestinal development and immune function of neonates with intra-uterine growth restriction in a pig model. PLoS One 2016;11(6):e0157314.
108. Gutierrez-Castrellon P, Mora-Magana I, Diaz-Garcia L, et al. Immune response to nucleotide-supplemented infant formulae: systematic review and meta-analysis. Br J Nutr 2007;98(Suppl 1):S64–7.
109. Brenna JT, Varamini B, Jensen RG, et al. Docosahexaenoic and arachidonic acid concentrations in human breast milk worldwide. Am J Clin Nutr 2007; 85(6):1457–64.
110. Richard C, Lewis ED, Field CJ. Evidence for the essentiality of arachidonic and docosahexaenoic acid in the postnatal maternal and infant diet for the development of the infant's immune system early in life. Appl Physiol Nutr Metab 2016; 41(5):461–75.
111. Field CJ, Thomson CA, Van Aerde JE, et al. Lower proportion of CD45R0+ cells and deficient interleukin-10 production by formula-fed infants, compared with human-fed, is corrected with supplementation of long-chain polyunsaturated fatty acids. J Pediatr Gastroenterol Nutr 2000;31(3):291–9.
112. Zhang P, Lavoie PM, Lacaze-Masmonteil T, et al. Omega-3 long-chain polyunsaturated fatty acids for extremely preterm infants: a systematic review. Pediatrics 2014;134(1):120–34.
113. Ustundag B, Yilmaz E, Dogan Y, et al. Levels of cytokines (IL-1beta, IL-2, IL-6, IL-8, TNF-alpha) and trace elements (Zn, Cu) in breast milk from mothers of preterm and term infants. Mediators Inflamm 2005;2005(6):331–6.
114. Trend S, de Jong E, Lloyd ML, et al. Leukocyte populations in human preterm and term breast milk identified by multicolour flow cytometry. PLoS One 2015; 10(8):e0135580.
115. Takahata Y, Takada H, Nomura A, et al. Detection of interferon-gamma-inducible chemokines in human milk. Acta Paediatr 2003;92(6):659–65.

116. Gao X, McMahon RJ, Woo JG, et al. Temporal changes in milk proteomes reveal developing milk functions. J Proteome Res 2012;11(7):3897–907.
117. Field CJ, Van Aerde JE, Robinson LE, et al. Effect of providing a formula supplemented with long-chain polyunsaturated fatty acids on immunity in full-term neonates. Br J Nutr 2008;99(1):91–9.
118. Ewaschuk JB, Unger S, O'Connor DL, et al. Effect of pasteurization on selected immune components of donated human breast milk. J Perinatol 2011;31(9):593–8.
119. O'Connor DL, Ewaschuk JB, Unger S. Human milk pasteurization: benefits and risks. Curr Opin Clin Nutr Metab Care 2015;18(3):269–75.
120. Kuitunen M, Savilahti E. Mucosal IgA, mucosal cow's milk antibodies, serum cow's milk antibodies and gastrointestinal permeability in infants. Pediatr Allergy Immunol 1995;6(1):30–5.
121. Rognum TO, Thrane S, Stoltenberg L, et al. Development of intestinal mucosal immunity in fetal life and the first postnatal months. Pediatr Res 1992;32(2):145–9.
122. Saiman L. Risk factors for hospital-acquired infections in the neonatal intensive care unit. Semin Perinatol 2002;26(5):315–21.
123. Seidel BM, Schulze B, Schubert S, et al. Oral mucosal immunocompetence in preterm infants in the first 9 months of life. Eur J Pediatr 2000;159(10):789.
124. Miyara M, Sakaguchi S. Natural regulatory T cells: mechanisms of suppression. Trends Mol Med 2007;13(3):108–16.
125. Schelonka RL, Infante AJ. Neonatal immunology. Semin Perinatol 1998;22(1):2–14.
126. Carr R, Modi N. Haemopoietic colony stimulating factors for preterm neonates. Arch Dis Child Fetal Neonatal Ed 1997;76(2):F128–33.
127. Roncarolo MG. Immuno responses of cord blood cells. Bone Marrow Transplant 1998;22(Suppl 1):S55.
128. Trivedi HN, HayGlass KT, Gangur V, et al. Analysis of neonatal T cell and antigen presenting cell functions. Hum Immunol 1997;57(2):69–79.
129. Abughali N, Berger M, Tosi MF. Deficient total cell content of CR3 (CD11b) in neonatal neutrophils. Blood 1994;83(4):1086–92.
130. Bjorkqvist M, Jurstrand M, Bodin L, et al. Defective neutrophil oxidative burst in preterm newborns on exposure to coagulase-negative staphylococci. Pediatr Res 2004;55(6):966–71.
131. Buhrer C, Stibenz D, Graulich J, et al. Soluble L-selectin (sCD62L) umbilical cord plasma levels increase with gestational age. Pediatr Res 1995;38(3):336–41.
132. Lorant DE, Li W, Tabatabaei N, et al. P-selectin expression by endothelial cells is decreased in neonatal rats and human premature infants. Blood 1999;94(2):600–9.
133. Nupponen I, Pesonen E, Andersson S, et al. Neutrophil activation in preterm infants who have respiratory distress syndrome. Pediatrics 2002;110(1 Pt 1):36–41.
134. Schuller SS, Sadeghi K, Wisgrill L, et al. Preterm neonates display altered plasmacytoid dendritic cell function and morphology. J Leukoc Biol 2013;93(5):781–8.
135. Kohl S, Sigouroudinia M, Engleman EG. Adhesion defects of antibody-mediated target cell binding of neonatal natural killer cells. Pediatr Res 1999;46(6):755–9.
136. McDonald T, Sneed J, Valenski WR, et al. Natural killer cell activity in very low birth weight infants. Pediatr Res 1992;31(4 Pt 1):376–80.

137. Herrod HG, Cooke RJ, Valenski WR, et al. Evaluation of lymphocyte phenotype and phytohemagglutinin response in healthy very low birth weight infants. Clin Immunol Immunopathol 1991;60(2):268–77.

138. Walker JC, Smolders MA, Gemen EF, et al. Development of lymphocyte subpopulations in preterm infants. Scand J Immunol 2011;73(1):53–8.

139. Kaur K, Chowdhury S, Greenspan NS, et al. Decreased expression of tumor necrosis factor family receptors involved in humoral immune responses in preterm neonates. Blood 2007;110(8):2948–54.

140. Landor M. Maternal-fetal transfer of immunoglobulins. Ann Allergy Asthma Immunol 1995;74(4):279–83 [quiz: 284].

141. Mehta R, Petrova A. Biologically active breast milk proteins in association with very preterm delivery and stage of lactation. J Perinatol 2011;31(1):58–62.

142. Hsu YC, Chen CH, Lin MC, et al. Changes in preterm breast milk nutrient content in the first month. Pediatr Neonatol 2014;55(6):449–54.

143. Mastromarino P, Capobianco D, Campagna G, et al. Correlation between lactoferrin and beneficial microbiota in breast milk and infant's feces. Biometals 2014; 27(5):1077–86.

144. Montagne P, Cuilliere ML, Mole C, et al. Immunological and nutritional composition of human milk in relation to prematurity and mother's parity during the first 2 weeks of lactation. J Pediatr Gastroenterol Nutr 1999;29(1):75–80.

145. Velona T, Abbiati L, Beretta B, et al. Protein profiles in breast milk from mothers delivering term and preterm babies. Pediatr Res 1999;45(5 Pt 1):658–63.

146. Dawarkadas AM, Saha K, Mathur NB. A comparative study of cells and antimicrobial proteins in colostrum of mothers delivering pre- and full-term babies. J Trop Pediatr 1991;37(5):214–9.

147. Jain N, Mathur NB, Sharma VK, et al. Cellular composition including lymphocyte subsets in preterm and full term human colostrum and milk. Acta Paediatr Scand 1991;80(4):395–9.

148. Koenig A, de Albuquerque Diniz EM, Barbosa SF, et al. Immunologic factors in human milk: the effects of gestational age and pasteurization. J Hum Lact 2005; 21(4):439–43.

149. Polat A, Tunc T, Erdem G, et al. Interleukin-8 and its receptors in human milk from mothers of full-term and premature infants. Breastfeed Med 2016;11:247–51.

150. Meki A-RMA, Saleem T, Al-Ghazali M, et al. Interleukins-6, -8 and -10 and tumor necrosis factor-alpha and its soluble receptor I in human milk at different periods of lactation. Nutr Res 2003;23(1):845–55.

151. Collado MC, Santaella M, Mira-Pascual L, et al. Longitudinal study of cytokine expression, lipid profile and neuronal growth factors in human breast milk from term and preterm deliveries. Nutrients 2015;7(10):8577–91.

152. Nagashima K, Itoh K, Kuroume T. Levels of insulin-like growth factor I in full- and preterm human milk in comparison to levels in cow's milk and in milk formulas. Biol neonate 1990;58(6):343–6.

153. De Leoz ML, Gaerlan SC, Strum JS, et al. Lacto-N-tetraose, fucosylation, and secretor status are highly variable in human milk oligosaccharides from women delivering preterm. J Proteome Res 2012;11(9):4662–72.

154. Kovacs A, Funke S, Marosvolgyi T, et al. Fatty acids in early human milk after preterm and full-term delivery. J Pediatr Gastroenterol Nutr 2005;41(4):454–9.

155. Spevacek AR, Smilowitz JT, Chin EL, et al. Infant maturity at birth reveals minor differences in the maternal milk metabolome in the first month of lactation. J Nutr 2015;145(8):1698–708.

Necrotizing Enterocolitis and Human Milk Feeding
A Systematic Review

Nicole Theresa Cacho, DO, MPH[a],*, Leslie A. Parker, PhD, ARNP[b], Josef Neu, MD[c]

KEYWORDS

- Necrotizing enterocolitis • Human milk • Premature infant • Donor milk
- Exclusive human milk

KEY POINTS

- There is a lack of clear evidence that donor milk decreases the incidence of necrotizing enterocolitis (NEC) in preterm infants.
- An exclusive human milk diet may provide protection against NEC.
- A higher dose of human milk, particularly more than 50% of feedings, reduces the risk of NEC in preterm infants.

INTRODUCTION

Human milk (HM) is widely considered to be the optimal form of infant nutrition, and is endorsed by both national and international health organizations.[1] Because HM contains bioactive substances with bactericidal, immunomodulating, and intestinal maturation-inducing properties, the potential for improved health in premature infants is significant, especially for those born extremely premature. HM has been shown to significantly decrease complications associated with prematurity, including feeding intolerance, late-onset sepsis, and retinopathy of prematurity.[2,3] Other benefits

Disclosure: N.T. Cacho, L.A. Parker, and J. Neu all receive a grant funded by Medela. L.A. Parker and J. Neu are funded by the National Institutes of Health R15NR013566-01A1. J. Neu is on the Scientific Advisory Board for Medela and receives a research grant from Medela. He also serves on the Scientific Advisory Board for Infant Bacterial Therapeutics and is principal investigator for a multicenter safety phase trial.
[a] Division of Neonatology, Department of Pediatrics, University of Florida, 1600 Southwest Archer Road, HD-118, Gainesville, FL 32610, USA; [b] Biobehavioral Nursing Science, College of Nursing, University of Florida, PO Box 100187, HPNP 2227, Gainesville, FL 32610-0187, USA; [c] Division of Neonatology, Department of Pediatrics, University of Florida, 1600 Southwest Archer Road, HD-112, Gainesville, FL 32610, USA
* Corresponding author.
E-mail address: nicole.cacho@peds.ufl.edu

Clin Perinatol 44 (2017) 49–67
http://dx.doi.org/10.1016/j.clp.2016.11.009   perinatology.theclinics.com
0095-5108/17/© 2016 Elsevier Inc. All rights reserved.

include fewer rehospitalizations, improved neurodevelopmental outcomes,[4,5] as well as lower obesity rates and blood pressure and less insulin resistance in adolescence.[6,7] Moreover, studies of HM suggest reduction of the risk and severity of necrotizing enterocolitis (NEC).[8,9]

NEC is a potentially serious disease affecting approximately 7% of premature very low birth weight (VLBW) infants with an overall mortality of 20% to 30%, depending on disease severity and need for surgical intervention.[10,11] Complications are common and include intestinal strictures, short bowel syndrome, and an increased risk of neurodevelopmental delay.[12] Recent evidence suggests that provision of mother's own milk (MOM) may significantly reduce the incidence and severity of NEC and although these protective effects may be dose dependent, clarification regarding the dose necessary to provide protection is lacking.[8,9]

However, mothers of VLBW infants may be unable or unwilling to provide sufficient HM to meet their infant's nutritional needs.[8] In order to avoid exposing this vulnerable population to the potentially adverse effects of formula, the Section on Breastfeeding of the American Academy of Pediatrics now recommends that VLBW infants be fed donor HM (DHM) if MOM is unavailable.[1] Although the use of DHM in neonatal intensive care units (NICUs) has increased dramatically in recent years, questions remain regarding its impact on the incidence of NEC.[13,14]

Fortification of HM is indicated in VLBW infants to provide sufficient protein, calories, and other elements necessary to optimize growth.[1] At present, most NICUs use bovine-derived fortifiers, but HM-based fortifiers have recently been developed, allowing clinicians to provide infants an exclusively HM (EHM) diet.

Although evidence exists regarding the protective effects of MOM in reducing the risk of NEC in very premature infants, questions remain regarding whether DHM or an EHM diet provide the same protective benefits. In addition, clarification of the dose of HM required to reduce the risk of NEC is needed. Therefore, this article systematically identifies, investigates, and summarizes research on the association between DHM, an EHM diet, and dose of HM and the risk of NEC in premature infants.

METHODOLOGY
Search Strategy

A search was conducted in the electronic databases PubMed, Embase, CINAHL, and the Cochrane Database of Systematic Reviews using the search terms "Human Milk and Necrotizing Enterocolitis," "Donor Milk and Necrotizing Enterocolitis," "Breast Milk and Necrotizing Enterocolitis." Journal articles published between January 1, 2000, and June 30, 2016, were identified. The bibliographies of all articles included for data extraction were hand searched for additional eligible articles. Because of advancements in neonatology, including improvements in HM fortifiers and preterm formulas, an earlier initiation and attainment of full feedings, as well as a narrower diagnosis of NEC, the authors elected to limit the search to articles published after January, 2000.

Eligibility Criteria

Articles were considered eligible for the review if (1) they included premature infants who received HM feedings, (2) NEC was a primary or secondary outcome, and (3) they described original data-driven research. Animal studies, quality improvement projects, case reports, case series, guidelines, book chapters, and review articles were excluded from the review.

Data Extraction

Abstracts of articles identified by the initial search were screened for definite exclusion criteria and duplication. Remaining articles were then obtained and their full texts reviewed and examined for eligibility criteria. If uncertainty existed regarding an article's eligibility, the article was discussed by both reviewers and a decision was agreed on. For all final articles, each reviewer used a standard table to extract data, including information on population, study design, type and dose of HM provided, outcome, and level of evidence.

Level of Evidence

Level of evidence was determined using the Quality of Evidence grading scale from the Centre of Evidence-Based Medicine, Oxford, United Kingdom.[15] This method rates the quality of evidence based on a numerical scale (1–5) and an alphabetical scale (a–c). The level of evidence for this review focused on therapy or prevention, instead of diagnosis or prognosis. Each reviewer independently assessed and graded the level of evidence for each study and results were compared and discussed until agreement was reached.

Data Synthesis and Reporting

The type and dose of HM provided to infants was reported for each study. To facilitate data synthesis, the studies were grouped into 3 categories: studies investigating DHM, an EHM diet, and dose of HM (MOM and/or DHM).

RESULTS

The search revealed 24 studies that met inclusion criteria (**Fig. 1**).

Donor Human Milk

Six studies investigated the effect of DHM on the incidence of NEC, including 2 meta-analyses, 2 randomized controlled trials (RCTs), and 2 observational studies (**Table 1**).

Meta-analyses

Both meta-analyses reported a decreased risk of NEC when infants were fed a diet that consisted exclusively of DHM compared with formula.[16,17] Boyd and colleagues[16] in their analysis of 3 studies (2 RCTs and 1 observational study) published from 1983 to 1990 with a total sample size of 268 infants found a decreased incidence of NEC when infants were fed DHM (relative risk [RR], 0.21; 95% confidence interval [CI], 0.06–0.76). The second meta-analysis, by Quigley and colleagues,[17] analyzed 6 RCTs, including 869 infants, and also reported a decreased incidence of NEC (RR, 2.77; 95% CI, 1.40–5.46) in infants fed DHM. However, 4 of the 6 studies included in this meta-analysis were published in the 1980s. Notably, both meta-analyses found a significant decrease in NEC when infants received an exclusive diet of DHM compared with formula, but this benefit was lost when DHM was used as a supplement to MOM. In addition, only 2 studies included in either meta-analyses used fortified DHM and these studies reported no difference in the incidence of NEC between groups.

Randomized controlled trials

In contrast with the results of the meta-analyses, neither RCT reported a decreased incidence of NEC when premature infants received DHM compared with formula when MOM was unavailable.[9,18] Corpeleijn and colleagues,[18] in a multicenter double-blinded RCT of 373 premature VLBW infants stratified for gestational age,

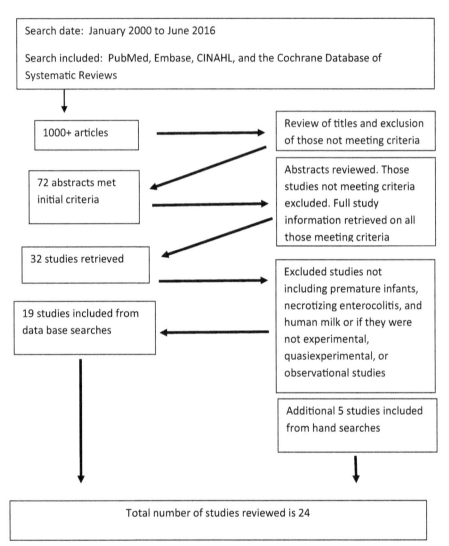

Fig. 1. Search strategies.

found no difference in the combined outcome of NEC, serious infection, and morbidity ($P = .37$). Although not powered to detect a significant difference, the incidence of NEC was 9.3% (DHM) versus 8.9% (formula) ($P = .99$). The high percentage of MOM provided to these infants (89.1% and 84.5%) in the DHM and formula groups respectively may have diluted the protective effect of DHM. Similarly, Schanler and colleagues[9] conducted a blinded RCT of 243 infants less than 30 weeks' gestation and found similar rates of NEC in infants who received DHM compared with formula when MOM was unavailable ($P = .27$). NEC was not the primary outcome of this study and thus there was insufficient power to accurately discern differences between groups. In addition, 21% of infants randomized to receive DHM were switched to the formula group because of poor weight gain, which again may have diluted the protective effects of DHM.

Table 1
Donor human milk

Author, Year of Publication, Type of Study, Country of Study Level of Evidence	Sample Size, Sample Characteristics, Study Characteristics, Duration of Intervention	Outcomes Measured	Results and Comments
Boyd et al,[16] 2006, systematic review, varied 1a[a]	N = 3 studies including 268 infants Duration: varied Compared diet of unfortified DHM vs formula	Incidence of NEC, death, infection, and growth	DHM was associated with a decreased incidence of NEC (RR, 0.21; 95% CI, 0.06–0.76). All studies were >25 y old
Chowning et al,[20] 2016, retrospective cohort, United States 2b	N = 550 infants <1500 g and < 35 wk Duration: not stated. Followed outcomes for entire hospitalization Compared DHM vs formula when MOM unavailable	Incidence of NEC and growth	DHM associated with a decreased incidence of NEC (13.5% vs 3.4%; P<.001); 23% of infants in the control group received DHM
Kantorowska et al,[19] 2016, retrospective cohort, United States 2b	N = 10,823 infants <1500 g from 22 hospitals Duration: not stated. Followed outcomes for 30 d Compared DHM vs formula when MOM unavailable	Breastfeeding at discharge and incidence of NEC	DHM associated with a decreased incidence of NEC from 5.7% to 2.9% (P = .0006). No information on confounding variables provided
Corpeleijn et al,[18] 2016, multicenter RCT, Netherlands 1b	N = 373 infants <1500 g stratified for birthweight Duration: birth to 10 d. Followed outcomes for 60 d Compared unfortified DHM vs formula when MOM unavailable	Composite outcome of NEC, serious infection, and mortality	DHM was not associated with a decrease in the composite outcome of NEC, serious infection and morbidity (P = .37), or NEC 9.3% (DHM) vs 8.9% (formula) (P = .99). Intake of MOM was high at 89.1% (DHM) vs 84.5% (formula)
Quigley & McGuire,[17] 2014, meta-analysis, varied 1a[a]	N = 6 RCTs including 869 infants Duration: varied Compared DHM vs formula	Incidence of NEC	DHM was associated with a decreased incidence of NEC (RR, 2.77; 95% CI, 1.40–5.46). Four of the 6 included studies were published in the 1980s and included unfortified DHM
Schanler et al,[9] 2005, RCT, United States 1b	N = 243 infants <30 wk stratified for gestational age Duration: 90 d or discharge. Followed outcomes from 50 mL/kg/d until 90 d or discharge Compared DHM vs formula when no MOM available	Late-onset sepsis and/or NEC	DHM was not associated with a decreased incidence of NEC (P = .27) or the composite of NEC and/or sepsis (P = .42); 21% of patients randomized to receive DHM were switched to the formula group because of poor growth

Abbreviations: CI, confidence interval; RR, relative risk.
[a] These studies may be considered a lower level of evidence because of outdated studies included in the systematic review and meta-analysis.

Observational studies

Both observational studies were retrospective and reported an association between DHM and a decreased risk of NEC.[19,20] Kantorowska and colleagues[19] conducted large cohort study of 10,823 VLBW infants from 22 hospitals and compared the incidence of NEC before and after a practice change to provision of DHM when MOM was unavailable; results showed a decreased incidence of NEC from 5.7% to 2.9% (*P* = .0006). However, limitations of this study included a lack of information regarding the amount of MOM consumed, feeding practices at each institution, and a comparison of confounding variables. In the second observational study, Chowning and colleagues[20] reported a decreased incidence of NEC (13.5% vs 3.4%; *P*<.001) following implementation of a DHM program. However, 13.5% was an unusually high incidence of NEC at this institution, which in previous years was typically between 5% and 7%. Thus, when the incidence of NEC was compared with the incidences from typical years, the findings were no longer significant. Furthermore, 23% of infants in the control group received DHM and baseline differences between groups were not reported. Neither study included a sample size calculation.

An Exclusive Human Milk Diet

Six studies examined the effect of an EHM diet on the incidence of NEC, including 1 meta-analysis, 2 RCTs, and 3 observational studies (**Table 2**).

Meta-analysis

The meta-analysis by Abrams and colleagues[21] included 2 RCTs and reported a lower risk of NEC (17% vs 5%; *P* = .002) and surgical NEC (12% vs 2%; *P* = .003) in those infants who received an EHM diet.

Randomized controlled trials

The 2 multicenter RCTs were from the same group and were included in the meta-analysis discussed earlier.[8,22] Sullivan and colleagues[8] stratified 207 infants less than 1250 g by birthweight and found that infants fed an EHM diet had lower rates of NEC (6% vs 16%; *P* = .02) and surgical NEC (1.4% vs 10%; *P* = .007) than infants who received bovine-based products when MOM was unavailable. Similarly, in a multicenter RCT of 53 infants whose mothers did not provide HM, Cristofalo and colleagues[22] found that infants randomized to receive an EHM diet had a lower rate of NEC, although this was not statistically significant (3% vs 21%; *P* = .08), and less surgical NEC (0% vs 17%; *P* = .04) than infants who received formula. However, the incidence of NEC in the formula group was higher than normally reported[11] and both studies were small, with NEC investigated as a secondary outcome.

Observational studies

Three retrospective cohort studies compared the incidence of NEC before and after implementation of a practice change from formula plus bovine-fortified MOM to an EHM diet.[23–25] Herrman and colleagues[23] found that infants fed an EHM diet were diagnosed with NEC earlier and at a younger postmenstrual age than those fed formula or bovine-fortified MOM but, notably, the incidence of NEC remained unchanged (3.8% vs 3.5%). In a multicenter cohort study of 1587 infants, Hair and colleagues[24] found than an EHM diet was associated with a decreased incidence of NEC, from 16.7% to 6.9% (*P* = .00001). However, infants who received EHM were significantly larger and more likely to have received antenatal steroids. In addition, differences in feeding practices between NICUs may have affected results. In the third cohort study, Assad and colleagues[25] reported an association between EHM and a lower incidence

Table 2
An exclusive human milk diet

Author, Year of Publication, Type of Study, Country of Study Level of Evidence	Sample Size, Sample Characteristics, Study Characteristics, Duration of Intervention	Outcomes Measured	Results and Comments
Abrams et al,[21] 2014, meta-analysis, United States and Austria 1a	N = 260 infants <1250 g and <30 wk Duration: until consumption of 4 oral feeds, discharge, or 91 d Compared an EHM diet with formula or HM fortified with a BBF	Mortality, NEC, growth, and duration of parenteral nutrition	An EHM diet was associated with a decreased incidence of NEC (17% vs 5%; $P = .002$) and NEC requiring surgery (12% vs 2%; $P = .003$). Analysis of 2 multicenter RCTs
Assad et al,[25] 2016, retrospective cohort, United States and Austria 2b	N = 293 infants <29 wk and/or ≤1500 g Duration: entire hospitalization Compared 5 groups: (1) EHM, (2) MOM with BBF, (3) MOM with BBF and formula, and (4) formula	Length of stay, episodes of feeding intolerance, time to full feeds. NEC was a secondary outcome	EHM associated with a lower incidence of NEC (1.1% vs 10%; $P<.011$). Infants were excluded from analysis if transferred before 34 wk
Cristofalo et al,[22] 2013, multicenter RCT, United States and Austria 1b	N = 53 infants ≤1250 g Duration: until consumption of 4 oral feeds, discharge, or 91 d. Compared EHM with formula	Duration of parenteral nutrition. Incidence of NEC was a secondary outcome	EHM was associated with less NEC (3% vs 21%; $P = .08$) and less NEC requiring surgery (0% vs 17%; $P = .04$). The incidence of NEC in the formula group was exceptionally high
Hair et al,[24] 2016, retrospective cohort, United States 2b	N = 1584 infants <1250 g from 22 hospitals Duration: entire hospitalization Compared an EHM with a diet of MOM fortified with BBF + formula	NEC and mortality	An EHM diet was associated with a decreased incidence of NEC (16.7% to 6.9%; $P = .00001$). Differences in feeding practices were evident between centers
Herrmann & Carroll,[23] 2014, retrospective cohort, United States 2b	N = 642 infants <33 wk Duration: birth to 33 wk. Outcomes measured for entire hospitalization Compared EHM diet with MOM with BBF + formula	Time to full feeds and NEC	There was no difference in the incidence of NEC (3.8% vs 3.5%); 9% of the EHM group did not receive an EHM diet. Infants were excluded from analysis if they died or were transferred to another hospital
Sullivan et al,[8] 2010, multicenter RCT, United States and Austria 1b	N = 207 infants ≤1250 g stratified by birthweight Duration: until consumption of 4 oral feeds, discharge, or 91 d of life Compared an EHM diet with a diet of MOM with BBF + formula	Duration of parenteral nutrition. NEC was a secondary outcome	An EHM diet was associated with a decreased incidence of NEC (6% vs 16%; $P = .02$) and less surgical NEC (1.4% vs 10%; $P = .007$). Baseline NEC incidence high

Abbreviation: BBF, bovine-based fortifier.

of NEC (1.1% vs 10%; $P<.011$). None of the included observational studies included a sample size determination.

Dose of Human Milk

Twelve studies examined the effect of specific doses of HM on the incidence of NEC, including 1 secondary analysis of the combined results of 2 RCTs, 2 RCTs (using an observational component), and 9 observational studies (**Table 3**).

Incremental increases in dose

Two studies reported an incremental decrease in the incidence of NEC as the dose of HM increased.[21,26] Abrams and colleagues[21] compared a diet of EHM with a diet of formula and bovine-fortified MOM and found that each 10% dose of a non-EHM diet increased the risk of medical and surgical NEC by 11.8% (95% CI, 0.2%–24.8%) and 21% (95% CI, 4.2%–39.6%) respectively. Similarly, in a post hoc analysis of a multicenter RCT of 1272 VLBW infants, Meinzen-Derr and colleagues[26] reported that the likelihood of NEC or death decreased by a factor of 0.83 (95% CI, 0.72, 0.97) for each 10% increase in MOM as a proportion of total diet. In addition, for every 100-mL/kg increase in MOM consumed during the first 14 days of life, the risk of NEC or death significantly decreased (hazard ratio [HR], 0.87; 95% CI, 0.77, 0.97).

Diet consisting of greater than 50% mother's own milk

The most commonly reported dose of MOM associated with a decreased incidence of NEC was at least 50% of the infant's total enteral intake.[9,18,20,27,28] Corpeleijn and colleagues[18] (2016) reported that infants who consumed at least 50% of their diet as MOM experienced a decreased composite risk of serious infection, NEC, and mortality. Similarly, Schanler and colleagues[9] also found that consumption of a diet containing at least 50% MOM produced lower rates of late-onset sepsis and/or NEC. In addition, Sisk and colleagues grouped infants according to percentage of MOM consumed and found that those whose diet consisted of at least 50% MOM had the lowest incidence of NEC. In addition, although Corpeleijn and colleagues[27] (2012) reported a decreased composite risk of NEC, sepsis, and death with consumption of any MOM during the first 5 days of life (dose<50%, $P = .003$; dose>50%, $P<.001$), this protective effect only continued during day 6 to 10 when the dose of MOM exceeded 50% ($P<.001$). Although Furman and colleagues[28] found no difference in the incidence of NEC when infants were fed 1 to 24 mL/kg, 25 to 49 mL/kg, or greater than or equal to 50 mL/kg of MOM, because infants are generally fed between 120 and 150 mL/kg/d, the effect of a dose greater than 50% was not determined.

Number of days human milk consumed

Chowning and colleagues[20] reported that, when infants received HM (DHM or MOM) on more than 90% of hospital days, they had a lower incidence of NEC ($P = .005$) but also experienced significantly less growth ($P<.01$).[20] However, when they received HM on more than 50% of hospital days, they continued to have a lower incidence of NEC (13.5% vs 3.4%; $P<.001$) without an associated decrease in growth. Kimak and colleagues,[29] in a case-control study of 1028 infants, found that those who received less than 7 days of HM (unclear whether it was MOM or DHM) were significantly more likely to develop NEC than those who received more than 7 days of HM. Although infants were matched for birth weight, other potential cofounding variables, including gestational age and illness severity, were not considered.

Table 3
Dose of human milk

Author, Year of Publication, Type of Study, Country of Study Level of Evidence	Sample Size, Sample Characteristics, Study Characteristics, Duration of Intervention, Dose	Outcomes Measured	Results and Comments
Abrams et al,[21] 2014, secondary analysis of a meta-analysis, United States and Austria 1b	N = 260, infants <1250 g and >30 wk Duration: until consumption of 4 oral feeds, discharge, or 91 d Dose: percentage of diet as EHM	Mortality, NEC, growth, and duration of parenteral nutrition	Every 10% increase in diet other than EHM increased the risk of NEC 11.8% (95% CI, 0.2%–24.8%), and the risk of surgical NEC by 21% (95% CI, 4.2%–39.6%). The percentage of diet other than EHM was a significant predictor of NEC (P = .047) and surgical NEC (P = .01)
Chowning et al,[20] 2016, retrospective cohort, United States 2b	N = 550 infants <1500 g and <35 wk Duration: not stated. Followed outcomes for entire hospitalization Dose: percentage of hospital days infants consumed HM (0%, <50%, >50%, or >90%)	Incidence of NEC and growth	Infants who received ≥50% of HM feeds compared with <50% had lower rates of NEC (P<.001) and mortality (P = .017)
Corpeleijn et al,[18] 2016, multicenter RCT, Netherlands 2b	N = 373 infants <1500 g Duration: first 60 d of life Dose: compared 0%, 0.01%–50%, and >50% of MOM	Composite outcome of serious infection, NEC, and mortality	>50% of total feeds consisting of MOM was associated with a reduced risk of the composite outcome. Intake of MOM was high in both groups: 89.1% in the DHM group and 84.5% in the formula group

(continued on next page)

Table 3
(continued)

Author, Year of Publication, Type of Study, Country of Study, Level of Evidence	Sample Size, Sample Characteristics, Study Characteristics, Duration of Intervention, Dose	Outcomes Measured	Results and Comments
Corpeleijn et al,[27] 2012, retrospective cohort, Netherlands 2b	N = 349 infants weighing <1500 g. Duration: first 10 d. Followed outcomes for 60 d. Dose: 0.01%–50% MOM vs 50.01%–100% MOM	Incidence of late-onset sepsis, NEC, and/or mortality	Any intake of MOM in the first 5 d was associated with a decreased incidence of NEC, sepsis, and/or mortality (HR in 0.01%–50% MOM, 0.49; 95% CI, 0.28, 0.87; HR in the category 50.01%–100% MOM, 0.50; 95% CI, 0.22, 0.65). MOM was only protective during days 6–10 if >50% of feeds were MOM (HR, 0.37; 95% CI, 0.22, 0.65)
Furman et al,[28] 2003, prospective cohort, United States 2b	N = 119 infants <33 wk weighing 600–1499 g. Duration: 4 wk. Dose: mean daily intake of MOM of 1–24, 25–49, and ≥50 mL/kg/d	Incidence of NEC and late-onset sepsis	No difference in the incidence of NEC based on the amount of MOM received
Kimak et al,[29] 2015, case-control study, Brazil 3b	N = 1028 infants weighing 750–1499 g. Duration: birth to 30 d. Dose: all feeds as HM (unclear whether it was DHM or MOM) for <7 d vs ≥7 d	Incidence of NEC	Infants who received <7 d of HM were at 4-fold higher risk of NEC (P = .02)
Maayan-Metzger et al,[31] 2012, retrospective cohort, Israel 2b	N = 400 infants ≤32 wk. Duration: first month of life. Dose: MOM only, formula only, mainly MOM, mainly formula, equal formula and MOM	Incidence of NEC, retinopathy of prematurity, bronchopulmonary dysplasia, and late-onset sepsis	Only and mainly MOM had significantly less NEC (P = .044) compared with only and mainly formula

Study	Population/Dose/Duration	Outcome	Results
Meinzen-Derr et al,[26] 2009, retrospective cohort, United States 2b	N = 1272 infants weighing between 401 and 1000 g Duration: first 14 d of life Dose: amount of MOM consumed as a proportion of total nutritional intake (enteral plus parenteral nutrition)	Incidence of NEC or death	A higher proportion of MOM was associated with a decreased risk of NEC (HR, 0.83; 95% CI, 0.72, 0.96). Infants who received 100% of their total enteral nutrition as MOM experienced a decreased risk of NEC or death (HR, 0.85; 95% CI, 0.60, 1.19)
Montjaux-Regis et al,[30] 2011, prospective cohort, France 2b	N = 55 infants <32 wk Duration: from initiation of enteral feeds to 1400 g and/or 32 wk Dose: <20%, 20%–80%, or >80% of MOM	Growth feeding intolerance (including NEC) and infection were secondary outcomes	Infants with NEC consumed significantly less MOM (P = .03) but there was no difference in the incidence of NEC between groups (P = .23). Extensive exclusion criteria excluded 75% of infants
Schanler et al,[9] 2005, observational component of an RCT, United States 1b	N = 243 infants <30 wk Duration: 90 d or discharge Dose: >50% of total feeds consisting of MOM	Incidence of late-onset sepsis and/or NEC	Dose: >50% of total feeds consisting of MOM. Dose: >50% of total feeds consisting of MOM was associated with fewer episodes of LOS and/or NEC; 21% of infants received only MOM
Sisk et al., 2007,[58] prospective cohort, United States 2b	N = 202 infants weighing 700–1500 g Duration: until discharge Dose: <50% vs ≥50% MOM	Incidence of NEC	Intake of total feeds consisting of >50% MOM was associated with a lower risk of NEC (Odds ratio, 0.17; 95% CI, 0.04–0.68; P = .01)
Stout et al,[32] 2008, case-control, United States 3b	N = 231 infants admitted to the NICU Duration: first week of life Dose: (1) HM only, (2) formula only, and (3) HM + formula. Unclear whether HM was MOM or MOM and/or DHM	Risk factors and feeding practices associated with NEC	Infants diagnosed with NEC were less likely to have been fed HM only (P = .003)

Abbreviations: HR, hazard ratio; LOS, late-onset sepsis.

No specific dose identified

Three additional studies reported an association between a higher dose of HM and a decreased incidence of NEC but did not specify the dose required to potentially provide protection.[28,30–32] Montjaux-Regis and colleagues[30] grouped 55 infants according to percentage of MOM consumed (<20%, 20%–80%, or >80%) and although no difference in NEC existed between groups, infants diagnosed with NEC received significantly less MOM (P = .03). Exclusion criteria were broad and included severe intraventricular hemorrhage, respiratory distress requiring mechanical ventilation, and intense phototherapy, potentially excluding a significant number of infants at high risk for developing NEC. Maayan-Metzger and colleagues[31] divided infants' diet in the first month after birth into 5 categories: MOM only, formula only, mainly MOM, mainly formula, and equal parts formula and MOM. In a subgroup analysis comparing only and mainly MOM with only and mainly formula, infants in the MOM groups were significantly less likely to be diagnosed with NEC (P = .044) but the specific volume of MOM that infants received was not reported. Moreover, Stout and colleagues[32] matched 21 cases of NEC with 6100 controls and reported that infants with NEC were less likely to have been fed exclusive HM (type of HM not reported) (P = .003) and were more likely to have been fed exclusively formula (P = .019). Infants fed a mixture of HM and formula were no less likely to be diagnosed with NEC (P = .399). However, this study only included cases of NEC occurring in the first week of life and included both term infants and infants with underlying congenital heart disease, which may represent a disease fundamentally different from classic NEC, which typically occurs following the first 1 to 2 weeks of life and affects predominately premature infants.[10,32–37]

DISCUSSION

This systematic review summarizes the evidence regarding the association of DHM, an EHM diet, and different HM doses with the incidence of NEC in premature infants. There is (1) a lack of clear evidence that DHM decreases the incidence of NEC, (2) preliminary evidence that an EHM diet may provide protection against NEC, and (3) consistent evidence that a higher dose of MOM reduces the risk of NEC.

One consideration that needs to be taken into account for all NEC-related studies is the criteria used to diagnose NEC in all the studies reported in this review. The high baseline incidence of NEC in some studies may partially have been a result of inclusion of infants without confirmed stage 2 NEC. This problem in the diagnosis of this disease is common and future studies will need to use strict diagnostic criteria.

DHM as a substitute for MOM in extremely premature infants has rapidly gained acceptance following recommendations by the American Academy of Pediatrics, the European Society of Pediatric Gastroenterology and Nutrition, and the World Health Organization.[1,38,39] There is a lack of clear evidence that DHM significantly decreases the incidence of NEC in premature infants. Both meta-analyses included in this review predominately contained research published more than 25 years ago that compared the benefits of unfortified DHM versus formula.[16,17] Fortification of HM is now considered standard of care, potentially decreasing the clinical relevance of these results.[1] In addition, DHM was investigated as a supplement to MOM rather than an exclusive diet, and the risk of NEC was similar to infants fed formula. Because a significant percentage of mothers provide HM to their infants for at least a portion of their hospital stay, the clinical relevance of these results are again questionable.[40] Heterogeneity between studies, lack of sample size estimates, and no comparison of potentially confounding factors in some studies may also have affected results.

Because an EHM diet limits exposure to the bovine-based products present in traditional HM fortifiers, it may provide protection against NEC and this review found preliminary evidence of an association between an EHM diet and a decreased incidence of NEC. However, none of the included studies were sufficiently powered to determine differences in the incidence of NEC, nor was there a direct comparison of an EHM diet with a diet of HM fortified with a bovine-based fortifier.

The protective effect of MOM against NEC seems to be dose dependent, with a dose of greater than 50% providing the greatest benefit. However, the observational and retrospective nature of included studies may have biased results and the lack of a consistent dose of MOM made meaningful comparisons between studies difficult. In addition, inclusion of infants with diagnoses other than classic NEC may have altered results.

Donor Human Milk

The underlying cause of NEC is poorly understood but seems multifactorial and is strongly associated with prematurity. Intestinal mucosal injury and inflammation as well as the presence of abnormal intestinal colonization are theorized as contributory factors in its development.[10,41] MOM may be protective against NEC through its bactericidal, immunologic, antioxidant, and antiinflammatory properties.[42] In addition, MOM contains commensal bacteria that may reduce the risk of NEC by promoting less pathologic intestinal colonization, as well as diminishing the intestinal inflammatory response to pathogenic bacteria and toxins.[43,44]

DHM differs from MOM, potentially diminishing its protective properties.

Holder pasteurization, performed to decrease or eliminate bacteria and viruses, also destroys or significantly decreases many of the protective elements in MOM, including lysozymes, secretory immunoglobulin A, growth factors, lactoferrin, and commensal bacteria.[45,46] DHM is often donated by mothers of term or older infants and is thus different from the HM from mothers of preterm infants in the presence and level of protective components, including cytokines, growth factors, and lactoferrin.[47,48] In addition, the beneficial effects of MOM may be unique to the specific mother-infant dyad, thereby providing maximum protection to the mother's own infant.[49]

Adequate growth and nutrition are known to improve the neurodevelopmental outcome of VLBW infants and therefore optimal nutritional support in the NICU is critical.[50] Because of its diminished protein content and decreased fat absorption caused by inactivation of bile salt–stimulating lipase by pasteurization, DHM may not provide sufficient nutrition for optimal growth and development.[46,51] Several studies have reported decreased growth compared with infants fed formula or MOM,[9,30,51] and additional nutritional supplementation may be necessary to optimize growth.[52] In contrast, an EHM diet seems to promote appropriate growth, possibly related to the ability to ultraconcentrate nutrients in HM-based fortifiers.[8,21,24,25]

Exclusive Human Milk Diet

Because HM contains insufficient kilocalories, protein, calcium, and phosphorus for premature infant growth, fortification with either bovine or HM-based fortifier is necessary.[1] Bovine-based fortifiers may promote an environment conducive to the development of NEC by promoting secretion of proinflammatory substances, including cytokines that can stimulate or intensify the inflammatory response, increase oxidative stress, and increase intestinal permeability.[53,54] Although several studies, including a meta-analysis of 14 individual studies, have shown fortification with bovine-based products to improve growth without increasing the risk of complications, including NEC, this review found evidence that an EHM diet may reduce the risk of NEC.[55–57]

Dose of Human Milk

In term infants, higher doses of MOM have been shown to reduce the incidence of acute otitis media, upper respiratory tract infections, gastroenteritis, type 1 diabetes, and leukemia.[1] Results of this review suggest that protection against NEC may also be dose dependent, with consumption of more than 50% of the total feeds providing the greatest protection.[9,18,20,27,58] The cause of this dose-dependent response is unclear and may be related to either more protection provided through a greater intake of MOM or less exposure to formula.[21,26,29,30]

A higher dose of MOM has also been associated with a decreased incidence of other neonatal morbidities, such as late-onset sepsis,[2,9,18,27,31,59] as well as improved neurodevelopmental outcomes at 18 and 30 months.[4,60] Similarly to the results of this review, a dose of at least 50% of feeds seems to offer the greatest protection.[9,28,61] Furthermore, there may be a critical time period after birth during which MOM is most protective.[2,28,58,59] Thus it may be more important for infants to receive higher doses of MOM during the first 14 to 28 days following birth compared with lower doses throughout their hospitalization.

Limitations of the Review

Many studies included in this review were observational and/or retrospective, which potentially reduced the reliability of the results. In addition, heterogeneity between studies, including population, timing of initiation and duration of the type or dose of HM feedings, individual NICU feeding practices, and uncertainty regarding whether HM consisted of MOM only or a mixture of MOM and DHM, made comparisons difficult. Inclusion of term infants, infants with congenital heart disease, and those diagnosed in the first week of life may have limited the ability to generalize from the results. Furthermore, although standardized feeding protocols have been associated with a reduced incidence of NEC,[56–58] not all studies included a standardized feeding protocol in their methodology. Moreover, several studies excluded infants from analysis if they were transferred to other institutions, died, or were diagnosed with NEC within 2 weeks of birth, again potentially limiting the ability to generalize from the study results. In addition, no study was adequately powered to detect differences in the incidence of NEC.

Potential Cost Savings

NEC increases cost of care by US$43,818 to $73,700 and by US$186,200 when surgery is required, with total hospital costs of US$6.5 million per year.[62,63] The estimated effect of suboptimal HM feedings on the cost of NEC is US$27.1 million in direct medical costs and US$563,655 in indirect nonmedical costs,[64] with each additional milliliter per kilogram per day of MOM an infant receives during the first 28 days of life reducing hospital costs by US$534.[64] Minimal information exists regarding the cost-saving potential of either a DHM-based or an EHM-based diet. Both DHM and HM fortifiers are expensive, with DHM costing US$281 to $590 per infant depending on the amount of MOM available.[65] Although a retrospective study of 293 infants found cost savings of up to US$106,968 per infant when fed an EHM diet after accounting for the cost of DHM and HM fortifier,[25] additional research is needed to fully elucidate the cost-saving potential of DHM and an EHM diet.

Increasing Consumption of Mother's Own Milk

Evidence strongly suggests that MOM reduces the risk of NEC in VLBW infants. However, maintaining a sufficient breast milk supply is challenging for mothers of premature infants, necessitating supplementation with either DHM or formula. Increasing the amount of MOM infants receive during their hospitalization requires the assistance of health care workers, particularly NICU-specific lactation consultants and peer counselors.[66,67] Investigating strategies used by mothers successful in maintaining a sufficient breast milk supply may uncover motivational and/or supportive methods that can be included in strategies focused on improving lactation success in this population.[61] Interventions to support initiation and maintenance of lactation should include encouraging mothers to provide MOM; prioritizing the initiation, establishment, and maintenance of lactation; and the use of innovative lactation technologies to identify and solve lactation problems in this population.[61] In addition, determining baseline information concerning breast milk production in mothers of very premature infants is necessary to establish whether implementation of policies and procedures in individual NICUs is successful.

SUMMARY

This systematic review summarizes the evidence regarding whether DHM and/or an EHM diet decrease the incidence of NEC, and the dose of HM necessary to reduce the risk of NEC in premature infants. There is a lack of clear evidence that DHM decreases the incidence of NEC, preliminary evidence that an EHM diet may provide protection against NEC, and consistent evidence that a higher dose of MOM reduces the risk of NEC. Additional research regarding the protection afforded by DHM and EHM, as well as research elucidating the exact dose and type of HM (DHM, MOM, and or EHM) to reduce the risk of NEC, is needed.

Best practices

What is the current practice?

HM and NEC
    Give exclusive HM in the form of MOM as the standard of care
    If MOM is unavailable, consider donor breast milk instead
    As a supplement to a high percentage of MOM, donor breast milk or formula may both be safe

What changes in current practice are likely to improve outcomes?

Provide early lactation support to mothers of all infants in NICUs

Optimize the dose of HM (preferentially MOM) given as a percentage of feeds with a goal of greater than or equal to 50%

Track volume of breast milk that mothers of VLBW infants are producing and provide lactation support to assist with increasing and maintaining breast milk supply

Rating for the strength of the evidence
    Lack of clear evidence that DHM decreases the incidence of NEC. Preliminary evidence that an EHM diet may provide protection against NEC. Consistent evidence that a higher dose of MOM reduces the risk of NEC.

REFERENCES

1. Section on Breastfeeding. Breastfeeding and the use of human milk. Pediatrics 2012;129(3):e827–41.
2. Patel AL, Johnson TJ, Engstrom JL, et al. Impact of early human milk on sepsis and health-care costs in very low birth weight infants. J Perinatol 2013;33(7): 514–9.
3. Bharwani SK, Green BF, Pezzullo JC, et al. Systematic review and meta-analysis of human milk intake and retinopathy of prematurity: a significant update. J Perinatol 2016;36(11):913–20.
4. Vohr BR, Poindexter BB, Dusick AM, et al. Beneficial effects of breast milk in the neonatal intensive care unit on the developmental outcome of extremely low birth weight infants at 18 months of age. Pediatrics 2006;118(1):e115–23.
5. Isaacs EB, Fischl BR, Quinn BT, et al. Impact of breast milk on intelligence quotient, brain size, and white matter development. Pediatr Res 2010;67(4):357–62.
6. Singhal A, Cole TJ, Fewtrell M, et al. Breastmilk feeding and lipoprotein profile in adolescents born preterm: follow-up of a prospective randomised study. Lancet 2004;363(9421):1571–8.
7. Singhal A, Cole TJ, Lucas A. Early nutrition in preterm infants and later blood pressure: two cohorts after randomised trials. Lancet 2001;357(9254):413–9.
8. Sullivan S, Schanler RJ, Kim JH, et al. An exclusively human milk-based diet is associated with a lower rate of necrotizing enterocolitis than a diet of human milk and bovine milk-based products. J Pediatr 2010;156(4):562–7.e1.
9. Schanler RJ, Lau C, Hurst NM, et al. Randomized trial of donor human milk versus preterm formula as substitutes for mothers' own milk in the feeding of extremely premature infants. Pediatrics 2005;116(2):400–6.
10. Neu J, Walker WA. Necrotizing enterocolitis. N Engl J Med 2011;364(3):255–64.
11. Horbar JD, Carpenter JH, Badger GJ, et al. Mortality and neonatal morbidity among infants 501 to 1500 grams from 2000 to 2009. Pediatrics 2012;129(6): 1019–26.
12. Picciolini O, Montirosso R, Porro M, et al. Neurofunctional assessment at term equivalent age can predict 3-year neurodevelopmental outcomes in very low birth weight infants. Acta Paediatr 2016;105(2):e47–53.
13. Parker MG, Barrero-Castillero A, Corwin BK, et al. Pasteurized human donor milk use among US level 3 neonatal intensive care units. J Hum Lact 2013;29(3): 381–9.
14. Hagadorn JI, Brownell EA, Lussier MM, et al. Variability of criteria for pasteurized donor human milk use: a survey of U.S. Neonatal Intensive Care Unit Medical Directors. JPEN J Parenter Enteral Nutr 2016;40(3):326–33.
15. Oxford Centre for Evidence-Based Medicine—levels of evidence 2009. Available at: http://www.cebm.net/oxford-centre-evidence-based-medicine-levels-evidence-march- 2009. Accessed May 4, 2016.
16. Boyd CA, Quigley MA, Brocklehurst P. Donor breast milk versus infant formula for preterm infants: systematic review and meta-analysis. Arch Dis Child Fetal Neonatal Ed 2007;92(3):F169–75.
17. Quigley M, McGuire W. Formula versus donor breast milk for feeding preterm or low birth weight infants. Cochrane Database Syst Rev 2014;4:CD002971.
18. Corpeleijn WE, de Waard M, Christmann V, et al. Effect of donor milk on severe infections and mortality in very-low-birth-weight infants: the Early Nutrition Study randomized clinical trial. JAMA Pediatr 2016;170(7):654–61.

19. Kantorowska A, Wei JC, Cohen RS, et al. Impact of donor milk availability on breast milk use and necrotizing enterocolitis rates. Pediatrics 2016;137(3): e20153123.
20. Chowning R, Radmacher P, Lewis S, et al. A retrospective analysis of the effect of human milk on prevention of necrotizing enterocolitis and postnatal growth. J Perinatol 2016;36(3):221–4.
21. Abrams SA, Schanler RJ, Lee ML, et al. Greater mortality and morbidity in extremely preterm infants fed a diet containing cow milk protein products. Breastfeed Med 2014;9(6):281–5.
22. Cristofalo EA, Schanler RJ, Blanco CL, et al. Randomized trial of exclusive human milk versus preterm formula diets in extremely premature infants. J Pediatr 2013; 163(6):1592–5.e1.
23. Herrmann K, Carroll K. An exclusively human milk diet reduces necrotizing enterocolitis. Breastfeed Med 2014;9(4):184–90.
24. Hair AB, Peluso AM, Hawthorne KM, et al. Beyond necrotizing enterocolitis prevention: improving outcomes with an exclusive human milk-based diet. Breastfeed Med 2016;11(2):70–4.
25. Assad M, Elliott MJ, Abraham JH. Decreased cost and improved feeding tolerance in VLBW infants fed an exclusive human milk diet. J Perinatol 2016;36(3): 216–20.
26. Meinzen-Derr J, Poindexter B, Wrage L, et al. Role of human milk in extremely low birth weight infants' risk of necrotizing enterocolitis or death. J Perinatol 2009; 29(1):57–62.
27. Corpeleijn WE, Kouwenhoven SM, Paap MC, et al. Intake of own mother's milk during the first days of life is associated with decreased morbidity and mortality in very low birth weight infants during the first 60 days of life. Neonatology 2012; 102(4):276–81.
28. Furman L, Taylor G, Minich N, et al. The effect of maternal milk on neonatal morbidity of very low-birth-weight infants. Arch Pediatr Adolesc Med 2003; 157(1):66–71.
29. Kimak KS, de Castro Antunes MM, Braga TD, et al. Influence of enteral nutrition on occurrences of necrotizing enterocolitis in very-low- birth-weight infants. J Pediatr Gastroenterol Nutr 2015;61(4):445–50.
30. Montjaux-Regis N, Cristini C, Arnaud C, et al. Improved growth of preterm infants receiving mother's own raw milk compared with pasteurized donor milk. Acta Paediatr 2011;100(12):1548–54.
31. Maayan-Metzger A, Avivi S, Schushan-Eisen I, et al. Human milk versus formula feeding among preterm infants: short-term outcomes. Am J Perinatol 2012;29(2): 121–6.
32. Stout G, Lambert DK, Baer VL, et al. Necrotizing enterocolitis during the first week of life: a multicentered case-control and cohort comparison study. J Perinatol 2008;28(8):556–60.
33. Lin PW, Stoll BJ. Necrotising enterocolitis. Lancet 2006;368(9543):1271–83.
34. Yee WH, Soraisham AS, Shah VS, et al. Incidence and timing of presentation of necrotizing enterocolitis in preterm infants. Pediatrics 2012;129(2):e298–304.
35. Grave GD, Nelson SA, Walker WA, et al. New therapies and preventive approaches for necrotizing enterocolitis: report of a research planning workshop. Pediatr Res 2007;62(4):510–4.
36. Gordon PV. The little database that could: Intermountain Health Care and the uphill quest for prevention of term necrotizing enterocolitis. J Perinatol 2007;27(7): 397–8.

37. Pickard SS, Feinstein JA, Popat RA, et al. Short- and long-term outcomes of necrotizing enterocolitis in infants with congenital heart disease. Pediatrics 2009;123(5):e901–6.

38. Arslanoglu S, Corpeleijn W, Moro G, et al. Donor human milk for preterm infants: current evidence and research directions. J Pediatr Gastroenterol Nutr 2013; 57(4):535–42.

39. Guidelines on optimal feeding of low birth-weight infants in low- and middle-income countries. Geneva (Switzerland): World Health Organization; 2011.

40. Parker LA, Sullivan S, Krueger C, et al. Effect of early breast milk expression on milk volume and timing of lactogenesis stage II among mothers of very low birth weight infants: a pilot study. J Perinatol 2012;32(3):205–9.

41. Mai V, Young CM, Ukhanova M, et al. Fecal microbiota in premature infants prior to necrotizing enterocolitis. PLoS One 2011;6(6):e20647.

42. Rogier EW, Frantz AL, Bruno ME, et al. Secretory antibodies in breast milk promote long-term intestinal homeostasis by regulating the gut microbiota and host gene expression. Proc Natl Acad Sci U S A 2014;111(8):3074–9.

43. Neu J, Mihatsch WA, Zegarra J, et al. Intestinal mucosal defense system, Part 1. Consensus recommendations for immunonutrients. J Pediatr 2013;162(3 Suppl): S56–63.

44. Hunt KM, Foster JA, Forney LJ, et al. Characterization of the diversity and temporal stability of bacterial communities in human milk. PLoS One 2011;6(6):e21313.

45. Ewaschuk JB, Unger S, O'Connor DL, et al. Effect of pasteurization on selected immune components of donated human breast milk. J Perinatol 2011;31(9): 593–8.

46. Peila C, Moro GE, Bertino E, et al. The effect of holder pasteurization on nutrients and biologically-active components in donor human milk: a review. Nutrients 2016;8(8) [pii:E477].

47. Mehta R, Petrova A. Biologically active breast milk proteins in association with very preterm delivery and stage of lactation. J Perinatol 2011;31(1):58–62.

48. Castellote C, Casillas R, Ramirez-Santana C, et al. Premature delivery influences the immunological composition of colostrum and transitional and mature human milk. J Nutr 2011;141(6):1181–7.

49. Hassiotou F, Hepworth AR, Metzger P, et al. Maternal and infant infections stimulate a rapid leukocyte response in breastmilk. Clin Transl Immunology 2013; 2(4):e3.

50. Ehrenkranz RA, Dusick AM, Vohr BR, et al. Growth in the neonatal intensive care unit influences neurodevelopmental and growth outcomes of extremely low birth weight infants. Pediatrics 2006;117(4):1253–61.

51. Dritsakou K, Liosis G, Valsami G, et al. Improved outcomes of feeding low birth weight infants with predominantly raw human milk versus donor banked milk and formula. J Matern Fetal Neonatal Med 2016;29(7):1131–8.

52. Colaizy TT, Carlson S, Saftlas AF, et al. Growth in VLBW infants fed predominantly fortified maternal and donor human milk diets: a retrospective cohort study. BMC Pediatr 2012;12:124.

53. Koivusalo A, Kauppinen H, Anttila A, et al. Intraluminal casein model of necrotizing enterocolitis for assessment of mucosal destruction, bacterial translocation, and the effects of allopurinol and N-acetylcysteine. Pediatr Surg Int 2002;18(8): 712–7.

54. Friel JK, Diehl-Jones B, Cockell KA, et al. Evidence of oxidative stress in relation to feeding type during early life in premature infants. Pediatr Res 2011;69(2): 160–4.

55. Brown JV, Embleton ND, Harding JE, et al. Multi-nutrient fortification of human milk for preterm infants. Cochrane Database Syst Rev 2016;(5):CD000343.
56. Shah SD, Dereddy N, Jones TL, et al. Early secretory antibodies in breast milk promote long-term intestinal homeostasis by regulating the gut microbiota and host gene expression. J Pediatr 2016;174:126–31.e1.
57. Tillman S, Brandon DH, Silva SG. Evaluation of human milk fortification from the time of the first feeding: effects on infants of less than 31 weeks gestational age. J Perinatol 2012;32(7):525–31.
58. Sisk PM, Lovelady CA, Dillard RG, et al. Early human milk feeding is associated with a lower risk of necrotizing enterocolitis in very low birth weight infants. J Perinatol 2007;27(7):428–33.
59. Patel A, Engstrom J, Goldman J, et al. Dose response benefits of human milk in extremely low birth weight premature infants [abstract]. Pediatric Academic Socities 2008.
60. Vohr BR, Poindexter BB, Dusick AM, et al. Persistent beneficial effects of breast milk ingested in the neonatal intensive care unit on outcomes of extremely low birth weight infants at 30 months of age. Pediatrics 2007;120(4):e953–9.
61. Meier PP, Engstrom JL, Patel AL, et al. Improving the use of human milk during and after the NICU stay. Clin Perinatol 2010;37(1):217–45.
62. Bisquera JA, Cooper TR, Berseth CL. Impact of necrotizing enterocolitis on length of stay and hospital charges in very low birth weight infants. Pediatrics 2002;109(3):423–8.
63. Johnson TJ, Patel AL, Bigger HR, et al. Cost savings of human milk as a strategy to reduce the incidence of necrotizing enterocolitis in very low birth weight infants. Neonatology 2015;107(4):271–6.
64. Colaizy TT, Bartick MC, Jegier BJ, et al. Impact of optimized breastfeeding on the costs of necrotizing enterocolitis in extremely low birthweight infants. J Pediatr 2016;175:100–5.e2.
65. Carroll K, Herrmann KR. The cost of using donor human milk in the NICU to achieve exclusively human milk feeding through 32 weeks postmenstrual age. Breastfeed Med 2013;8(3):286–90.
66. Oza-Frank R, Bhatia A, Smith C. Combined peer counselor and lactation consultant support increases breastfeeding in the NICU. Breastfeed Med 2013;8(6):509–10.
67. Meier PP, Engstrom JL, Rossman B. Breastfeeding peer counselors as direct lactation care providers in the neonatal intensive care unit. J Hum Lact 2013;29(3):313–22.

Neurodevelopmental Outcomes of Preterm Infants Fed Human Milk

A Systematic Review

Beatrice E. Lechner, MD[a,b,*], Betty R. Vohr, MD[a,b]

KEYWORDS

- Human milk • Neurodevelopmental • Brain • Donor milk • Outcomes

KEY POINTS

- Human milk (HM) contains the precursors of the n-3 and n-6 long-chain polyunsaturated fatty acids (LC-PUFA), especially docosahexaenoic acid and arachidonic acid, which play an important role in neurogenesis.
- Preterm infants derive a developmental benefit from HM.
- There is evidence to support the beneficial effects of HM on brain, visual, and cognitive development from infancy to adolescence.
- Volume of breast milk consumed is an important predictor of cognitive outcomes.

This article covers the benefits contributing to improved neurodevelopmental outcomes. A systematic evaluation of peer-reviewed studies published in PubMed was conducted. Terms of interest were prematurity, human milk (HM), donor milk benefits, neurodevelopmental outcomes, and brain.

There have been several recent papers summarizing the importance of nutrition for early brain development and developmental outcomes.[1,2] Although the evidence for the association of HM and improved medical outcomes[3,4] is clear, the relationship with neurodevelopmental outcomes has at times been controversial, and it has been implied that improved outcomes are related more to higher maternal education and socioeconomic status rather than nutrients found in HM.[5] The evidence is clearer for preterm infants with randomized trials demonstrating decreased rates

Disclosure Statement: The authors have nothing to disclose.
[a] Department of Pediatrics, Women and Infants Hospital of Rhode Island, 101 Dudley Street, Providence, RI 02905, USA; [b] Department of Pediatrics, Alpert School of Medicine, Brown University, 222 Richmond Street, Providence, RI 02903, USA
* Corresponding author. Department of Pediatrics, Women and Infants Hospital of Rhode Island, 101 Dudley Street, Providence, RI 02905.
E-mail address: blechner@wihri.org

Clin Perinatol 44 (2017) 69–83
http://dx.doi.org/10.1016/j.clp.2016.11.004
0095-5108/17/© 2016 Elsevier Inc. All rights reserved.

of sepsis and necrotizing enterocolitis and 2 weeks shorter duration of care in the neonatal intensive care unit (NICU).[4,6–8] Because these neonatal morbidities are associated with adverse neurodevelopmental outcomes, this is one mechanism by which the use of HM is associated with improved neurodevelopment in the premature infant. There is additional evidence, however, that HM is associated with more optimal brain development. HM contains the n-3 and n-6 fatty acids linolenic acid and linoleic acid, which are precursors of the n-3 and n-6 long-chain polyunsaturated fatty acids (LC-PUFA). LC-PUFAs, especially docosahexaenoic acid (DHA) and arachidonic acid (AA), play an important role in neurogenesis. Evidence for the benefit of supplementation with LC-PUFA prenatally and in formula, however, is inconclusive.[9–12]

There are emerging studies, however, supporting the effects of HM on brain development. Deoni and colleagues[13] used MRI to assess white matter microstructure of 133 children between 10 months and 4 years of age who were either exclusively HM fed a minimum of 3 months, exclusively formula fed, or received a mixture of HM and formula. They identified that HM-fed children exhibited increased white matter development in later maturing frontal and association brain regions and found positive associations between white matter microstructure and breastfeeding duration in several brain regions. They also reported higher receptive language scores and vision reception scores among the infants exclusively breast fed. Isaacs and colleagues,[14] using MRI and long-term follow-up, reported in a group of 50 adolescents that percent expressed HM was associated with higher verbal intelligence for the cohort, and for boys with all intelligence quotient (IQ) scores, total brain volume and white matter volume. Their study supports the beneficial effects of HM on brain and cognitive development. Kafouri and colleagues[15] showed that exclusive breastfeeding was associated with increased cortical thickness of the superior and inferior parietal lobules and breastfeeding was associated with variations in the thickness of the parietal cortex in a sample of 512 adolescents. They also reported an association of breastfeeding duration with full scale and performance IQ at ages 12 to 18 years.

This article focuses on neurodevelopmental outcomes in preterm infants fed HM. Discussed are the components of breast milk and their role in neurodevelopment, studies of outcomes during infancy, childhood and adolescence, the role of maternal and infant nutritional supplementation during breastfeeding, and the challenges of studying the role of breastfeeding and breast milk provision in neurodevelopmental outcomes.

COMPONENTS OF BREAST MILK AND NEURODEVELOPMENT

The mechanisms by which breast milk contributes to improved neurodevelopmental outcomes have not yet been fully explored. Components of HM that have received significant attention are LC-PUFA. These components have been implicated in improved cognitive[16] and visual development[17] in infants.

Another, more recent, emerging body of evidence suggests that HM oligosaccharides, (the HM "glycobiome") support the establishment of a healthy neonatal gut microbiome.[18] In turn, necrotizing enterocolitis, which is a risk factor for poor neurodevelopmental outcomes in premature infants,[19] is associated with abnormal neonatal gut microbiome, or "dysbiosis."[20,21] Thus, although there is no direct evidence linking HM oligosaccharides to neurodevelopmental outcomes in preterm infants, a case is made for their indirect contribution to improved cognitive outcomes via the necrotizing enterocolitis pathway.

OUTCOME STUDIES
Infancy: Newborn to 2 Years

The following section reviews studies published since 2000, which includes volume of HM provided. Studies are summarized in **Table 1**. Feldman and Eidelman[22] conducted a study in which volume of HM in the NICU was recorded, infant feeds were videotaped for mother-infant interaction, maternal depression was evaluated, and the Bayley II[23] was administered at 6 months corrected age (CA). Mother-infant dyads were divided into groups based on volume of HM (substantial, intermediate, and minimal). Mothers who provided more breast milk initiated more affectionate touch and their infants were more alert. In adjusted analyses, infants with the greatest volume of HM had greater motor maturity and range of state on the Brazelton examination[24] at the time of discharge and higher Bayley Mental Development Index (MDI) and Psychomotor Development Index (PDI) scores at 6 months CA. Maternal affectionate touch was also related to motor maturity and infant alertness and moderated the effects of HM on cognitive development. Infants with both the highest volume of HM and high maternal touch had the highest cognitive scores. These data indicate that HM and maternal interactive behaviors impact on early developmental outcomes (**Table 2**).

Volume of HM was also examined in preterm infants less than 2000 g by Blaymore Bier and colleagues.[25] Infants were administered the Alberta Infant Motor Scale at 3, 7, and 12 months CA and the Bayley MDI at 12 months CA. In analyses adjusted for maternal Peabody Picture Vocabulary Scores, and days of oxygen, the HM group had higher Alberta Infant Motor Scale scores at 3 and 12 months and a higher MDI at 12 months.

Pinelli and colleagues[26] examined the influence of breast milk consumption, as a dose response, in very-low-birth-weight (VLBW) infants (<1500 g) on neurodevelopmental outcomes at 6 and 12 months CA. Mothers recorded the 24-hour volume of expressed milk once per week in the hospital. At each follow-up visit, the volume of a single feeding was assessed by prebreastfeeding and postbreastfeeding test weights. The Bayley Scales of Infant Development II was administered. After controlling for sociodemographic and infant variables, VLBW infants showed no statistically significant effect of predominantly breastfeeding compared with predominantly formula feeding on neurodevelopmental outcomes to 12 months. The most significant predictor of MDI scores at 6 and 12 months CA was birth weight, in which higher birth weights predicted higher MDI scores. Although the group differences were not statistically significant, there was a small advantage for infants who received mother's milk.

O'Connor and colleagues[27] examined data collected in a previous randomized controlled trial assessing the benefit of supplementing nutrient-enriched formulas for LBW infants with AA and DHA. If HM was fed before hospital discharge, it was fortified to 22 to 24 kcal/oz. As infants were weaned from HM, they were fed nutrient-enriched formula with or without arachidonic and DHAs. Infants were categorized into four mutually exclusive feeding groups: (1) predominantly HM until term CA, (2) greater than or equal to 50% energy from HM before discharge ($\geq$50% HM), (3) less than 50% of energy from HM before hospital discharge, or (4) predominantly formula fed to term (PFF-T). The PFF-T infants weighed approximately 500 g more at term CA than did predominantly HM until term infants, which lasted until 6 months CA. Between 2 and 6 months infants in the HM groups had higher Teller acuity card scores. There were no differences between the study groups in Bayley MDI and PDI scores. However, there was a positive association between duration of HM feeding and the Bayley MDI at 12 months CA ($P = .032$ full model) after controlling for the confounding

Table 1
Studies during infancy: between newborn and 2 years of age

Author	Population	Birth Years	Age	Test		Outcome					
Feldman & Eidelman,[22] 2003	86 infants <1750 g	1996–1999	At discharge and 6 mo	Bayley II	6m	Substantial	Intermediate	Minimal			P
					MDI	94.2 ± 9	91.7 ± 7	90.5 ± 8			<.05
					PDI	85.8 ± 11	78.6 ± 13	78.0 ± 12			<.01
Blaymore Bier et al,[25] 2002	39 infants <2000 g	1996–1999	7 and 12 mo	Bayley II	12m	HM	Formula				P
					MDI	100 ± 12	91 ± 10				<.05
Pinelli et al,[26] 2003	148 infants <1500 g	2008–2009	6 and 12 mo	Bayley II	12m	>80%	<80%				P
					MDI	98 ± 15	91 ± 12				NS
					PDI	78 ± 15	77 ± 14				NS
O'Connor et al,[27] 2003	463 infants 750–1800 g	1996–1998	12 mo	Bayley II		PHM-T	≥50% HM-T	<50% HM-T	PFF-T		Adjust. P
					MDI	93.1 ± 15	95 ± 13	91.6 ± 11	92.9 ± 13		
					PDI	86.8 ± 15	84.6 ± 15	86.5 ± 15	88.1 ± 15		
Vohr et al,[28] 2006	1035 infants <1000 g	1999–2001	18–22 mo	Pentiles of HM vol. Bayley II		≤20th	20–40th	40–60th	60–80th	>80th	Adjust. P
					MDI	74.2	76.9	78.3	90.4	97.3	.004
					PDI	80.2	82.7	84.2	84.4	89.4	.003
					BRS	44.8	52.1	50.1	51.8	58.8	.028
Furman et al,[5] 2004	98 infants <1500 g	1997–1999	20 mo	HM mL/kg/d Bayley II		None	1–24 mL	25–29 mL	≥50 mL		Adjusted P
					MDI	80 ± 16	70 ± 14	75 ± 14	85 ± 21		NS
					PDI	80 ± 16	75 ± 19	71 ± 17	76 ± 16		NS

Abbreviations: BRS, Behavior Rating Scale; MDI, Bayley Mental Development Index; NS, not significant; PDI, Psychomotor Development Index; PFF, predominantly formula fed; PFF-T, predominantly formula fed until term; PHM-T, predominantly HM until term.

Table 2
Studies in childhood: ages 2 years to 12 years

Author	Population	Birth Years	Age	Test	Outcome		
					Parameter estimate	Standard error	Adjusted P value
Vohr et al,[29] 2007	773 infants NICHD 401–1000 g	Oct 1999–Jun 2001	30 m CA	Bayley II MDI PDI Total behavioral score	0.59 pts per 10 mL[a] 0.56 pts per 10 mL[a] 0.99% per 10 mL[a]	0.17 0.21 0.33	.0005 .0092 .0028
Rozé et al,[30] 2012	2925 infants LIFT (<33 wk) France EPIPAGE (22–32 wk) France	Jan 2003–Jun 2008 1997	2 y 5 y	Ages and Stages Questionnaire KABC	Association between breastfeeding at time of discharge and nonoptimal neurodevelopmental performance[b] OR (95% CI) LIFT 0.53 (0.39–0.73) EPIPAGE 0.44 (0.33–0.60)		P value .001 .001
Beaino et al,[33] 2011	1503 infants EPIPAGE (22–32 wk) France	1997	5 y	KABC MPC Mild cognitive deficiency[f] Severe cognitive deficiency[g]	Breast milk % OR (95% CI) 15% 0.54 (0.39–0.76) 4% 0.25 (0.14–0.44)	No breast milk % OR 23% 1.00[c] 13% 1.00[c]	
Tanaka et al,[34] 2009	38 infants VLBW Japan	1999–2000	5 y	KABC MPC Simultaneous processing Sequential processing Day-Night Test KRISP Motor Planning Test SDQ	Breast milk 100.9 ± 14.6 99.3 ± 13.8 106.7 ± 14.5 14.1 ± 1.4 17.2 ± 0.8 18.8 ± 5.3 11.0 ± 1.2	Formula 94.5 ± 11.8 94.6 ± 15.9 94.7 ± 11.6[c] 11.1 ± 0.9[c] 15.0 ± 1.4[d] 12.0 ± 3.9[c] 13 ± 3.9[c,e]	

(continued on next page)

Table 2
(continued)

Author	Population	Birth Years	Age	Test	Outcome		
					No breast milk	Expressed breast milk	Direct breastfeeding
Smith et al,[39] 2003	439 infants <1500 g	1991–1993	6–8 y	Overall intellectual function			
				KABC MPC	92.3 (15.3)	94.2 (17.3)	102.8 (15.2)[j]
				Verbal ability			
				PPVT-III	92.6 (17.2)	94.1 (18.6)	102.7 (16.5)[j]
				CELF-3	88.5 (21.6)	89.5 (22.9)	102.4 (19.4)[j]
				Memory			
				CVLT short-term recall	43.8 (11.2)	44.5 (12.0)	46.4 (11.6)
				CVLT delayed recall	5.9 (3.7)	6.2 (3.2)	6.4 (3.0)
				Visual-spatial skill			
				WRAVMA matching	89.8 (15.5)	91.6 (17.0)	98.1 (17.2)[j]
				KABC gestalt closure	9.7 (3.0)	9.7 (3.0)	9.9 (3.0)
				Visual-motor skill			
				WRAVMA drawing	90.6 (13.5)	94.5 (16.7)	97.7 (14.6)[i]
				KABC triangle completion	9.1 (2.5)	9.9 (3.0)	10.6 (3.0)[i]
				Fine motor skill			
				WRAVMA pegboard	91.1 (20.2)	89. (20.4)	97.6 (17.1)[h]

Author	Population	Birth Years	Age	Test	Duration of breastfeeding					
					Not breastfed	<4 mos	4–7 mos	8+ mos	β value	P value
Horwood et al,[40] 2001	280 infants VLBW	1986 New Zealand	7–8 y	WISC-R						
				Verbal IQ	96.1	98.1	100.1	102.1	0.12	<.05
				Performance IQ	99.6	100.8	102.1	103.3	0.08	>.15

Source	Population	Dates	Age	Test	Results
Johnson et al,[42] 2011	811 infants EPICure <26 wk United Kingdom and Ireland	March–December 1995	11 y	WIAT-II[UK] Reading Mathematics	**Any breast milk given (univariate)** — Reading: Coefficient 13.48 (95% CI 5.79–21.16) P .001. **Any breast milk given (multiple regression)** — Reading: Coefficient 7.3 (95% CI 1.3–13.3) P .02; Mathematics: Coefficient 10.99 (95% CI 2.99–18.98) P .007
Elgen et al,[43] 2003	131 LBW infants 130 healthy control infants <2000 g Norway	April 1, 1986–August 8, 1988	11 y	WISC-R (excluding cerebral palsy, blindness, deafness, multiple malformations, and chromosomal aberrations)	Mean IQ: No breast milk 88 ± 13, Breast milk 97 ± 13, P = .01. Regression coefficient for lack of breast milk −5.8 (−11 to −1) P = .02. After controlling for parental education, lack of breast milk no longer significant

Abbreviations: CI, confidence interval; KABC, Kaufman Assessment Battery for Children; KRISP, Kansas Reflection Impulsivity Scale for Children; MPC, Mental Processing Composite; NICHD, National Institute of Child Health and Human Development; OR, odds ratio; VLBW, very low birth weight; WISC-R, Wechsler Intelligence Scale for Children–Revised.

a Breast milk.
b Nonoptimal neurodevelopment: KABC Mental Composite Processing <85 at 5 years in EPIPAGE cohort; Age and Stages Questionnaires score <220 at 2 years of corrected age in LIFT cohort.
c P<.05.
d P<.01.
e The lower score is better in the SDQ test.
f Mild cognitive deficiency MPC 70–85 compared with no cognitive deficiency MPC ≥85.
g Severe cognitive deficiency MPC ≤70 compared with no cognitive deficiency MPC ≥85.
h P<.01.
i P<.001.
j P<.0001.

variables of home environment and maternal intelligence. Infants with chronic lung disease fed greater than or equal to 50% HM until term CA had a mean Bayley PDI 11 points higher at 12 months CA compared with infants PFF-T (P = .033 full model). These findings indicate that despite a slower early growth rate, HM-fed LBW infants have development at least comparable with that of infants fed nutrient-enriched formula and that some subgroups of HM-fed LBW infants may have enhanced development.

In a National Institute of Child Health and Human Development (NICHD) Neonatal Research Network study,[28] nutrition data including enteral and parenteral feeds were collected prospectively, and follow-up assessments of 1035 extremely low birth weight (ELBW) infants at 18 months CA were performed. Total volume of HM feeds (milliliter per kilogram per day) during hospitalization was calculated. There were 775 (75%) infants in the HM and 260 (25%) infants in the no-HM group. Energy intakes of 107.5 kg/day and 105.9 kg/day did not differ between groups. After adjustment for confounders including maternal age, education, marital status, race/ethnicity, and the other standard covariates, children in the HM group were more likely to have a Bayley MDI greater than or equal to 85, higher mean Bayley PDI, and higher Bayley Behavior Rating Scale percentile scores for orientation/engagement, motor regulation, and total score. Multivariate analyses, adjusting for confounders, confirmed a significant independent association of HM on all four primary outcomes: (1) the mean Bayley MDI, (2) PDI, (3) Behavior Rating Scale, and (4) incidence of rehospitalization. For every 10 mL/kg/d increase in HM ingestion, the MDI increased by 0.53 points, the PDI increased by 0.63 points, the Behavior Rating Scale percentile score increased by 0.82 points, and the likelihood of rehospitalization decreased by 6%. Infants were divided into five quintiles of HM ingestion. Therefore, the impact of HM ingestion for infants in the highest quintile (110 mL/kg/d) on the Bayley MDI would be 10 × 0.53, or 5.3 points. This suggests that an increase of five points potentially would decrease costs by decreasing the number of ELBW children who require special education services. The societal implications of a five-point difference (one-third of an standard deviation) in IQ are substantial. The potential long-term benefit of receiving HM in the NICU for ELBW infants may be to optimize cognitive potential and reduce the need for special education services.

Not every study examining HM volume has identified independent effects of HM on developmental outcomes. The effect of maternal milk feeding during the first 4 weeks of life on neurodevelopmental outcomes at 20 months CA of singleton VLBW (<1.5 kg) infants was examined by Furman and colleagues.[5] Ninety-eight VLBW infants born were followed to 20 months CA. HM intake was calculated as both mean milliliters per kilogram per day and graded doses. Outcomes included the MDI and PDI, and rates of cerebral palsy and of overall neurodevelopmental impairment. After adjusting for neonatal and social risk, results revealed no effect of maternal milk on outcomes. MDI was predicted by social and neonatal risk, and PDI, cerebral palsy, and neurodevelopmental impairment were predicted by neonatal risk. In contrast to the NICHD study, HM volume in the first 4 weeks rather than during the entire hospitalization was available. Only 32 of the 98 infants received at least 50 mL/kg/d through week 4 of life. Overall, the studies from birth to 2 years of larger cohorts support that after adjusting for confounders, greater volume of HM during the NICU stay is beneficial for cognitive development of preterm infants.

Childhood: 2 Years to 12 Years

This section reviews studies published since 2001 describing neurodevelopmental outcomes of premature infants during childhood. In a follow-up study to the NICHD

Neonatal Research Network cohort assessed at 18 months CA discussed previously,[28] 30-month CA follow-up assessments were completed on ELBW infants.[29] The 30-month interim history, neurodevelopmental outcomes, and growth parameters were analyzed. For every 10 mL/kg/d increase in breast milk, the Bayley mental developmental index increased by 0.59 points, the psychomotor developmental index increased by 0.56 points, the total behavior percentile score increased by 0.99 points, and the risk of rehospitalization between discharge and 30 months decreased by 5%. There were no differences in growth parameters or cerebral palsy. Thus, the beneficial effects of ingestion of breast milk in the NICU seen at 18 months CA persisted at 30 months CA in a vulnerable ELBW population.

Rozé and colleagues[30] evaluated neurodevelopmental outcomes in two preterm cohorts in France: the LIFT cohort of less than 33 week gestational age infants at 2 years of age, and the EPIPAGE cohort of 22 to 32 week gestational age infants at 5 years of age. The Ages and Stages Questionnaire[31] was applied at 2 years and the Kaufman Assessment Battery for Children (KABC)[32] at 5 years. At both ages, they found a significant association between breastfeeding at time of discharge and nonoptimal neurodevelopmental performance. Breastfeeding decreased the risk of nonoptimal neurodevelopmental performance. Nonoptimal neurodevelopmental performance was defined as a KABC Mental Processing Composite (MPC) score of less than 85 at 5 years or an Ages and Stages Questionnaires score less than 220 at 2 years of CA.

Another analysis of the EPIPAGE cohort,[33] using the MPC component of the KABC test,[32] demonstrated that the odds for mild and severe cognitive deficiency at 5 years of age are decreased in children who received breast milk at hospital discharge. Mild cognitive deficiency, defined as an MPC score of 70 to 85 compared with no cognitive deficiency MPC greater than or equal to 85, was associated with low social status and lack of breastfeeding at discharge, whereas severe cognitive deficiency, defined as an MPC score of less than or equal to 70, was associated with the medical factors of the presence of cerebral lesions on ultrasound and being small for gestational age, in addition to the social factors of low social status, lack of breastfeeding at discharge, and a high number of siblings.

In a Japanese cohort of VLBW preterm infants,[34] multiple tests were administered at 5 years of age, including the KABC,[32] Day-Night Test,[35] Kansas Reflection Impulsivity Scale for Preschoolers,[36] Motor Planning Test,[37] and the Strength and Difficulties Questionnaire.[38] On each of these tests, except for two out of three subtests within the KABC, children whose feeding had consisted of at least 80% breast milk during the first month of life scored significantly higher than the control group. In this study, DHA levels in red blood cell membranes at 4 weeks of age were significantly higher in the breastfed group compared with the control group.

Moving beyond the preschool age, Smith and colleagues[39] evaluated the connection between breastfeeding and cognitive outcomes in a cohort of school-aged (ages 6–8 years) former VLBW children in the United States. They tested children using a battery of tests including the KABC for overall intellectual function and various tests of verbal ability, memory, visual-spatial skill, visual-motor skill, and fine motor skill. Children were categorized into three groups according to whether they received no breast milk, expressed breast milk, or direct breastfeeding. The study's findings indicated that direct breastfeeding is associated with better outcomes in all test categories except for memory. However, these differences are reduced when confounding variables, such as maternal verbal ability, home environment, and socioeconomic status, are accounted for. After regression analysis to adjust for these variables, only visual-motor skill remained significant. This study is well designed in that it attempts to analyze an often overlooked yet significant component of the debate on the benefits of breastfeeding for premature infants. It is important to point out that the provision of expressed maternal breast milk to a preterm infant and the direct breastfeeding of the infant are not interchangeable and potentially equally beneficial activities. Current literature on the benefits of breastfeeding to the neurodevelopmental outcomes of ELBW and VLBW infants often does not clearly differentiate between the two feeding methods. Although there is a paucity of necessary data on subject, it is reasonable to hypothesize that significant differences exist between the effect of expressed maternal breast milk fed by bottle and direct breastfeeding. The likely positive effects of direct breastfeeding may be mediated directly by the oral motor stimulation and skin-to-skin experience that is not attained by bottle feeding expressed breast milk, or they may be mediated by social confounding variables that are similar to the variables that are associated with mothers who choose to provide breast milk compared with those who do not. Additionally, the positive effects of direct breastfeeding may be mediated by the fact that handling, such as refrigeration, freezing, thawing, and warming up of expressed breast milk, which may lead to the loss of active factors, is avoided. Either way, this is an area of research in which future studies are necessary to inform clinical care of preterm infants.

In a VLBW birth cohort in New Zealand, Horwood and colleagues[40] studied the impact of the duration of breastfeeding on neurodevelopmental outcomes. Wechsler Intelligence Scale for Children—Revised (WISC-R)[41] verbal IQ and performance IQ testing was performed at 7 to 8 years of age, demonstrating that both measures were positively associated with duration of breast milk feeding. When confounding covariates were controlled for, verbal IQ was still significantly correlated with breast milk feeding duration. Children breast fed for 8 months or longer had adjusted mean verbal IQ scores that were six (0.36) points higher than the scores of those who did not receive breast milk. However, performance IQ was no longer significant. Confounding variables included maternal education level, two-parent families, higher income families, non-Polynesian ethnicity, and the absence of maternal smoking during pregnancy.

To study school achievement in later childhood, Johnson and colleagues[42] assessed infants born at less than 26 weeks in the United Kingdom and Ireland and enrolled in the EPICure study at 11 years of age for educational outcomes. At 11 years, the WIAT-II[UK] was used to assess academic achievement. On univariate analysis, children who had received any breast milk as a neonate scored significantly higher in reading and mathematics than children who had not received any breast milk. On multiple regression analysis, including the assessment of 30 months CA neurodevelopmental testing, the difference remained significant in reading. Thus, the authors found that the provision of breast milk as a neonate was an independent predictor of educational outcomes at 11 years.

In another study looking at late childhood outcomes in infants born at less than 2000 g in Norway, WISC-R[41] testing was performed at 11 years of age.[43] Children with cerebral palsy, blindness, deafness, multiple malformations, and chromosomal abnormalities were excluded. Mean IQ was significantly higher in infants who had received breast milk, but this increase did not remain significant once the confounding variable of parental education was controlled for. In summary, the effects of any breast milk feeding during the neonatal period and the duration of breastfeeding display effects on cognition well into preschool and school age. Although confounding social variables play a significant role in these effects, an effect of breastfeeding is sustained into childhood even when confounding covariates are accounted for, as is the case with each of the reviewed studies except for the Japanese and UK/Irish cohort.

Adolescence: 13 Years to 19 Years

Few studies exist examining the link between HM and long-term neurodevelopmental outcomes of preterm infants into adolescence. Isaacs and colleagues[14] studied the correlation between breast milk feeding, brain size, white matter development, and IQ in a cohort of ex-preterm adolescents at the mean age of 15 years and 9 months. They calculated the percentage of expressed breast milk feedings in 50 adolescents and performed brain MRI scans to calculate total brain volume and white and gray matter volume. The WISC-III or Wechsler Adult Intelligence Scale-III test was administered. The authors found that the percentage of expressed breast milk in the NICU correlated significantly with the verbal IQ component in all adolescents and with all IQ scores, total brain volume, and white matter volume in boys. Significant relationships were not seen in girls or with gray matter. These findings suggest not only that the effects of breast milk feeding in the NICU are sustained through adolescence, but also that breast milk likely has selective effects on the white matter compared with gray matter and being gender specific.

MATERNAL AND INFANT NUTRITIONAL SUPPLEMENTATION

In recent years, attention has been focused not only on the role that the breast milk components DHA and AA play in the development of the brain and vision, but also on novel approaches to supplementation of these LC-PUFAs to positively influence neurodevelopmental outcomes in preterm infants.

Henriksen and colleagues[44] demonstrated in very preterm infants that neonatal supplementation of either mother's own expressed breast milk or donor milk with DHA and AA from 1 week of life until hospital discharge was associated with higher problem-solving and recognition memory scores at 6 months CA. On cognitive testing at 20 months chronologic age in the same population, supplemented children demonstrated higher attention capacity scores.[45]

Other studies suggest that supplementing either breastfeeding mothers or the formula in formula-fed infants is associated with improved neurodevelopmental outcomes in preterm infants in a gender-specific manner.[46] In this study, DHA supplementation of less than 33 week infants was associated with an increase in MDI scores of female infants but not male infants. At 26 months, 3 years, and 5 years language development and behavior was the same in supplemented and nonsupplemented children in the same cohort.[47]

Isaacs and colleagues[48] also found gender-specific improved outcomes. In this study, former preterm girls who received LC-PUFA supplementation demonstrated higher literacy scores at 9 years of age. Also, LC-PUFA-supplemented children who had received only formula during infancy displayed higher cognitive scores compared with their nonsupplemented counterparts, whereas LC-PUFA-supplemented children who had received breast milk did not. This observation suggests that the mechanism of action of LC-PUFA supplementation may be that it replaces LC-PUFA in formula that is already naturally occurring in breast milk, thus in essence attempting to make formula more like breast milk.

Similarly, Tanaka and colleagues[49] showed that fortifying breast milk and formula with sphingomyelin was associated with increased neurobehavioral scores at 18 months CA.

Other studies did not find a difference in infant visual acuity in full-term infants at 4 months of age whose mothers had received DHA supplementation during pregnancy,[50] or improved cognitive or language development at 18 months of age[51] or at 4 years of age.[52]

THE CHALLENGES OF STUDYING BREASTFEEDING AND COGNITION: THE INTERACTION BETWEEN PARENTAL SOCIAL FACTORS AND BREASTFEEDING

A major challenge of studying the effects of breastfeeding on infant neurodevelopmental outcomes is that confounding variables, such as parental IQ, socioeconomic status, and parental stimulation, play a significant role in infant neurodevelopment and the choice to breastfeed.

As Lucas and colleagues[53] showed almost 30 years ago, women who choose to provide their premature infant with breast milk are a population that is distinct from women who choose not to. Women who choose to provide breastmilk are more likely to be well educated, married, primiparous, and aged 20 years or older.

Additionally, there is a paucity of high-quality studies. Although many studies show an improvement in cognitive outcomes in breastfed infants, few studies display appropriate study design, sample size, data collection, and control for confounding variables.[54] Many of the studies that control for confounding variables of breastfeeding, including those discussed here in detail, show improved neurodevelopmental outcome measures for breastfed infants in the raw data. However, in some studies the improvement is no longer significant once parental education level, IQ, home environment/stimulation, and socioeconomic factors are controlled for. Although multiple studies do demonstrate sustained improvement in cognition, the effect size is smaller than the nonadjusted data. Other studies have shown that although breastfeeding is associated with an increase in IQ in children, this increase is no longer present if confounders, such as maternal IQ or the child's social environment, are adjusted for (Gale and Martyn, 1996;[55] Jacobson and colleagues, 1999;[56] Der and colleagues, 2006[57]).

In a systematic meta-analysis of the long term effects of breastfeeding, Horta and Victora[58] found that although residual confounding by socioeconomic status needs to be taken into account when interpreting studies, breastfeeding was nonetheless associated with an increase in 3.5 points in normalized test scores in the pooled analyses of all studies reviewed, and 2.2 points when only high-quality studies were included. The authors conclude that there is strong evidence of a causal effect of breastfeeding on IQ, but the magnitude of the effect is small.

SUMMARY

Because preterm infants are already at high risk for neurodevelopmental delays and abnormalities, any intervention that has the potential to increase cognitive ability, even if the effect size is small, is a significant tool. Thus, encouraging and supporting mothers to pump breast milk and to breastfeed in the NICU and beyond is of paramount importance in the quest to improve neurodevelopmental outcomes of preterm infants.

REFERENCES

1. Fox SE, Levitt P, Nelson CA 3rd. How the timing and quality of early experiences influence the development of brain architecture. Child Dev 2010;81:28–40.
2. Cusick SE, Georgieff MK. The role of nutrition in brain development: the golden opportunity of the "first 1000 days". J Pediatr 2016;175:16–21.
3. Furman L, Taylor G, Minich N, et al. The effect of maternal milk on neonatal morbidity of very low-birth-weight infants. Arch Pediatr Adolesc Med 2003;157: 66–71.
4. Abrams SA, Schanler RJ, Lee ML, et al. Greater mortality and morbidity in extremely preterm infants fed a diet containing cow milk protein products. Breastfeed Med 2014;9:281–5.

5. Furman L, Wilson-Costello D, Friedman H, et al. The effect of neonatal maternal milk feeding on the neurodevelopmental outcome of very low birth weight infants. J Dev Behav Pediatr 2004;25:247–53.
6. Sullivan S, Schanler RJ, Kim JH, et al. An exclusively human milk-based diet is associated with a lower rate of necrotizing enterocolitis than a diet of human milk and bovine milk-based products. J Pediatr 2010;156:562–7.e1.
7. Meinzen-Derr J, Poindexter BB, Donovan EF, et al. The role of human milk feedings in risk of late-onset sepsis. Pediatr Res 2004;55:393A.
8. Cristofalo EA, Schanler RJ, Blanco CL, et al. Randomized trial of exclusive human milk versus preterm formula diets in extremely premature infants. J Pediatr 2013; 163:1592–5.e1.
9. Delgado-Noguera MF, Calvache JA, Bonfill Cosp X. Supplementation with long chain polyunsaturated fatty acids (LCPUFA) to breastfeeding mothers for improving child growth and development. Cochrane Database Syst Rev 2010;(12):CD007901.
10. Simmer K. Long-chain polyunsaturated fatty acid supplementation in infants born at term. Cochrane Database Syst Rev 2001;(4):CD000376.
11. O'Connor DL, Weishuhn K, Rovet J, et al, Post-Discharge Feeding Study Group. Visual development of human milk-fed preterm infants provided with extra energy and nutrients after hospital discharge. JPEN J Parenter Enteral Nutr 2012;36: 349–53.
12. Hurtado JA, Iznaola C, Pena M, et al. Effects of maternal omega-3 supplementation on fatty acids and on visual and cognitive development. J Pediatr Gastroenterol Nutr 2015;61:472–80.
13. Deoni SC, Dean DC 3rd, Piryatinsky I, et al. Breastfeeding and early white matter development: a cross-sectional study. Neuroimage 2013;82:77–86.
14. Isaacs EB, Fischl BR, Quinn BT, et al. Impact of breast milk on intelligence quotient, brain size, and white matter development. Pediatr Res 2010;67:357–62.
15. Kafouri S, Kramer M, Leonard G, et al. Breastfeeding and brain structure in adolescence. Int J Epidemiol 2013;42:150–9.
16. Agostoni C, Trojan S, Bellu R, et al. Neurodevelopmental quotient of healthy term infants at 4 months and feeding practice: the role of long-chain polyunsaturated fatty acids. Pediatr Res 1995;38:262–6.
17. Carlson SE, Werkman SH, Rhodes PG, et al. Visual-acuity development in healthy preterm infants: effect of marine-oil supplementation. Am J Clin Nutr 1993;58: 35–42.
18. Zivkovic AM, German JB, Lebrilla CB, et al. Human milk glycobiome and its impact on the infant gastrointestinal microbiota. Proc Natl Acad Sci U S A 2011;108(Suppl 1):4653–8.
19. Hintz SR, Kendrick DE, Stoll BJ, et al. Neurodevelopmental and growth outcomes of extremely low birth weight infants after necrotizing enterocolitis. Pediatrics 2005;115:696–703.
20. Azcarate-Peril MA, Foster DM, Cadenas MB, et al. Acute necrotizing enterocolitis of preterm piglets is characterized by dysbiosis of ileal mucosa-associated bacteria. Gut Microbes 2011;2:234–43.
21. Elgin TG, Kern SL, McElroy SJ. Development of the neonatal intestinal microbiome and its association with necrotizing enterocolitis. Clin Ther 2016;38: 706–15.
22. Feldman R, Eidelman AI. Direct and indirect effects of breast milk on the neurobehavioral and cognitive development of premature infants. Dev Psychobiol 2003;43:109–19.

23. Bayley N. Bayley scales of infant development-II. San Antonio (TX): Psychological Corporation; 1993.
24. Lester BM, Tronick EZ, Brazelton TB. The neonatal intensive care unit network neurobehavioral scale procedures. Pediatrics 2004;113:641–67.
25. Blaymore Bier J, Oliver T, Ferguson AE, et al. Human milk improves cognitive and motor development of premature infants during infancy. J Hum Lact 2002;18:261–367.
26. Pinelli J, Saigal S, Atkinson SA. Effect of breastmilk consumption on neurodevelopmental outcomes at 6 and 12 months of age in VLBW infants. Adv Neonatal Care 2003;3:76–87.
27. O'Connor DL, Jacobs J, Hall R, et al. Growth and development of premature infants fed predominantly human milk, predominantly premature infant formula, or a combination of human milk and premature formula. J Pediatr Gastroenterol Nutr 2003;37:437–46.
28. Vohr BR, Poindexter BB, Dusick AM, et al. Beneficial effects of breast milk in the neonatal intensive care unit on the developmental outcome of extremely low birth weight infants at 18 months of age. Pediatrics 2006;118:e115–23.
29. Vohr BR, Poindexter BB, Dusick AM, et al. Persistent beneficial effects of breast milk ingested in the neonatal intensive care unit on outcomes of extremely low birth weight infants at 30 months of age. Pediatrics 2007;120:e953–9.
30. Rozé JC, Darmaun D, Boquien CY, et al. The apparent breastfeeding paradox in very preterm infants: relationship between breast feeding, early weight gain and neurodevelopment based on results from two cohorts, EPIPAGE and LIFT. BMJ Open 2012;2:e000834.
31. Bricker D, Squires J. Ages and stages questionnaires: a parent-completed, child-monitoring system. Baltimore (MD): Paul H. Brookes Publishing Co; 1999.
32. Kaufman NL. Kaufman assessment battery for children, second edition (KABC-II). San Antonio (TX): Pearson; 2004.
33. Beaino G, Khoshnood B, Kaminski M, et al. Predictors of the risk of cognitive deficiency in very preterm infants: the EPIPAGE prospective cohort. Acta Paediatr 2011;100:370–8.
34. Tanaka K, Kon N, Ohkawa N, et al. Does breastfeeding in the neonatal period influence the cognitive function of very-low-birth-weight infants at 5 years of age? Brain Dev 2009;31:288–93.
35. Gerstadt CL, Hong YJ, Diamond A. The relationship between cognition and action: performance of children 3 1/2-7 years old on a Stroop-like day-night test. Cognition 1994;53:129–53.
36. O'Donnell JP, Paulsen KA, McGann JD. Matching familiar figures test: a unidimensional measure of reflection-impulsivity? Percept Mot Skills 1978;47:1247–53.
37. Harvey JM, O'Callaghan MJ, Mohay H. Executive function of children with extremely low birthweight: a case control study. Dev Med Child Neurol 1999;41:292–7.
38. Goodman R. Psychometric properties of the strengths and difficulties questionnaire. J Am Acad Child Adolesc Psychiatry 2001;40:1337–45.
39. Smith MM, Durkin M, Hinton VJ, et al. Influence of breastfeeding on cognitive outcomes at age 6-8 years: follow-up of very low birth weight infants. Am J Epidemiol 2003;158:1075–82.
40. Horwood LJ, Darlow BA, Mogridge N. Breast milk feeding and cognitive ability at 7-8 years. Arch Dis Child Fetal Neonatal Ed 2001;84:F23–7.
41. Wechsler D. Wechsler Intelligence Scale for Children—Revised. New York: The Psychological Corporation; 1974.

42. Johnson S, Wolke D, Hennessy E, et al. Educational outcomes in extremely preterm children: neuropsychological correlates and predictors of attainment. Dev Neuropsychol 2011;36:74–95.
43. Elgen I, Sommerfelt K, Ellertsen B. Cognitive performance in a low birth weight cohort at 5 and 11 years of age. Pediatr Neurol 2003;29:111–6.
44. Henriksen C, Haugholt K, Lindgren M, et al. Improved cognitive development among preterm infants attributable to early supplementation of human milk with docosahexaenoic acid and arachidonic acid. Pediatrics 2008;121:1137–45.
45. Westerberg AC, Schei R, Henriksen C, et al. Attention among very low birth weight infants following early supplementation with docosahexaenoic and arachidonic acid. Acta Paediatr 2011;100:47–52.
46. Makrides M, Gibson RA, McPhee AJ, et al. Neurodevelopmental outcomes of preterm infants fed high-dose docosahexaenoic acid: a randomized controlled trial. JAMA 2009;301:175–82.
47. Smithers LG, Collins CT, Simmonds LA, et al. Feeding preterm infants milk with a higher dose of docosahexaenoic acid than that used in current practice does not influence language or behavior in early childhood: a follow-up study of a randomized controlled trial. Am J Clin Nutr 2010;91:628–34.
48. Isaacs EB, Ross S, Kennedy K, et al. 10-year cognition in preterms after random assignment to fatty acid supplementation in infancy. Pediatrics 2011;128:e890–8.
49. Tanaka K, Hosozawa M, Kudo N, et al. The pilot study: sphingomyelin-fortified milk has a positive association with the neurobehavioural development of very low birth weight infants during infancy, randomized control trial. Brain Dev 2013;35:45–52.
50. Smithers LG, Gibson RA, Makrides M. Maternal supplementation with docosahexaenoic acid during pregnancy does not affect early visual development in the infant: a randomized controlled trial. Am J Clin Nutr 2011;93:1293–9.
51. Makrides M, Gibson RA, McPhee AJ, et al. Effect of DHA supplementation during pregnancy on maternal depression and neurodevelopment of young children: a randomized controlled trial. JAMA 2010;304:1675–83.
52. Makrides M, Gould JF, Gawlik NR, et al. Four-year follow-up of children born to women in a randomized trial of prenatal DHA supplementation. JAMA 2014; 311:1802–4.
53. Lucas A, Cole TJ, Morley R, et al. Factors associated with maternal choice to provide breast milk for low birthweight infants. Arch Dis Child 1988;63:48–52.
54. Jain A, Concato J, Leventhal JM. How good is the evidence linking breastfeeding and intelligence? Pediatrics 2002;109:1044–53.
55. Gale CR, Martyn CN. Breastfeeding, dummy use, and adult intelligence. Lancet 1996;347:1072–5.
56. Jacobson SW, Chiodo LM, Jacobson JL. Breastfeeding effects on intelligence quotient in 4- and 11-year-old children. Pediatrics 1999;103:e71.
57. Der G, Batty GD, Deary IJ. Effect of breast feeding on intelligence in children: prospective study, sibling pairs analysis, and meta-analysis. BMJ 2006;333:945.
58. Horta BL, Victora CG. Long-term effects of breastfeeding: a systematic review. Geneva, Switzerland: World Health Organization; 2013.

Should Women Providing Milk to Their Preterm Infants Take Docosahexaenoic Acid Supplements?

CrossMark

Berthold Koletzko, MD, PhD

KEYWORDS

- Arachidonic acid • Eicosapentaenoic acid • Docosahexaenoic acid
- Polyunsaturated fatty acids • Very low-birth-weight infants

KEY POINTS

- Human milk globally has a mean DHA content of 0.3% of fatty acids, with large variation along with different maternal DHA intakes from fish and seafood.
- Breastfeeding usually meets DHA needs of term infants (100 mg/d) but not the much higher requirements of very low birthweight infants (VLBWI).
- To match intrauterine DHA accretion, VLBWI require a human milk DHA content of about 1% that is achievable by maternal supplementation with 3 g/d tuna oil.
- A high milk DHA supply to VLBWI may enhance early visual and cognitive development and reduce adverse events include severe developmental delay, bronchopulmonary dysplasia, necrotizing enterocolitis and allergies.

The supply, metabolism, and biological effects of the omega-3 (n-3) and the omega-6 (n-6) essential polyunsaturated fatty acids (PUFA) during pregnancy, infancy, and childhood have received considerable attention and have been addressed in numerous research studies, as recently reviewed.[1–4] The essential fatty acids n-6 linoleic acid (18:2n-6, LA) and n-3 alpha-linolenic acid (18:3n-3, ALA) found in plants and vegetable oils are the precursors of the biologically active long-chain polyunsaturated fatty acids (LC-PUFA). The quantitatively predominant LC-PUFA are n-6 arachidonic

The work of the author is financially supported in part by the Commission of the European Community, the 7th Framework Programme Early Nutrition (FP7-289346), the Horizon 2020 Research and Innovation Programme DYNAHEALTH (No 633595), and the European Research Council Advanced Grant META-GROWTH (ERC-2012-AdG, no. 322605). This article does not necessarily reflect the views of the Commission and in no way anticipates the future policy in this area.
Division of Metabolism and Nutritional Medicine, Dr. von Hauner Children's Hospital, University of Munich Medical Center, Ludwig-Maximilians-Universität Munich, Campus Innenstadt Lindwurmstrasse 4, D-80337 Munich, Germany
E-mail address: office.koletzko@med.lmu.de

0095-5108/17/© 2016 The Author. Published by Elsevier Inc. This is an open access article under the CC BY-NC-ND license (http://creativecommons.org/licenses/by-nc-nd/4.0/).

acid (ARA, 20:4n-6), n-3 eicosapentaenoic acid (20:5n-3, EPA), and n-3 docosahexa-enoic acid (DHA, 22:6n-3). During both pregnancy and infancy, n-6 and n-3 LC-PUFA are accreted in relatively large amounts in fetal and infant tissues. Particularly high concentrations are found in the brain gray matter and in the rod outer segments of the retina and have been related to functional development, such as cognition and visual acuity.[4] Some LC-PUFA, including n-6 dihomo-gamma-linolenic acid (20:3n-6), ARA, EPA, and DHA, also serve as precursors of eicosanoids and docosanoids, such as prostaglandins, prostacyclins, leukotrienes, and resolvins. In low concentrations, eicosanoids and docosanoids are powerful regulators of numerous physiologic processes, such as cardiovascular function and the early postnatal closure of the ductus arteriosus Botalli, thrombocyte aggregation and bleeding time, inflammation and immunity, and others. In fact, the early availability of LC-PUFA has been associated with immune functions and the likelihood of the development of allergies and infections.[1]

LC-PUFA either can be provided preformed via the placenta or the dietary sources, such as human milk, or can be endogenously synthesized from the precursors LA and ALA by consecutive desaturation and chain elongation. However, in humans, the conversion rates are rather low. It was estimated that only 0.1% to 10% of the precursor fatty acids are converted to LC-PUFA, with a particularly low rate of synthesis for DHA.[5–7] The rates of conversion are also very variable depending on genotypes of the fatty acid desaturase (FADS) gene cluster. Individuals with certain genetic haplotypes have extremely low rates of ARA and DHA synthesis and thus depend even more on the supply of preformed LC-PUFA to maintain plasma and tissue levels.[1,8–12] In infants, and particularly in preterm infants, the rates of parent PUFA conversion to LC-PUFA are considered insufficient to achieve biochemical and functional normality.[13,14]

In utero, ARA and DHA are supplied preformed to the fetus by way of an active and preferential materno-fetal transport across the placenta that have been measured in vivo using fatty acids labeled with stable isotopes.[15,16] The underlying mechanisms of this active materno-fetal LC-PUFA transfer have been partly explored.[17–19] Fatty acids from maternal lipoproteins are released by 2 lipases expressed in placental tissue, lipoprotein lipase (LPL) and endothelial lipase (EL). LPL hydrolyses triglycerides, whereas EL is a phospholipase with little triacylglycerol lipase activity. EL continues to be expressed toward the end of pregnancy, whereas LPL is virtually absent in the trophoblast. In addition, maternal circulating NEFA non-esterified fatty acids (NEFA) are mediated by membrane-bound proteins expressed in the trophoblast, including FABPpm (fatty acid binding protein plasma membrane), p-FABPpm (placental plasma membrane fatty acid-binding protein), FAT/CD36 (fatty acid translocase), and FATP (fatty acid transport proteins) -1 to -6.[17,19] In the cytosol, fatty acids are bound to fatty acid binding proteins (FABPs), leading to interaction with subcellular organelles, including the endoplasmic reticulum, mitochondria, lipid droplets, and peroxisomes. FABPs are also likely to function in the nucleus through the delivery of specific ligands to nuclear transcription factors, such as the peroxisome proliferator-activated receptors. This complex system achieves an active placental materno-fetal transfer of ARA and particularly of DHA. Given that intrauterine growth and body composition are generally considered the reference that postnatal care of preterm infants should match as much as feasible, it appears prudent to aim at approaching the degree of intrauterine provision of preformed LC-PUFA with postnatal nutritional regimens.

After birth, breastfed infants always receive preformed ARA and DHA with human milk lipids. The milk fatty acid composition is modified by maternal diet, lipolysis of body fat stores that markedly contribute to milk fat synthesis, maternal genotype, and stage of lactation.[11,20,21] Around the world, human milk provides a relatively stable ARA supply around 0.5% of milk fatty acids, whereas DHA is found at a mean level of 0.3% but shows much more variation primarily due to differences in maternal intake of dietary DHA sources, such as fish and seafood.[21,22] Full breastfeeding usually meets the recommended intakes for term-born infants of 140 mg ARA/d and 100 mg DHA/d,[1,23] but not the higher recommended intakes for preterm infants. Although the milk of mothers of preterm women contains slightly higher amounts of LC-PUFA,[24] the recommended DHA supply of very low-birth-weight infants can only be met through human milk if women obtain a markedly increased DHA intake. The human milk DHA content is linearly related to the maternal DHA intake, as the author documented in a supplementation study of well-nourished mothers who fully breastfed their infants born at term (**Fig. 1**).[25]

LONG-CHAIN POLYUNSATURATED FATTY ACIDS SUPPLY TO PRETERM INFANTS

Increasing DHA provision to preterm infants through DHA supplements to the lactating mother needs to be justified by indications for a benefit for clinical outcome. The recent systematic review of the Early Nutrition Academy on the roles of prenatal and postnatal LC-PUFA included studies in preterm infants published until 2013.[1] The LC-PUFA provision to preterm infants was also evaluated in a meta-analysis of available studies[26] and in recent reviews.[2,27] Most of the available studies in preterm infants evaluated DHA supplies with human milk or formula of about 0.2% to 0.3% of fat, as often provided to healthy infants born at term. However, this level of supply is not sufficient to achieve the estimated daily intrauterine deposition of DHA of 43 mg/kg body weight, which occurs along with an even higher ARA deposition of about 212 mg/kg.[28] It has been estimated that the intrauterine DHA

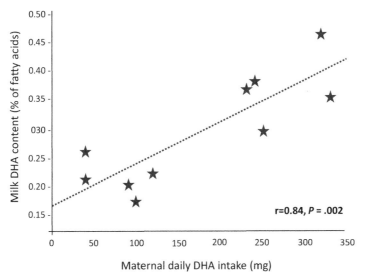

Fig. 1. The DHA content in mature human milk is linearly related to the DHA intake of the breastfeeding mother. Data from a randomized supplementation trial. (*Adapted from* Fidler N, Sauerwald T, Pohl A, et al. Docosahexaenoic acid transfer into human milk after dietary supplementation: a randomized clinical trial. J Lipid Res 2000;41(9):1376–83.)

accretion rate may be matched postnatally in preterm infants by a DHA provision amount to 1% of human milk or formula fat.[29] This approach has been evaluated in randomized trials that studied the addition of LC-PUFA–rich oils to human milk[30] or the supplementation of mothers providing human milk with LC-PUFA–rich marine oil.[31–34]

Visual and Cognitive Development

The Cochrane meta-analysis by Schulzke and colleagues[26] found no benefit of an added LC-PUFA supply to preterm infants on cognitive outcomes at the age of 12 to 18 months in 4 of 7 studies included in this meta-analysis. Of interest, the 3 studies that found such benefits used the newer version II of the "Bayley Scales of Infant Development," which raises the question whether the older version of the Bayley test or other tests might not be as sensitive to detect effects. Visual acuity was not found to be influenced by LC-PUFA supply.[26]

Of particular interest are the findings of 2 large studies providing much higher DHA amounts with milk and hence approaching more closely the levels of intrauterine supply. Henriksen and colleagues[30] randomized 141 very low-birth-weight infants to an intervention adding an LC-PUFA–rich algal oil, mixed with soy oil and medium-chain triglyceride oil. The intervention provided an added 32 mg of DHA and 31 mg of ARA per 100 mL of human milk and started at 1 week after birth, with continuation until discharge from the hospital, which occurred on average after 9 weeks. Cognitive development was evaluated at 6 months of age by the "Ages and Stages Questionnaire" and event-related potentials, a measure of brain correlates related to recognition memory. At the 6-month follow-up, the investigators found a better performance of the intervention group on the problem-solving subscore, compared with the control group (53.4 vs 49.5 points). There was also a nonsignificant trend to a higher total score (221 vs 215 points). The event-related potential data revealed that infants in the intervention group had significantly lower responses after the standard image, compared with the control group (8.6 vs 13.2). Further follow-up to the age of 8 years did not indicate any significant differences at school age with regards to brain structure, cognition, and behavior.[35,36]

Makrides and coworkers[29] performed a very large randomized multicenter trial enrolling as many as 657 preterm infants who were provided with a conventional (0.35%) or high (1%) DHA supply from day 2 to 4 of life until term. The higher DHA provision was achieved by supplementation of women providing human milk with a daily dose of 3 g of tuna oil, or by a preterm formula with increased DHA content, along with about 0.5% ARA.[31–34] No adverse effects of supplementation were observed in the infants. The higher DHA supply improved visual acuity development at the corrected age of 4 months, with an acuity that was 1.4 cycles per degree higher than in the control group (**Table 1**).[37] The Bayley test of infant development (version II) was applied at an age of 18 months, corrected for gestational age. Although no significant benefit of the intervention was detected in the total study population, improved cognitive development was found in girls, and in the group of smaller infants with a birth weight less than 1250 g (see **Table 1**). Probably of even greater clinical importance, the rate of children with severe developmental retardation (Mental Development Index <70) was reduced by half (see **Table 1**). Later follow-up to the age of 7 years did not indicate any significant differences at school age with regards to cognition, behavior, and visual function.[38–40]

Effects on Other Outcomes

In the previously cited trial with 657 preterm infants provided with conventional (0.35%) or high (1%) levels of DHA in the milk supplied, the occurrence of chronic

Table 1
Providing preterm infants with milk with a higher docosahexaenoic acid dose (about 1% of fatty acids, compared with 0.3%) improved early visual function and reduced markedly abnormal developmental outcomes at age 18 months

	High DHA (≈1%)	Standard DHA (≈0.3%)	Significance
Visual acuity (cycles per degree), aged 4 mo (corrected for gestational age)			
	9.6 (3.7)	8.2 (1.8)	$P = .025$
Mental development index (MDI), aged 18 mo (corrected for gestational age)			
Girls	99.1(13.9)	94.4 (17.5)	$P = .03$
Boys	91.3 (14.0)	91.9 (17.2)	n.s.
Markedly abnormal development index (MDI), aged 18 mo (corrected for gestational age)			
MDI <70	17 (5%)	35 (11%)	$P = .03$
MDI <85	64 (20%)	90 (27%)	$P = .08$

Note: Later follow-up did not indicate any significant developmental differences at school age.
Abbreviation: n.s., not significant.
Data from Makrides M, Gibson RA, McPhee AJ, et al. Neurodevelopmental outcomes of preterm infants fed high-dose docosahexaenoic acid a randomized controlled trial. JAMA 2009;301(2):175–82.

lung disease (bronchopulmonary dysplasia, BPD), defined by the need for oxygen treatment at a postmenstrual age of 36 weeks, was reduced by high DHA supply in boys (relative risk [RR]: 0.67, 95% confidence interval [CI]: 0.47–0.96; $P = .03$) and in all infants with a birth weight of less than 1250 g (RR: 0.75, 95% CI: 0.57–0.98; $P = .04$).[32] Because this was a secondary endpoint, a new trial to revisit this important effect has been initiated.[41] A meta-analysis including 18 randomized controlled trials found that n-3 LC-PUFA supply was not associated with a decreased risk of BPD in all studied preterm infants, but trials that included only infants born at 32 weeks or less found a trend toward reduced BPD (pooled RR 0.88, 95% CI 0.74–1.05, 7 studies, n = 1156 infants) along with a reduction in the risk of necrotizing enterocolitis (pooled RR 0.50, 95% CI 0.23–1.10, 5 studies, n = 900 infants).[42]

The previously cited large preterm trial[29,32] providing either 0.3% or 1% of milk fatty acids as DHA also evaluated the incidence of atopic conditions up to the age of 18 months. There was no effect on duration of respiratory support, admission length, or home oxygen requirement. There was a reduction in reported hay fever in all infants in the high-DHA group at either 12 or 18 months (RR: 0.41, 95% CI: 0.18–0.91; $P = .03$) and at either 12 or 18 months in boys (RR: 0.15, 95% CI: 0.03–0.64; $P = .01$), whereas there was no effect on asthma, eczema, or food allergy. A recent *Cochrane Review* evaluated published data on effects of prenatal or postnatal n-3 LC-PUFA supplementation to women during pregnancy or the or breastfeeding period on allergy outcomes in their children.[43] Although the data were derived from a limited number of informative randomized trials, an added n-3 LC-PUFA supply reduced the risk of any medically diagnosed, immunoglobulin E (IgE)-mediated allergy in children aged 12 to 36 months (risk ratio 0.66, 95% CI 0.44–0.98) but not after the age of 36 months. Food allergies were no different after the age of 1 year, but a clear reduction was seen for infants. Also, medically diagnosed IgE-mediated eczema was reduced by maternal n-3 LC-PUFA supply at the age of 1 to 3 years but not at other ages.[43] These data point to possible benefits of a higher n-3 LC-PUFA supply in early life on allergic and atopic disorders.

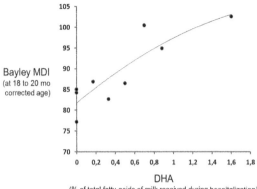

Fig. 2. Dose-response relationship between milk DHA supply to preterm infants and the Mayley Mental Development Index (Baley MDI) at age 18 to 20 months, corrected for gestational age. (*From* Lapillonne A. Enteral and parenteral lipid requirements of preterm infants. In: Koletzko B, Poindexter B, Uauy R, editors. Nutritional care of preterm infants. Scientific basis and practical guidelines. Basel (Switzerland): Karger; 2014. p. 90; with permission.)

SUMMARY

Based on the available data, a high milk DHA supply to very low-birth-weight infants and to extremely low-birth-weight infants at levels that support tissue accretion rates similar to the high rates of intrauterine deposition has the potential to enhance the early visual and cognitive development, and to reduce the occurrence of adverse events, such as severe developmental delay, BPD, necrotizing enterocolitis, and allergic manifestations in infancy and early childhood. Lapillonne[44] described the dose-response relationship between the level of DHA in the milk provided to preterm infants and the achieved mental development (**Fig. 2**) and concluded that a DHA intake near 1% of fatty acid supply is desirable. Based on current knowledge, DHA should always be supplied to young infants along with ARA, which human milk always provides.[45]

Current recommendations stipulate for very low-birth-weight infants a daily DHA supply of at least 18 mg but preferably 55 to 60 mg/kg body weight ($\approx$ 1% of total fatty acid supply) and a daily ARA supply of at least 18 mg but preferably 35 to 45 mg/kg ($\approx$ 0.6–0.75%).[1,27] It is possible that subgroups of preterm infants achieve greater benefits, for example, more immature infants or those with lower birth weights, as well as infants with genotypes predicting a low rate of endogenous LC-PUFA formation. Women providing milk to their very low or extremely low birth-weight infants can achieve the desirable DHA content in their milk by taking a supplement of 3 g tuna oil per day ($\approx$ 1% of total fatty acid supply).[29]

ACKNOWLEDGMENTS

The authors' work is financially supported in part by the Commission of the European Communities, Projects Early Nutrition (FP7-289346), DYNAHEALTH (H2020-633595) and LIFECYCLE (H2020-SC1-2016-RTD), and the European Research Council Advanced Grant META-GROWTH (ERC-2012-AdG 322605). Additional support from the German Ministry of Education and Research, Berlin (Grant Nr. 01 GI 0825), the German Research Council (Ko 912/12-1) is gratefully acknowledged.

REFERENCES

1. Koletzko B, Boey CC, Campoy C, et al. Current information and Asian perspectives on long-chain polyunsaturated fatty acids in pregnancy, lactation and infancy. Systematic review and practice recommendations from an Early Nutrition Academy workshop. Ann Nutr Metab 2014;65(1):i49–80.
2. Lapillonne A, Moltu SJ. Long chain polyunsaturated fatty acids and clinical outcomes of preterm infants. Ann Nutr Metab 2016;69(Suppl 1):36–44.
3. Makrides M, Best K. DHA and preterm birth. Ann Nutr Metab 2016;69(Suppl 1): 23–8.
4. Calder PC. Docosahexaenoic acid. Ann Nutr Metab 2016;69(Suppl 1):7–21.
5. Vermunt SH, Mensink RP, Simonis AM, et al. Effects of age and dietary n-3 fatty acids on the metabolism of [13C]-alpha-linolenic acid. Lipids 1999;34(Suppl): S127.
6. Pawlosky RJ, Hibbeln JR, Novotny JA, et al. Physiological compartmental analysis of alpha-linolenic acid metabolism in adult humans. J lipid Res 2001;42(8): 1257–65.
7. Brenna JT. Efficiency of conversion of alpha-linolenic acid to long chain n-3 fatty acids in man. Curr Opin Clin Nutr Metab Care 2002;5(2):127–32.
8. Lattka E, Klopp N, Demmelmair H, et al. Genetic variations in polyunsaturated fatty acid metabolism—implications for child health? Ann Nutr Metab 2012; 60(Suppl 3):8–17.
9. Glaser C, Lattka E, Rzehak P, et al. Genetic variation in polyunsaturated fatty acid metabolism and its potential relevance for human development and health. Matern Child Nutr 2011;7(Suppl 2):27–40.
10. Koletzko B, Lattka E, Zeilinger S, et al. Genetic variants of the fatty acid desaturase gene cluster predict amounts of red blood cell docosahexaenoic and other polyunsaturated fatty acids in pregnant women: findings from the Avon Longitudinal Study of Parents and Children. Am J Clin Nutr 2011;93(1):211–9.
11. Lattka E, Rzehak P, Szabo E, et al. Genetic variants in the FADS gene cluster are associated with arachidonic acid concentrations of human breast milk at 1.5 and 6 mo postpartum and influence the course of milk dodecanoic, tetracosenoic, and trans-9-octadecenoic acid concentrations over the duration of lactation. Am J Clin Nutr 2011;93(2):382–91.
12. Steer CD, Lattka E, Koletzko B, et al. Maternal fatty acids in pregnancy, FADS polymorphisms, and child intelligence quotient at 8 y of age. Am J Clin Nutr 2013;98(6):1575–82.
13. Uauy R, Castillo C. Lipid requirements of infants: implications for nutrient composition of fortified complementary foods. J Nutr 2003;133(9):2962S–72S.
14. Uauy R, Dangour AD. Fat and fatty acid requirements and recommendations for infants of 0-2 years and children of 2-18 years. Ann Nutr Metab 2009;55(1–3):76–96.
15. Gil-Sanchez A, Larque E, Demmelmair H, et al. Maternal-fetal in vivo transfer of [13C]docosahexaenoic and other fatty acids across the human placenta 12 h after maternal oral intake. Am J Clin Nutr 2010;92(1):115–22.
16. Larque E, Demmelmair H, Berger B, et al. In vivo investigation of the placental transfer of (13)C-labeled fatty acids in humans. J Lipid Res 2003;44(1):49–55.
17. Larque E, Ruiz-Palacios M, Koletzko B. Placental regulation of fetal nutrient supply. Curr Opin Clin Nutr Metab Care 2013;16(3):292–7.
18. Prieto-Sanchez MT, Ruiz-Palacios M, Blanco-Carnero JE, et al. Placental MFSD2a transporter is related to decreased DHA in cord blood of women with treated gestational diabetes. Clin Nutr 2016. [Epub ahead of print].

19. Larque E, Pagan A, Prieto MT, et al. Placental fatty acid transfer: a key factor in fetal growth. Ann Nutr Metab 2014;64(3–4):247–53.
20. Del Prado M, Villalpando S, Elizondo A, et al. Contribution of dietary and newly formed arachidonic acid to human milk lipids in women eating a low-fat diet. Am J Clin Nutr 2001;74(2):242–7.
21. Koletzko B, Agostoni C, Bergmann R, et al. Physiological aspects of human milk lipids and implications for infant feeding: a workshop report. Acta Paediatr 2011; 100(11):1405–15.
22. Brenna JT, Varamini B, Jensen RG, et al. Docosahexaenoic and arachidonic acid concentrations in human breast milk worldwide. Am J Clin Nutr 2007;85(6): 1457–64.
23. EFSA-Panel-on-Dietetic-Products. Scientific opinion on nutrient requirements and dietary intakes of infants and young children in the European Union. EFSA J 2013; 11(10):3408.
24. Genzel-Boroviczeny O, Wahle J, Koletzko B. Fatty acid composition of human milk during the 1st month after term and preterm delivery. Eur J Pediatr 1997; 156(2):142–7.
25. Fidler N, Sauerwald T, Pohl A, et al. Docosahexaenoic acid transfer into human milk after dietary supplementation: a randomized clinical trial. J Lipid Res 2000;41(9):1376–83.
26. Schulzke SM, Patole SK, Simmer K. Long-chain polyunsaturated fatty acid supplementation in preterm infants. Cochrane Database Syst Rev 2011;2:CD000375.
27. Koletzko B, Poindexter B, Uauy R, editors. Nutritional care of preterm infants. Basel (Switzerland): Karger; 2014.
28. Kuipers RS, Luxwolda MF, Offringa PJ, et al. Fetal intrauterine whole body linoleic, arachidonic and docosahexaenoic acid contents and accretion rates. Prostaglandins Leukot Essent Fatty Acids 2012;86(1–2):13–20.
29. Makrides M, Gibson RA, McPhee AJ, et al. Neurodevelopmental outcomes of preterm infants fed high-dose docosahexaenoic acid a randomized controlled trial. JAMA 2009;301(2):175–82.
30. Henriksen C, Haugholt K, Lindgren M, et al. Improved cognitive development among preterm infants attributable to early supplementation of human milk with docosahexaenoic acid and arachidonic acid. Pediatrics 2008;121(6):1137–45.
31. Atwell K, Collins CT, Sullivan TR, et al. Respiratory hospitalisation of infants supplemented with docosahexaenoic acid as preterm neonates. J Paediatr Child Health 2013;49(1):E17–22.
32. Manley BJ, Makrides M, Collins CT, et al. High-dose docosahexaenoic acid supplementation of preterm infants: respiratory and allergy outcomes. Pediatrics 2011;128(1):e71–7.
33. Collins CT, Makrides M, Gibson RA, et al. Pre- and post-term growth in pre-term infants supplemented with higher-dose DHA: a randomised controlled trial. Br J Nutr 2011;105(11):1635–43.
34. Smithers LG, Gibson RA, McPhee A, et al. Effect of two doses of docosahexaenoic acid (DHA) in the diet of preterm infants on infant fatty acid status: results from the DINO trial. Prostaglandins, Leukot Essent Fatty Acids 2008;79(3–5): 141–6.
35. Almaas AN, Tamnes CK, Nakstad B, et al. Diffusion tensor imaging and behavior in premature infants at 8 years of age, a randomized controlled trial with long-chain polyunsaturated fatty acids. Early Hum Dev 2016;95:41–6.
36. Almaas AN, Tamnes CK, Nakstad B, et al. Long-chain polyunsaturated fatty acids and cognition in VLBW infants at 8 years: an RCT. Pediatrics 2015;135(6):972–80.

37. Smithers LG, Gibson RA, McPhee A, et al. Higher dose of docosahexaenoic acid in the neonatal period improves visual acuity of preterm infants: results of a randomized controlled trial. Am J Clin Nutr 2008;88(4):1049–56.

38. Smithers LG, Collins CT, Simmonds LA, et al. Feeding preterm infants milk with a higher dose of docosahexaenoic acid than that used in current practice does not influence language or behavior in early childhood: a follow-up study of a randomized controlled trial. Am J Clin Nutr 2010;91(3):628–34.

39. Collins CT, Gibson RA, Anderson PJ, et al. Neurodevelopmental outcomes at 7 years' corrected age in preterm infants who were fed high-dose docosahexaenoic acid to term equivalent: a follow-up of a randomised controlled trial. BMJ open 2015;5(3):e007314.

40. Molloy CS, Stokes S, Makrides M, et al. Long-term effect of high-dose supplementation with DHA on visual function at school age in children born at <33 wk gestational age: results from a follow-up of a randomized controlled trial. Am J Clin Nutr 2016;103(1):268–75.

41. Collins CT, Gibson RA, Makrides M, et al. The N3RO trial: a randomised controlled trial of docosahexaenoic acid to reduce bronchopulmonary dysplasia in preterm infants < 29 weeks' gestation. BMC Pediatr 2016;16:72.

42. Zhang P, Lavoie PM, Lacaze-Masmonteil T, et al. Omega-3 long-chain polyunsaturated fatty acids for extremely preterm infants: a systematic review. Pediatrics 2014;134(1):120–34.

43. Gunaratne AW, Makrides M, Collins CT. Maternal prenatal and/or postnatal n-3 long chain polyunsaturated fatty acids (LCPUFA) supplementation for preventing allergies in early childhood. Cochrane Database Syst Rev 2015;(7):CD010085.

44. Lapillonne A. Enteral and parenteral lipid requirements of preterm infants. In: Koletzko B, Poindexter B, Uauy R, editors. Nutritional care of preterm infants. Scientific basis and practical guidelines. Basel (Switzerland): Karger; 2014. p. 82–98.

45. Koletzko B, Carlson SE, van Goudoever JB. Should infant formula provide both omega-3 DHA and omega-6 arachidonic acid? Ann Nutr Metab 2015;66:137–8.

Human Milk—Treatment and Quality of Banked Human Milk

Jean-Charles Picaud, MD, PhD[a,b,c,d,e,*], Rachel Buffin, MD[a,b]

KEYWORDS

- Prematurity • Milk banking • Donor milk • Pasteurization • Nutrition • Infection
- Breastfeeding • Milk

KEY POINTS

- Donor human milk (DHM) is beneficial for the health of preterm infants, and it is essential that human milk banks deliver a safe and high-quality DHM.
- Low temperature (62.5°C) long time (30 minutes) pasteurization offers the best compromise between microbiological safety and immunologic quality of DHM.
- Not all pasteurizers are equivalent to apply well-controlled temperature, and regular strict quality control is necessary.
- New techniques have been proposed, such as high temperature short time, high-pressure processing, or UV irradiation, which have been tested in experimental conditions.
- When devices usable in human milk banks will be available, it will be necessary to test these new methods in real conditions.

INTRODUCTION

Breast milk is a unique bioactive substance essential to the development of the newborn's immature immune and digestive systems. In preterm infants, there are specific benefits related to human milk (HM) that helps to reduce significantly the risk of digestive intolerance, necrotizing enterocolitis, late onset sepsis, bronchopulmonary dysplasia, and retinopathy of prematurity.[1–6] It has also a long-term positive impact on cognitive development and metabolism and cardiovascular health at adult age.[7] Therefore, HM nutrition is one of most cost-effective interventions that allow

Disclosure Statement: The authors have no commercial or financial conflicts of interest to disclose and do not declare any funding sources.
[a] Neonatal Unit, Hôpital de la Croix-Rousse, Lyon F-69004, France; [b] Rhone-Alpes Auvergneregional Human Milk Bank, Hôpital de la Croix-Rousse, Lyon F-69004, France; [c] Lyon Sud Charles Merieux School of Medicine, Université Claude Bernard Lyon 1, Pierre-Bénite F-69310, France; [d] Rhone-Alpes Human Nutrition Research Center, Hôpital Lyon Sud, Pierre-Bénite F-69310, France; [e] European Milk Bank Association (EMBA), Milano, Italy
* Corresponding author. Department of Neonatology, Hôpital de la Croix-Rousse, Lyon, France.
E-mail address: jean-charles.picaud@chu-lyon.fr

Clin Perinatol 44 (2017) 95–119
http://dx.doi.org/10.1016/j.clp.2016.11.003
0095-5108/17/© 2016 Elsevier Inc. All rights reserved.

perinatology.theclinics.com

promoting childhood and adult health.[8] Mothers who delivered prematurely often experience significant difficulties in breastfeeding their infant. Furthermore, because preterm neonates are not able to breastfeed during the first weeks of life, they are at greatest risk of not receiving HM.

Breast milk from their own mother (MOM) is the first option for these newborns. When this is not possible, the next best option is donor human milk (DHM) from a human milk bank (HMB).[9,10] In 2010, the European Society for Pediatric Gastroenterology, Hepatology, and Nutrition advocated the use of HM for preterm infants as standard practice, provided it is fortified with added nutrients where necessary to meet requirements.[11] The presence of HMB is useful to help provide most preterm babies with HM. It improves the exposure to HM during hospitalization and breastfeeding rates at discharge.[12–14]

DONOR HUMAN MILK TO FEED PRETERM INFANTS

When fresh MOM is not available, preterm infants benefit from receiving DHM rather than a preterm formula.[5] For example, gastric emptying is faster and digestive tolerance is better in children fed with pasteurized breast milk than in infants fed a preterm formula.[15] In a recent randomized trial, Cossey and colleagues[16] reported no difference in either the digestive tolerance or the prevalence of necrotizing enterocolitis in preterm infants fed fresh versus pasteurized MOM, confirming previously reported results.[17] Indeed, the prevention of necrotizing enterocolitis by HM passes mainly through its effects on gut maturation,[18,19] and breast milk components that have a maturational effect are apparently not destroyed by pasteurization.[20,21]

The protective effect of HM against late onset sepsis in preterm infants is related to the presence of immunologic factors, most of which are sensitive to storage, freezing, and pasteurization. However, pasteurized milk retains the ability to inhibit bacterial growth even if it is slightly reduced when compared with fresh milk.[22] Two randomized trials showed no significant difference in the prevalence of late onset sepsis among preterm infants fed fresh or pasteurized HM.[16,23] Other nonrandomized studies report similar findings.[24,25] Then, available evidence suggests that pasteurized HM retains a part of its anti-infective properties and could be as effective as fresh milk to protect premature infants against infections.

Pasteurization has no significant effect on nutrients that are essential to support postnatal growth, such as energy, protein, or zinc contents.[26,27] However, it has been suggested that the pasteurization of milk could have a negative effect on growth of preterm infants, via reduced intestinal fat absorption related to destruction of bile salts–stimulated lipase (BSSL).[28,29] However, Andersson and colleagues[28] observed a nonsignificant reduction of fat absorption and no effect on weight gain in preterm infants fed pasteurized HM. The absence of significant effect on growth could be partly explained because the HM is not the only source of lipase and also because heat treatment of HM increases significantly the amount of free fatty acids that is known to be better absorbed in the digestive system.[30] Moreover, the observational study from Montjaux-Régis and colleagues[29] has compared infants fed unpasteurized MOM or mature donor milk. As the protein content of milk from mothers delivering prematurely is higher in than mature milk provided by donors, it is likely that these investigators identified the effect of HM composition rather than the effect of pasteurization[31] (**Fig. 1**). In a case-control study, Giuliani and colleagues[24] found no significant difference in weight gain between premature infants receiving MOM or pasteurized milk. The only randomized trial comparing the growth of premature infants receiving fresh versus pasteurized MOM reported no difference in weight

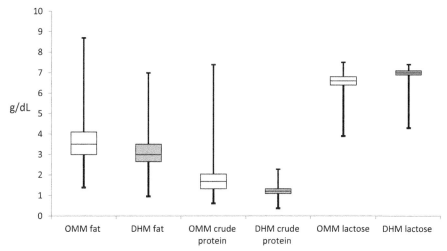

Fig. 1. Crude protein, fat, lactose, and energy content (median, P25, P75, minimum, and maximum values) assessed by a near infrared analyzer (Miris 3rd generation, Sweden) in MOM (N = 1350 samples) and DHM (N = 860 samples) treated in Auvergne Rhone-Alpes Regional Human Milk Bank. Twelve particularly high protein values above 4g/dL, obtained in OMM from twelve different mothers, 24 to 40 days after delivery. OMM, own mother's milk.

gain during hospitalization.[16] Thus, DHM is able to support postnatal growth, as fresh milk, as soon as it is fortified appropriately.

There are data suggesting an association between the consumption of HM during hospitalization and further cognitive development of very low-birth-weight infants.[2,32] Furthermore, it has been shown that, in premature infants exhibiting poor postnatal growth (weight-for-age z-score at −1.4 SD at discharge), cognitive development is better if they received breast milk during hospitalization.[33] Heat treatment applied to donor milk does not affect its fatty acid profile.[34,35] To date, there are no studies comparing the psychomotor development of preterm infants fed fresh versus pasteurized milk, but there is no rationale suggesting that it could impact long-term development.

Therefore, from the evidence available, it can be considered that DHM is beneficial for health and development of preterm infants. It is absolutely essential to provide preterm recipients with a safe and high-quality DHM, that is, without pathogens and preserving as much as possible its immunologic and nutritional properties.

MILK BANKS TO DELIVER SAFE AND HIGH-QUALITY DONOR HUMAN MILK

The first HMB opened in Vienna (Austria) in 1909 and soon after in Boston, Massachusetts, in 1910. In Europe, most HMBs opened during the second part of the twentieth century, and there are now 210 banks in 2016 (http://www.europeanmilkbanking.com). After the closing of many HMBs in North America during the 1980s, due to AIDS, they are now reopening, and the number is regularly increasing in North America and worldwide (https://www.hmbana.org/locations).

HMBs are established to recruit and screen breast milk donors, collect, treat (bacteriologic screening, pasteurization, storage), and distribute the donated HM. In most countries, it concerns only DHM, but in some countries, it concerns also MOM, notably when the mother is positive for cytomegalovirus (CMV), when the collection has not been performed in good hygienic conditions, or when the milk has been stored for more than 48 to 96 hours[36–38] (**Fig. 2**). Another role of HMBs is to promote/support breastfeeding in mothers of hospitalized preterm infants and among prospective donors.

HMBs rely on a donor breastfeeding population to ensure adequate supply. Donors are mothers who delivered often at term and give their extra milk for vulnerable hospitalized babies. Sometimes mothers who delivered preterm and produce enough milk to cover the needs of their own baby want to give the milk surplus to the HMB when their baby is discharged to home (**Fig. 3**). The DHM will be given to hospitalized preterm infants under medical prescription. This altruistic act, based on the

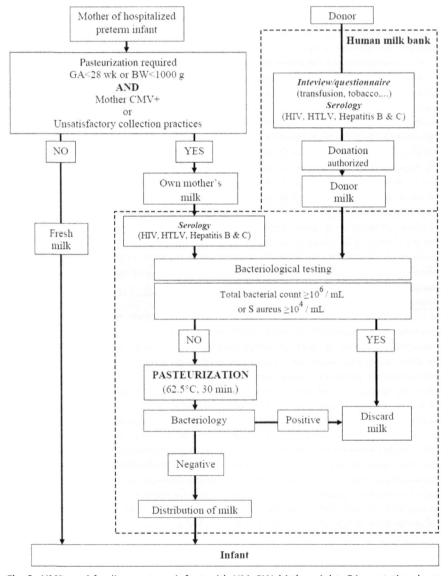

Fig. 2. HMBs and feeding preterm infant with HM. BW, birth weight; GA, gestational age.

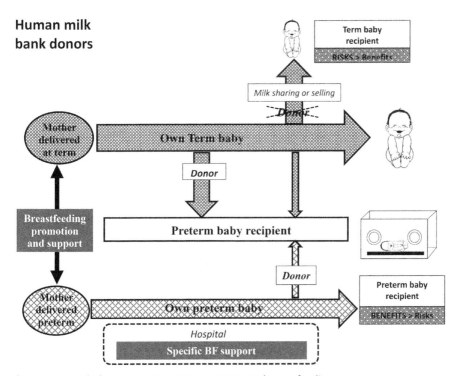

Fig. 3. Preterm baby can receive MOM or DHM. BF, breast feeding.

comprehension of the specific benefits of HM for preterm infants, is completely different from the mothers who give (or sell) their extra milk to another mother who delivered a healthy term baby who cannot get enough milk from his/her mother (see **Fig. 3**). The latter should not be considered "donors," which is applicable only for mothers giving their extra milk to HMBs to help sick babies and therefore have been carefully screened for health problems. Furthermore, some critical issues with bacteriologic safety and cow's milk protein content in such exchanged milk have been recently reported.[39–42]

To provide safe, high-quality DHM, a high-level quality assurance and strict tracking are required in HMBs. As the number of HMBs expands worldwide, universal common core practices are required, but there is not yet enough evidence for each practice, which leaves the field open to a significant heterogeneity.[43] More and more work is being done in each country to elaborate consensus statements based on evidence, otherwise on experience.[38,44–51] It concerns "traditional" milk banks, but other types of milk banks are settled over the world. Some "milk banks" are organized to collect, store, and distribute MOM.[52,53] These milk banks are installed in-hospital and are working only to provide infants hospitalized in the same hospital with MOM. In some countries such as Muslim countries, it may be difficult to build HMBs because of religious and cultural fear about milk kinship, and a model of HMB appropriate for these settings has been proposed.[54] In Brazil, there are more than 200 mother/baby centers for donor milk donation and lactation support. In settings where there is no access to pasteurizers, flash pasteurization has been proposed.[38] However, only the treatment and quality of milk treated in "traditional" milk banks are discussed later because it is the most common model.

To deliver safe and high-quality DHM, care must be taken in the process at all steps: selection of donors, collection, storage, treatment, and distribution. For example, the donors should be well informed to understand their responsibility in avoiding bacteriologic contamination, and therefore, milk discarding in the HMB due to bacteriologic count above the limit.[45,47,51] The present article discusses the treatment of HM. For the other steps, see Ben T. Hartmann's article, "Ensuring Safety in Donor Human Milk Banking in Neonatal Intensive Care," in this issue.

Treatment of HM should inactivate bacteria, viruses, and other potential pathogens while limiting the impact on the milk's protective elements or nutrients, such as proteins, antibodies, enzymes, and vitamins. Furthermore, the method should be usable in the setting of HMBs treating significant amounts of milk each day. To date, the best compromise is represented by Holder pasteurization, but new techniques have been proposed recently and will probably become available in the next years.

TREATMENT OF HUMAN MILK IN MILK BANKS
Low-Temperature Long-Time Pasteurization

The most common practice is a low-temperature (62.5°C) long-time (30 minutes), pasteurization (LTLT) known as "Holder" pasteurization. Pasteurization has long been the standard method to extend the shelf-life of dairy products and to reduce the risk of food-borne pathogens. This technique was first published by Nicolas Appert in 1831, developed by Louis Pasteur in 1865 for the pasteurization of beer, and used by the dairy industry to protect the bovine milk from *Mycobacterium bovis*. The milk was heated in trays that were called "Holders."

As LTLT offers the best compromise between microbiological safety and preservation of some important milk components, most of HMBs worldwide uses this reference technique.[38,44–51]

Impact of LTLT on components useful for nutrition and anti-infectious properties of HM has been extensively evaluated, mostly in experimental conditions.

Effect of low-temperature long-time pasteurization on microorganisms, bactericidal activity, cytokines, immunoglobulins, lactoferrin, and lysozyme

Safe HM from the HMB should not contain pathogens but should also retain antibacterial capacity and preserve immune proteins such as immunoglobulins, lactoferrin, and lysozyme contributing to the protection of the neonate against infection. HM has its own microbiota, which supports the development of gut microbiota in term infants.[55] However, in preterm infants with an immature immune system, it is not acceptable to propose HM-containing pathogens.[56] LTLT kills most pathogenic bacteria found in breast milk.[57] LTLT does not destroy sporulated bacteria such as *Bacillus cereus*, which is pathogenic in immunocompromised patients, including preterm infants.[58,59] It has been shown that *B cereus* spores in raw milk are the major source of *B cereus* in pasteurized milk.[60] Detection of *B cereus* in pasteurized milk justifies postpasteurization testing for any flora and, to the authors' knowledge, no severe infection related to pasteurized milk has been reported, even if suspected.[61] The main source of *B cereus* is usually found in the environment of infected or contaminated preterm infants.[62,63]

As heavily contaminated milk can theoretically contain enterotoxins and thermostable enzymes even after pasteurization, most HMBs test for total viable microbial content and other undesirable microbes such as *Staphylococcus aureus* (± Enterobacteriaceae in some countries) before pasteurization.[64] Milk is discarded when total viable microorganisms are greater than 10^4 colony forming units (CFU)/mL, *S aureus* greater than 10^4 CFU/mL, and Enterobacteriaceae greater than 10^4 CFU/mL (**Table 1**). Most countries recommend also microbiological testing after pasteurization, to monitor for

Table 1

Testing for microbial contamination of human milk before pasteurization in human milk banks according to guidelines published in 5 different countries

France	UK	North America	Italy	South Africa
2008	2010–2012	2013	2008–2010	2011
Testing of *subbatches* (donations from the same donor) and *batches* • In some HM banks, *sub-batches are tested* for total aerobic flora and kept in quarantine (+4°C) while waiting for the results. 　○ Total aerobic flora $\geq 10^6$ CFU/mL? 　　■ Yes → Subbatches are destroyed 　　■ No → Subbatches are grouped in batches and tested for total aerobic flora and *S aureus* before being pasteurized: 　○ If total aerobic flora $\geq 10^6$ CFU/mL or *S aureus* $\geq 10^4$ CFU/mL? 　　■ Yes → discard batches 　　■ No → deliver batches • In some HM banks, *subbatches are not tested*, and then batches undergo the same bacteriologic testing before being packed in bottles and pasteurized. The batches are discarded if total aerobic flora $\geq 10^5$ CFU/mL or *S aureus* $\geq 10^4$ CFU/mL. In all cases, while waiting for the results of testing, the milk is kept at + 4°C for 48 h or pasteurized immediately, frozen, and kept in quarantine until its compliance has been proven.	Test a sample from each batch of pooled donor milk for microbial contamination and discard if samples exceed a count of: • Total viable microorganisms $\geq 10^5$ CFU/mL or • Enterobacteriaceae $\geq 10^4$ CFU/mL or • *S aureus* $\geq 10^4$ CFU/mL	No testing	Testing • At the first donation • When the donor does not seem to guarantee the appropriate hygienic conditions • In any case, periodically in a random manner The milk is discarded if it contains: • Total viable bacteria $> 10^5$ CFU/mL or • Enterobacteriaceae $> 10^4$ CFU/mL or • *S aureus* $> 10^4$ CFU/mL	Testing for microbial contamination should be done on an aliquot of milk from the first donation of each donor mother. If any contamination is found, milk must be discarded and milk from the donor mother must be rechecked with the subsequent donation. For community-based banks, a simpler test which is used by all the Brazilian Breastmilk Banks is known as titratable acidity

contamination introduced after the pasteurization process or pasteurization failure. Safety of donor milk recipients is ensured by discarding milk if any microbial content is found (**Table 2**). There is no consensus on bacteriologic methods, but it is recommended to discard milk with any pathogen as the anti-infective properties of HM are modified by heat treatment. Such prepasteurization and postpasteurization microbiological screening results in approximately 10% to 30% of milk being discarded.[65,66] A strict application of the Hazard Analysis Critical Control Point principles during collection, storage, and pasteurization of donor milk is useful to reduce the amount of milk discarded.

Such microbiological testing of HM ensures bacteriologic safety of the final product delivered to preterm babies. Viral safety is ensured by selecting the donors through an interview and by testing the mothers for pathogenic viruses (HIV, hepatitis B and C, human T-cell leukemia virus type [HTLV]) before accepting that they can donate their milk. This screening is particularly important because LTLT destroys most high-risk viruses such as HIV, CMV, human papillomaviruses, herpes viruses, HTLV, but not hepatitis B virus.[67–72]

LTLT leads to the loss of some biologically active milk components and cells that are crucial for the defense against infections, such as immunoglobulins, leukocytes, secretory immunoglobulin A (IgAs), total IgAs, IgM, IgG, lactoferrin, lysozyme, lymphocytes, and cytokines.[20,73–75]

After LTLT around 40% of IgA is retained.[74–78] However, other studies have presented a higher IgA retention, ranging between 60% and 80%,[68,79–83] and even 100% was reported by some investigators.[83] Summary of main effects of LTLT on milk components is presented in **Table 3**.[84–113] These discrepancies could be explained by several factors, such as the time for reaching exact temperature, the time for cooling, and the volume of HM processed. Indeed, in most experimental studies that evaluated the effect of LTLT, only small aliquots (40 μL to 10 mL) were treated,[21,75,76,113] which is still much lower than the volume of milk usually processed in HMBs (100–250 mL). In such real conditions, higher loss of HM components is expected to occur due to the longer time needed to reach the desired temperature in the center of the container. It is crucial to ensure that the exposition of milk to high temperature is not too prolonged, because it could alter immunologic properties of milk.[80] Different devices are marketed to perform LTLT pasteurization, using water in different conditions, or air. The exposure to high temperature may be prolonged and/or excessive with some devices (Buffin 2016, personal data). Therefore, each pasteurizer should undergo regular quality control performed by each HMB to be sure that the increase in temperature or the temperature plateau is not too prolonged and that cooling is rapid enough. It requires the presence of temperature probes in some of the milk bottles undergoing pasteurization. The number of probes and where they have to be positioned into the pasteurizers are not clearly defined by the manufacturers, and until recently, some manufacturers did not even propose any probe in their device. Based on published data and daily experience of the 36 milk banks over the French territory, the French Human Milk Bank Association recently proposed that much stricter quality control should be done regularly on pasteurizers (**Fig. 4**). It should be noted that most studies evaluating the effect of pasteurization on microbial or immune content in HM used in vitro methodology based on special devices to mimic the pasteurizer, but it is required to perform this type of study in real conditions, using pasteurizers that underwent quality control. When studies were performed using pasteurizers, no study presented any information about the quality control of the device used.

Lactoferrin is bacteriostatic because it inhibits the growth of iron-dependent pathogens by reducing free iron availability, but it is also bactericidal through bactericidal

Table 2

Testing of pasteurized human milk for microbial contamination in human milk banks according to guidelines published in 5 countries

France	United Kingdom	USA & Canada	Italy	South Africa
2008	2010–2012	2013	2008–2010	2011
Systematic testing for any microbial contamination Test: 0.5 mL of undiluted milk on blood agar and incubation 48 h at 37°C. • Any batch with positive testing is destroyed. • A documented analysis is performed in order to find the causes of recurrent contamination. • Milk bottles are placed in quarantine after pasteurization and cooling and while waiting for the results of the testing. • Milk bottles can be either stored at +4°C for no more than 48 hours and frozen at −18°C or frozen immediately at −18°C.	*Regular testing* • At least once a month or every 10 cycles, depending on which comes first, or • On an ad-hoc basis if any new processes, equipment, or staff are introduced, or if there are concerns about any part of the process.	Bottle of milk used for testing should be chosen *randomly* and discarded after use Entire bottle of milk randomly selected from a batch or sample aliquots (100 µL of milk on sheep blood agar plates or plate count agar, results in CFU/100 µL) Any bacteriologic growth is unacceptable for heat-processed milk Aerobic or standard plate <1 CFU/100 µL • Dispense >5 CFU/100 µL • Discard Between 0.5 and 5 CFU/100 µL • "Indeterminate" Test 2 additional bottles from the batch (same procedure) If negative: Dispense If positive: Discard	*Regular testing* • Once a month, or • Every 10 pasteurization cycles, or • When there are concerns about the processing. The milk must be discarded in case of any kind of bacterial growth.	*Systematic testing* for microbial contamination. Test: 1 mL of milk: enumeration of E coli and coliform colonies on Petrifilm EC plates. Test: 100 µL of each sample to be plated onto McConkey agar and incubated for 24 h at 37°C. The following day a semiquantitative count will be performed. Only if required, will any suspicious colonies be further identified. If any contamination is found, milk must be discarded and milk from the donor mother must be rechecked with the subsequent donation.

Table 3
Summary of main effects of low time low temperature ("Holder") pasteurization on milk components

Component	→	↑	↓	∅	Ref.
Proteins					
Total protein content	X	—	—	—	84,85
Protein quality					
Available lysine	—	—	Xa	—	86,87
Free amino acids					
Cystine, taurine, methionine,	X	—	—	—	88,89
Arginine, leucine, glutamine	—	X	—	—	88,89
Aspartate	—	—	X	—	89
Bioactive peptides	X	—	—	—	26
Enzymes					
Amylase	—	—	X	—	68,87,90
Lipase, LPL, alkaline phosphatase	—	—	—	X	90
Immunoglobulins					
IgA, IgAs, IgG, IgM IgG4	—	—	X	—	77,82,91–95
Lactoferrine	—	—	Xa	—	79,80,83,92,93,95
Lyzozyme and lyzozyme activity	—	—	Xa	—	68,74,76,77,80,82,83,92,95,96
Lipids					
Total fat	X	—	—	—	30,34,84,85,90,97
Free fatty acids	—	X	—	—	30
Fatty acids 18:1, 18:3, 12:0, 14:0, 18:0	Xa	—	—	—	34,35,89,90,98–101
Other fatty acids	X	—	—	—	30,98,100,101
Saccharides					
Glucose	Xa	—	—	—	94,102
Lactose, oligosaccharides, GAG	X	—	—	—	84,85,94,97,102–104
Vitamins					
E, B2, B3, B5, B12, Biotin	X	—	—	—	93,105
C, D, B6	—	—	X	—	99,106,107
A, C, α-γ-δ-tocopherols	—	—	Xa	—	35,94,97,100,108
Zinc, Copper, Iron	X	—	—	—	97,109
Growth factors					
EGF, TGF-ß1, TGF-ß2, MCP-1	X	—	—	—	20,94,110
GM-CSF	—	X	—	—	94
EPO, HB-EGF, IGF-1, IGF-BP~2 & ~3	—	—	Xa	—	97,100,108
Hormones					
Leptine	X	—	—	—	79
Insuline, adiponectine	—	—	X	—	111
Cytokines					
IL-2, -4, -5, -12, -13, -17	X	—	—	—	35,94,100
IL-8, -7	—	Xa	—	—	94,100
IL-1ß, -6, -10, TNF-α, INF-γ	—	—	Xa	—	35,94,108

(continued on next page)

Table 3 (continued)					
Component	→	↑	↓	∅	Ref.
Oxidative stress markers					
Malonedialdehyde	X	—	—	—	112
Glutathione, GPA, TAC	—	—	X	—	112
Bactericial activity	—	X	—	—	113
Cells					
Lymphocytes	—	—	X	—	91
Macrophages	—	X	—	—	96
Electrolytes and minerals	X	—	—	—	78
Osmolality	X	—	—	—	78

Abbreviations: →, No/minor change; ↑, increase; ↓, decrease; ∅, Destruction; GAG, glycaminogly-cans; GPA, glutathione peroxidase activity; LPL, lipoprotein lipase; TAC, total antioxidant capacity; TNF, tumor necrosis factor.
 [a] Discordant results; requires further studies.

peptides resulting from the digestion of lactoferrin. There are some discrepancies in the results of studies that evaluated the effect of LTLT on lactoferrin. Depending on the study and the technique used for measurement of lactoferrin concentration, it was shown that about 10% to 65% of lactoferrin is retained after

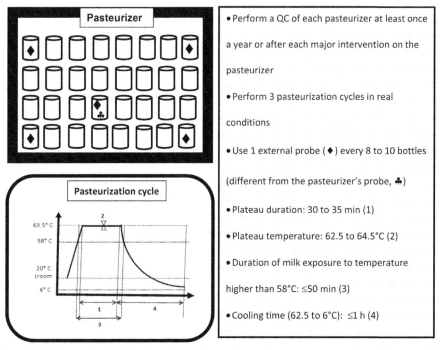

Fig. 4. Quality control (QC) parameters to be performed on each pasteurizer device used in HMB according to the French Human Milk Bank Association.

LTLT.[79,80,83,92,93,95] Therefore, there are still unanswered questions about lactoferrin, but it seems that some lactoferrin remains after LTLT, and part of the activity could be retained in pasteurized HM despite reduction of its concentration (see **Table 1**).

Lysozyme has a very stable structure maintained by disulfide bonds and is therefore highly resistant to technological treatments. Most studies report that lysozyme activity is maintained after LTLT, but the proportion of lysozyme retained is quite variable (15%–80%).[68,76,77,79,80,82,83,92,114] Similar discrepancies were reported in regard to lysozyme activity[77,92] (see **Table 1**).

HM possesses bactericidal capacity that is reduced after thermal processing. Bactericidal capacity (against *Escherichia coli*) is preserved after LTLT pasteurization, but is less than in untreated milk. *E coli* growth is reduced 52% versus 70% in untreated milk.[113] Bactericidal capacity is, moreover, better preserved by LTLT than when using higher heating temperatures[113] (see **Table 1**).

Most cytokines in HM are anti-inflammatory and theoretically could help preterm infants presenting with infections. After LTLT, most cytokines are unaffected; some increase, and few decrease[35,94,100–108] (see **Table 1**). Clinical relevance of such a cytokine profile is unknown.

Effect on nutrients (protein, lipids, carbohydrates, vitamins), enzymes (lipase), antioxidant capacity, growth factors, and antioxidant capacity

Protein and energy (total fat, and lactose) are preserved or slightly reduced after LTLT. Oligosaccharides, vitamins A and E, lactose, long chain polyunsaturated fatty acids and epidermal growth factor are preserved by LTLT.[20,73,90,103,105,112] Recently, Gomes and colleagues[106] reported a small (10%–20%) reduction of the concentration of some vitamin D compounds after LTLT. After LTLT, there is a significant decrease in the concentrations of ascorbic acid plus dehydroascorbic acid, ascorbic acid, α-tocopherol, and γ-tocopherol.[99,107] Iron, copper, and zinc are slightly reduced by LTLT, but the concentration remains within the acceptable range required to cover the specific nutritional needs of newborn infants fed pasteurized HM[109] (see **Table 1**).

LTLT leads to the loss of lipase, alkaline phosphatase, and some growth factors.[20,73,112]

Milk fatty acids, including polyunsaturated long-chain fatty acids, are unaffected by LTLT, but completely inactivate the enzyme lipase.[90] BSSL is required for fat absorption by the small intestine. As the infant can synthetize and secrete small quantities of BSSL, the BSSL present in HM acts to supplement this deficiency. BSSL is inactivated at relatively low temperatures (45–55°C).[98] BSSL activity is completely lost after Holder pasteurization[87,115] (see **Table 1**).

LTLT has no effect on total protein content of HM, but could have an effect on protein quality, as reflected by a significant (−29%) decrease in available lysine content after HTST when compared with fresh milk.[86] In an additional study using a different technique to apply HTST, this finding was not confirmed.[87] Thus, further studies are requested. However, it has been shown that LTLT pasteurization does not affect protein digestibility because the profile of bioactive peptides released from HM proteins by gastrointestinal digestion was preserved after pasteurization[26] (see **Table 1**).

Antioxidants are present in HM[116,117] and are part of the natural defense system against the action of free radicals, which are related to necrotizing enterocolitis, retinopathy of prematurity, bronchopulmonary dysplasia, and other complications of prematurity. The total antioxidant capacity of HM is decreased after LTLT pasteurization due to the decrease in some components like glutathione[112] of HM implies a decrease in total antioxidant capacity of HM (see **Table 1**).

Other Techniques to Pasteurize Human Milk

New techniques consist of a thermal (high-temperature short-time pasteurization [HTST] and thermoultrasonic pasteurization), or nonthermal (high-pressure processing [HPP] and UV irradiation) pasteurization.

Higher-temperature short-time pasteurization

HTST may be more effective at retaining milk properties. The most frequently evaluated is HTST using a temperature of 72°C for 15 seconds,[68,86,87,93,113] but different temperatures (62–82°C) for different times (1–19 seconds) have been tested on HM.[20,118–120] Different experimental systems were used to obtain HTST[68,93,118,119] but have never been tested in HMB conditions, as there is not yet a marketed device.

Effect of higher-temperature short-time pasteurization on microorganisms, bactericidal activity, cytokines, immunoglobulins, lactoferrin, and lysozyme HTST is efficient to eradicate bacteria (E coli, S aureus, Staphylococcus agalactiae, coliforms, and total viable count), CMV, and enveloped viruses (HIV, hepatitis B and C).[68,118–120] Nonenveloped viruses, such as hepatitis A are not eradicated by HTST.[120]

In experimental conditions, the concentration of lactoferrin is significantly reduced following HTST,[76,87,93] but the proportion of lactoferrin retained is still twice higher (52% after 600 MPa for 15 minutes) than after LTLT pasteurization (20%).[76]

After HTST, around 40% IgA is retained, as reported after LTLT pasteurization.[76] Similar retention for IgG, but total destruction of IgM, was reported.[93,119]

The residual enzymatic activity of lysozyme is higher or maintained when compared with untreated HM.[76,118] One study using different HTST technique reported a decrease in lysozyme.[68]

HTST was reported to have no effect on HM cytokines.[20]

Bactericidal capacity of HM (against E coli) is preserved after HTST, but is less than in untreated milk and in milk treated by LTLT. E coli growth is reduced by 36% after HTST versus 70% in untreated milk.[113]

Effect on nutrients (protein, lipids, carbohydrates, vitamins), enzymes (lipase), antioxidant capacity, growth factors, and antioxidant capacity Similar to LTLT pasteurization, the HTST technique was first shown to inactivate the BSSL,[118] but a recent study suggests that the integrity of the BSSL and its activity are preserved after HTST.[87]

HTST was reported to have no effect on total protein, folic acid, vitamin B12, and vitamin C.[63,86,118] Some investigators reported an effect on protein quality as reflected by a significant, but modest (−14%), decrease in available lysine content after HTST when compared with fresh milk.[86]

HTST, like LTLT, reduces significantly the amount of alkaline phosphatase and lipase in HM.[63]

Total antioxidant capacity of HM is preserved after HTST.[112]

In summary, experimental data suggest that HTST is efficient to destroy most microorganisms, as LTLT, but is better at preserving biological quality of HM. It should be confirmed in HMB conditions.

High-pressure processing

HPP has been used to inactivate pathogenic microorganisms in solid and liquid foods.[121–123] This technology applies high hydrostatic high pressure (usually 400–800 MPa) for a short time. Changes in the chemical composition, color, and aroma related to pressurization are less than those caused by a heat treatment.[122] Different levels of pressure (200–900 MPa), during different times (1–120 minutes), were tested on HM.[35,75,77,81,82,107,119,124,125]

Effect of high-pressure processing on microorganisms, bactericidal activity, cytokines, immunoglobulins, lactoferrin, and lysozyme The effect of HPP depends on the type of bacteria. Gram-positive microorganisms are more resistant to pressure than gram-negative ones, but pressure resistance varies also within strains of the same species. The pressure required to achieve inactivation of gram-positive microorganisms (500–600 MPa) is higher than for gram-negative microorganisms (300–400 MPa). Vegetative forms of yeasts and molds are the most pressure sensitive.[126] Many studies on the inactivation of microorganisms by HPP have been performed in milk during the last few years and have generally demonstrated that it is possible to obtain milk with a microbiological quality comparable to that of milk pasteurized at 72°C for 15 seconds, depending on the microbiological quality of the milk,[127] but not comparable to sterilized milk due to HPP-resistant spores. The inactivation of bacterial spores using HPP conditions is very difficult.[128]

Not all the results obtained using this new technology are presently available because of pending patenting process, but preliminary data suggest that HPP, performed in specific conditions, could destroy vegetative flora, S aureus, bacterial spores, and viruses together with a much better preservation of lactoferrin, lysozyme, and lipase than after LTLT.[129]

Because there is a high level of structural diversity among viruses, the effect of pressure is variable.[126] Complete inactivation of hepatitis A virus can be achieved by treatment at 275 to 450 MPa for 5 minutes.[130] As pressure at 300 MPa damages the virus envelope and prevents the virus particles from binding to the cells, it has been suggested that HPP could inactivate Herpes simplex virus-1, CMV, and other enveloped viruses.[131–133] HPP inactivates HIV.[134]

There are very few studies published on the efficacy of HPP processing on HM, and the first report about HPP ability to inactivate 5 selected bacterial pathogens in HM is quite recent.[135] The efficacy on bacteria seems to be variable depending on pressure applied and duration of exposure to high pressures. The efficacy of HPP is great on Listeria monocytogenes, Enterobacteriaceae, and total viable count that are eradicated, but is less for E coli and S aureus.[81,135]

The effect of processing on the immune cells (leukocyte content) and immunoglobulins content (IgM, IgA, and IgG) was evaluated.[75] HPP (400 MPa for 3 or 6 minutes) maintained the original levels of immunoglobulins and preserves leukocytes of HM better than LTLT.[75] Only the treatment less than 300 MPa maintains certain levels of immunoglobulins (75% of IgM, 48% of IgA, 100% of IgG).[125]

In experimental conditions, after the application of pressures between 300 and 650 MPa for 30 minutes, 36% to 80% of IgA is retained, whereas it is 40% after LTLT.[76,77] In similar conditions, lysozyme activity increased by 20% to 40%, which is approximately the same as after LTLT pasteurization.[76,81] After the application of pressures between 300, 400, 500, and 600 MPa for 15 minutes, 91%, 77%, 66%, and 52% of lactoferrin was retained, whereas it was 20% after LTLT.[136]

HHP induces a minimal effect on the level of interleukin-12 (IL-12), IL-17, and interferon-γ (IFN-γ), but leukocytes are very sensitive to HHP.[125]

Effect on nutrients (protein, lipids, carbohydrates, vitamins), enzymes (lipase), antioxidant capacity, growth factors, and antioxidant capacity HPP influences the physicochemical properties of milk. It has significant effect on protein quality. HPP denatures whey proteins, affects the activity of native milk enzymes, and produces changes in casein micelles, with the subsequent solubilization of colloidal calcium phosphate.[137,138] In milk subjected to HPP, the casein micelles are disintegrated into smaller particles, which are accompanied by an increase of caseins and calcium phosphate levels in the serum phase of milk.[139] After pressure treatment up to 500 MPa at 25°C, β-lactoglobulin is the most easily denatured serum protein, and denaturation of the immunoglobulins occurs at the highest pressures and particularly at 50°C. Greater than 300 MPa, there is a significant impact on the structure of β-lactoglobulin.[140]

There are discrepancies about the effect on fatty acids. Moltó-Puigmartí and colleagues[107] reported no effect of high pressures (400–600 MPa), but another study reported that the content of fatty acids is affected by the highest pressure values (600 and 900 MPa).[125]

No changes in lactose were observed after pressurization (100–400 MPa for 10–60 minutes at 25°C), suggesting that no Maillard reaction or lactose isomerization occurs in milk after pressure treatment.[141]

Vitamin C and tocopherol are retained after HPP, contrary to LTLT pasteurization.[107]

In summary, experimental data suggest that HPP is efficient to destroy most microorganisms, as LTLT, but could be better at preserving biological quality of HM. It should be confirmed in HMB conditions.

Ultraviolet irradiation

UV irradiation, specifically UV-C, destroys microorganisms, such as bacteria, viruses, and yeasts, but its penetration capacity is low, which limits its use to liquid foods and flat surfaces.[142,143] Data are mostly experimental, but it has never been used in HMB to pasteurize large amounts of milk. Ultrasound processing or sonication is one of the alternative technologies that have been proposed for food processing with a reduced impact on nutritional content and overall food quality. Sonication alone is not very effective in killing bacteria in food and has been coupled with mild heating (thermo-ultrasonication).[144] A 2- to 8-minute treatment at 50°C of artificially contaminated HM inactivates bacteria such as E coli and Staphylococcus epidermidis, with a retention of secretory IgA, lysozyme, lactoferrin, and BSS: of 91%, 80%, 77%, and 45%, respectively,[144] which is lower than the approximately 20% retention for observed secretory IgA, lysozyme, lactoferrin, and 0% for BSSL, after Holder pasteurization. It also inactivates CMV.[145]

For the ultrasound processing and UV irradiation, data are mostly experimental, and the feasibility of routine use in an HMB has yet to be demonstrated. Although LTLT pasteurization is the reference method, both HPP and HTST are promising as devices that could be usable in the near future in the setting of HMB.[82,129,146]

Pasteurization method used depends on organization and financial resources. Some simple, low-cost techniques such as flash-heat pasteurization have been proposed in resource-limited settings.[147–150] The Human Milk Banking Association of South Africa recommends that, where there is no access to pasteurizers, milk can be pasteurized using the following method: Up to 120 mL of milk should be expressed into a clean 450- to 500-mL glass jar, placed in a 1-L aluminum Hart pot and cold water added sufficient to cover the level of milk by 2 finger widths. The pot containing water and jar should be placed in the middle of the heat source. After water reaches a rolling boil, the jar with the breast milk should be removed and allowed to cool. Flash heat should preferably be performed as soon after expression as possible, and then HM can be stored for 8 hours at room temperature.[38]

OTHERS POINTS RELATED TO THE QUALITY OF DONOR HUMAN MILK
Absence of Cow's Milk Protein in Banked Milk

Some HMBs test for the presence of cow's milk protein, because it happens that mothers add cow's milk to their own milk. However, there is a lack of a simple, low-cost, and efficient test. Furthermore, it seems to be particularly relevant outside the setting of HMBs, when mothers get money by selling their milk, but the issue of HM purchased via Internet is completely different from milk donation.[151] In most countries, donors are not paid or receive small financial compensation,[47,50] so that there is no real temptation to add cow's milk to their milk. As the test was used in France between 1999 and 2009, French HMBs Association performed a survey and was able to estimate that about 99,500 tests were performed in 17 HMBs during this period of time and less than 10 tests were positive (personal data). These cases were related to maternal psychiatric troubles, and the amount of cow's milk was so important that professionals working in the HMB easily detected the unusual white aspect of milk when compared with HM. Furthermore, preterm infants receive significant amounts of cow's milk protein because cow's milk–based fortifiers are widely used and well tolerated in most preterm infants. Some studies have suggested that HM-based fortifiers could help to improve digestive tolerance and reduce the risk of necrotizing enterocolitis, but these products are not widely available and are still very expensive. Furthermore, their efficacy is still to be demonstrated in settings where the basal risk of necrotizing enterocolitis is low (3%–5%).[151,152] However, the detection of cow's milk protein in DHM does not seem to be relevant anymore in HMBs.

Labeling Nutritional Content of Banked Milk

Assessing macronutrient content of DHM can be useful because HM composition is variable (see Francis B. Mimouni and colleagues' article, "Preterm Human Milk Macronutrient and Energy Composition: A Systematic Review and Meta-Analysis," in this issue), and not to assess the effect of pasteurization on nutrients' content of HM because it is very limited (see earlier discussion). The effect of pasteurization is much lesser than the effect of the mode of feeding (continuous, bolus), which may have a huge effect on fat content of HM. Fat losses have been reported to be as high as 50%.[84] Therefore, it is crucial that the staff supports suckling and breastfeeding in preterm infants. The earlier these babies will suck efficiently from breast, the earlier the feeding tube and syringes will be removed, which is crucial to avoid fat losses. Bedside assessment of milk composition has been proposed because of the great variability of HM protein and energy contents (see **Fig. 1**), because bedside techniques became available (see Gerhard Fusch and colleagues' article, ""Bed Side" Human Milk Analysis in the Neonatal Intensive Care Unit: A Systematic Review," in this issue), and because products such as specifically designed protein supplement became available to perform a targeted fortification of HM (see Francis B. Mimouni and colleagues' article, "The Use of Multinutrient Human Milk Fortifiers in Preterm Infants: A Systematic Review of Unanswered Questions," in this issue). In some facilities, milk is tested for nutritional content every 2 weeks, each day, or even more to perform individualized targeted fortification.[50,153] In most places it is not done yet due to a lack of resources (staff and reliable analyzers) and because there is no strong evidence, even if there are some indications from pilot studies that it could help.[153] However, as the DHM is a mature milk often collected after a few weeks of lactation, its variability is much less that the variability in protein and lipid content in milk from mothers who delivered preterm (see **Fig. 1**). There is a consensus to use individualized fortification, but no consensus on the way to do it: targeted or adjustable. The latest does not require prior milk analysis because it is based on the evaluation of individual protein status through measurement of serum urea.[154,155] However, assessment of milk composition in HMBs could be useful to propose a DHM labeled with information about its protein and energy contents.

SUMMARY

HMBs are essential for providing safe donor milk to vulnerable infants, such as very low-birth-weight infants. The collection, treatment, and distribution of donor milk require technical processes that are still differing depending on locations, organization, and resources. Universal core requirements and quality principles for all HMBs are required. These requirements are often based on consensus between health professionals in each country. Further research is needed to help build universally accepted recommendations.

REFERENCES

1. Rønnestad A, Abrahamsen TG, Medbo S, et al. Late-onset septicemia in a Norwegian national cohort of extremely premature infants receiving very early full human milk feeding. Pediatrics 2005;115:e269–76.
2. Vohr BR, Poindexter BB, Dusick AM, et al, National Institute of Child Health and Human Development National Research Network. Persistent beneficial effects of breast milk ingested in the neonatal intensive care unit on outcomes of extremely low birth weight infants at 30 months of age. Pediatrics 2007;120: e953–9.
3. Meinzen-Derr J, Poindexter B, Wrage L, et al. Role of human milk in extremely low birth weight infants' risk of necrotizing enterocolitis or death. J Perinatol 2009;29:57–62.
4. Manzoni P, Stolfi I, Pedicino R, et al, Italian Task Force for the Study and Prevention of Neonatal Fungal Infections, Italian Society of Neonatology. Human milk feeding prevents retinopathy of prematurity (ROP) in preterm VLBW neonates. Early Hum Dev 2013;89:S64–8.
5. Quigley M, McGuire W. Formula versus donor breast milk for feeding preterm or low birth weight infants. Cochrane Database Syst Rev 2014;(4):CD002971.
6. Zhou J, Shukla VV, John D, et al. Human milk feeding as a protective factor for retinopathy of prematurity: a meta-analysis. Pediatrics 2015;136:e1576–86.
7. Horta BL, Victora CG, World Health Organization. Long-term effects of breastfeeding: a systematic review. Geneva (Switzerland): WHO Library; 2013.
8. Underwood MA. Missed opportunities: the cost of suboptimal breast milk feeding in the neonatal intensive care unit. J Pediatr 2016;175:12–4.
9. Section on Breastfeeding. Breastfeeding and the use of human milk. Pediatrics 2012;129:e827–41.
10. Arslanoglu S, Corpeleijn W, Moro G, et al, ESPGHAN Committee on Nutrition. Donor human milk for preterm infants: current evidence and research directions. J Pediatr Gastroenterol Nutr 2013;57:535–42.
11. Agostoni C, Buonocore G, Carnielli VP, et al, ESPGHAN Committee on Nutrition. Enteral nutrient supply for preterm infants: commentary from the European Society of Paediatric Gastroenterology, Hepatology and Nutrition Committee on Nutrition. J Pediatr Gastroenterol Nutr 2010;50:85–91.
12. Arslanoglu S, Moro GE, Bellù R, et al. Presence of human milk bank is associated with elevated rate of exclusive breastfeeding in VLBW infants. J Perinat Med 2013;41:129–31.
13. Utrera Torres MI, Medina López C, Vázquez Román S, et al. Does opening a milk bank in a neonatal unit change infant feeding practices? A before and after study. Int Breastfeed J 2010;5:4.
14. Marinelli KA, Lussier MM, Brownell E, et al. The effect of a donor milk policy on the diet of very low birth weight infants. J Hum Lact 2014;30:310–6.

15. Perrella SL, Hepworth AR, Simmer KN, et al. Influences of breast milk composition on gastric emptying in preterm infants. J Pediatr Gastroenterol Nutr 2015; 60:264–71.
16. Cossey V, Vanhole C, Eerdekens A, et al. Pasteurization of mother's own milk for preterm infants does not reduce the incidence of late-onset sepsis. Neonatology 2013;103:170–6.
17. Schanler RJ, Lau C, Hurst NM, et al. Randomized trial of donor human milk versus preterm formula as substitutes for mothers' own milk in the feeding of extremely premature infants. Pediatrics 2005;116:400–6.
18. Rowland KJ, Choi PM, Warner BW. The role of growth factors in intestinal regeneration and repair in necrotizing enterocolitis. Semin Pediatr Surg 2013;22: 101–11.
19. Choi YY. Necrotizing enterocolitis in newborns: update in pathophysiology and newly emerging therapeutic strategies. Korean J Pediatr 2014;57:505–13.
20. Goelz R, Hihn E, Hamprecht K, et al. Effects of different CMV-heat-inactivation methods on growth factors in human breast milk. Pediatr Res 2009;65:458–61.
21. Groer M, Duffy A, Morse S, et al. Cytokines, chemokines, and growth factors in banked human donor milk for preterm infants. J Hum Lact 2014;30:317–23.
22. Van Gysel M, Cossey V, Fieuws S, et al. Impact of pasteurization on the antibacterial properties of human milk. Eur J Pediatr 2012;171:1231–7.
23. Narayanan I, Prakash K, Murthy NS, et al. Randomised controlled trial of effect of raw and Holder pasteurised human milk and of formula supplements on incidence of neonatal infection. Lancet 1984;2(8412):1111–3.
24. Giuliani F, Prandi G, Coscia A, et al. Donor human milk versus mother's own milk in preterm VLBWIs: a case control study. J Biol Regul Homeost Agents 2012;26: 19–24.
25. Stock K, Griesmaier E, Brunner B, et al. Pasteurization of breastmilk decreases the rate of postnatally acquired cytomegalovirus infections, but shows a non-significant trend to an increased rate of necrotizing enterocolitis in very preterm infants—a preliminary study. Breastfeed Med 2015;10:113–7.
26. Wada Y, Lönnerdal B. Bioactive peptides released from in vitro digestion of human milk with or without pasteurization. Pediatr Res 2015;77:546–53.
27. Peila C, Moro GE, Bertino E, et al. The effect of Holder pasteurization on nutrients and biologically-active components in donor human milk: a review. Nutrients 2016;8:477.
28. Andersson Y, Sävman K, Bläckberg L, et al. Pasteurization of mother's own milk reduces fat absorption and growth in preterm infants. Acta Paediatr 2007;96: 1445–9.
29. Montjaux-Régis N, Cristini C, Arnaud C, et al. Improved growth of preterm infants receiving mother's own raw milk compared with pasteurized donor milk. Acta Paediatr 2011;100:1548–54.
30. Lepri L, Del Bubba M, Maggini R, et al. Effect of pasteurization and storage on some components of pooled human milk. J Chromatogr B Biomed Sci Appl 1997;704:1–10.
31. Bauer J, Gerss J. Longitudinal analysis of macronutrients and minerals in human milk produced by mothers of preterm infants. Clin Nutr 2011;30:215–20.
32. Gibertoni D, Corvaglia L, Vandini S, et al. Positive effect of human milk feeding during NICU hospitalization on 24 month neurodevelopment of very low birth weight infants: an Italian cohort study. PLoS One 2015;10:e0116552.
33. Rozé JC, Darmaun D, Boquien CY, et al. The apparent breastfeeding paradox in very preterm infants: relationship between breast feeding, early weight gain and

neurodevelopment based on results from two cohorts, EPIPAGE and LIFT. BMJ Open 2012;2:e000834.

34. Fidler N, Sauerwald TU, Demmelmair H, et al. Fat content and fatty acid composition of fresh, pasteurized, or sterilized human milk. Adv Exp Med Biol 2001; 501:485–95.

35. Delgado FJ, Cava R, Delgado J, et al. Tocopherols, fatty acids and cytokines content of Holder pasteurized and high-pressure processed human milk. Dairy Sci Technol 2014;94:145–56.

36. Deutsch J, Haiden N, Hauer A, et al. Prävention von CMV-Infektionen bei Frühgeborenen durch Muttermilch. Monatsschr Kinderheilkd 2009;157:795–7.

37. ANSES - French Agency for Food, Environmental and Occupational Health & Safety. Hygiene recommendations for the preparation, handling and storage of feeding bottles. In AFSSA proceedings. 2005. Available at: http://nosobase. chu-lyon.fr/recommandations/afssa/2005_alimentation_AFSSA.pdf. Accessed December 7, 2016.

38. Human Milk Banking Association of South Africa. Guidelines for the Operation of a Donor Human Milk Bank in South Africa: best practice for the collection, storage and handling of human milk. 2011. Available at: http://www.hmbasa.org.za. Accessed August 31, 2016.

39. Keim SA, Hogan JS, McNamara KA, et al. Microbial contamination of human milk purchased via the Internet. Pediatrics 2013;132:e1227–35.

40. Nakamura K, Kaneko M, Abe Y, et al. Outbreak of extended-spectrum β-lactamase-producing Escherichia coli transmitted through breast milk sharing in a neonatal intensive care unit. J Hosp Infect 2016;92:42–6.

41. Picaud JC, Jarreau PH. For the French human milk bank association and the French Society of Neonatology. 2011. Could Facebook seriously impair the health of newborns? Available at: http://sdp.perinat-france.org/ADLF/risques-lies-a-l-echange-de-lait.php. Accessed August 31, 2016.

42. European Milk Bank Association. Milk sharing. A statement from the European Milk Bank Association (EMBA) and the Human Milk Banking Association of North America (HMBANA). 2015. Available at: http://europeanmilkbanking. com/joint-emba-and-hmbana-statement-on-milk-sharing-has-been-released/. Accessed December 7, 2016.

43. PATH. Strengthening human milk banking: a global implementation framework. Version 1.1. Seattle (WA): Bill & Melinda Gates Foundation Grand Challenges Initiative, PATH; 2013. Available at: https://www.path.org/publications/files/ MCHN_strengthen_hmb_frame_Jan2016.pdf.

44. Hartmann BT, Pang WW, Keil AD, et al. Australian Neonatal Clinical Care Unit. Best practice guidelines for the operation of a donor human milk bank in an Australian NICU. Early Hum Dev 2007;83:667–73.

45. French Human Milk Bank Association. The good practice rules for the collection, preparation, qualification, treatment, storage, distribution and dispensing on medical prescription of human milk by the milk banks. Available at: http://sdp. perinat-france.org/ADLF/files/lactarium_ guide_ bonnes_pratiques_5_janvier_ 2008_traduction_anglais.pdf. Accessed August 31, 2016.

46. Grøvslien AH, Grønn M. Donor milk banking and breastfeeding in Norway. J Hum Lact 2009;25:206–10.

47. National Institute for Health and Clinical Excellence. Donor breast milk banks: the operation of donor milk bank services. 2010. Available at: https://www. nice.org.uk/guidance/cg93/evidence/cg93-donor-breast-milk-banks-full-guideline3. Accessed August 31, 2016.

48. Arslanoglu S, Bertino E, Tonetto P, et al. Guidelines for the establishment and operation of a donor human milk bank. J Matern Fetal Neonatal Med 2010; 23:1–20.

49. Frischknecht K, Wälchli C, Annen C, et al. Recommandations pour l'organisation et le fonctionnement d'une banque de lait en Suisse. Paediatrica 2010;21:24–8.

50. Milknet. Guidelines for use of human milk and milk handling in Sweden 2011. Available at: http://neoforeningen.se/dokument/vardprogram/Milknet_english_ 2011.pdf. Accessed August 31, 2016.

51. Human Milk Bank Association of North America. Guidelines for the establishment and operation of a donor Human Milk Bank 2013. Available at: https:// www.hmbana.org/publications. Accessed August 31, 2016.

52. Hurst NM, Myatt A, Schanler RJ. Growth and development of a hospital-based lactation program and mother's own milk bank. J Obstet Gynecol Neonatal Nurs 1998;27:503–10.

53. Mizuno K, Sakurai M, Itabashi K. Necessity of human milk banking in Japan: questionnaire survey of neonatologists. Pediatr Int 2015;57:639–44.

54. Khalil A, Buffin R, Sanlaville D, et al. Milk kinship is not an obstacle to using donor human milk to feed preterm infants in Muslim countries. Acta Paediatr 2016;105:462–7.

55. Jeurink PV, van Bergenhenegouwen J, Jiménez E, et al. Human milk: a source of more life than we imagine. Benef Microbes 2013;4:17–30.

56. Tissières P, Ochoda A, Dunn-Siegrist I, et al. Innate immune deficiency of extremely premature neonates can be reversed by interferon-γ. PLoS One 2012;7:e32863.

57. Wills ME, Han VE, Harris DA, et al. Short-time low-temperature pasteurization of human milk. Early Hum Dev 1982;7:71–80.

58. Aires GS, Walter EH, Junqueira VC, et al. Bacillus cereus in refrigerated milk submitted to different heat treatments. J Food Prot 2009;72:1301–5.

59. Tuladhar R, Patole SK, Koh TH, et al. Refractory Bacillus cereus infection in a neonate. Int J Clin Pract 2000;54:345–7.

60. Lin S, Schraft H, Odumeru JA, et al. Identification of contamination sources of Bacillus cereus in pasteurized milk. Int J Food Microbiol 1998;43:159–71.

61. Decousser JW, Ramarao N, Duport C, et al. Bacillus cereus and severe intestinal infections in preterm neonates: putative role of pooled breast milk. Am J Infect Control 2013;41:918–21.

62. Balm MN, Jureen R, Teo C, et al. Hot and steamy: outbreak of Bacillus cereus in Singapore associated with construction work and laundry practices. J Hosp Infect 2012;81:224–30.

63. Hosein IK, Hoffman PN, Ellam S, et al. Summertime Bacillus cereus colonization of hospital newborns traced to contaminated, laundered linen. J Hosp Infect 2013;85:149–54.

64. Pardou A, Serruys E, Mascart-Lemone F. Human milk banking: influence of storage processes and of bacterial contamination on some milk constituents. Biol Neonate 1994;65:302–9.

65. Simmer K, Hartmann B. The knowns and unknowns of human milk banking. Early Hum Dev 2009;85:701–4.

66. Dewitte C, Courdent P, Charlet C, et al. Contamination of human milk with aerobic flora: evaluation of losses for a human milk bank. Arch Pediatr 2015;22: 461–7 [in French].

67. Orloff SL, Wallingford JC, McDougal JS. Inactivation of human immunodeficiency virus type I in human milk: effects of intrinsic factors in human milk and of pasteurization. J Hum Lact 1993;9:13–7.
68. Hamprecht K, Maschmann J, Müller D, et al. Cytomegalovirus (CMV) inactivation in breast milk: reassessment of pasteurization and freeze-thawing. Pediatr Res 2004;56:529–35.
69. Donalisio M, Cagno V, Vallino M, et al. Inactivation of high-risk human papillomaviruses by Holder pasteurization: implications for donor human milk banking. J Perinat Med 2014;42:1–8.
70. Bona C, Dewals B, Wiggers L, et al. Short communication: pasteurization of milk abolishes bovine herpes virus infectivity. J Dairy Sci 2005;88:3079–83.
71. Yamato K, Taguchi H, Yoshimoto S, et al. Inactivation of lymphocyte-transforming activity of human T-cell leukemia virus type 1 by heat. Jpn J Cancer Res 1986;77:13–5.
72. de Oliveira PR, Yamamoto AY, de Souza CB, et al. Hepatitis B viral markers in banked human milk before and after Holder pasteurization. J Clin Virol 2009;45:281–4.
73. Tully DB, Jones F, Tully MR. Donor milk: what's in it and what's not. J Hum Lact 2001;17:152–5.
74. Koenig A, de Albuquerque Diniz EM, Barbosa SF, et al. Immunologic factors in human milk: the effects of gestational age and pasteurization. J Hum Lact 2005;21:439–43.
75. Contador R, Delgado-Adámez J, Delgado FJ, et al. Effect of thermal pasteurization or high pressure processing on immunoglobulin and leukocyte contents of human milk. Int Dairy J 2013;32:1–5.
76. Mayayo C, Montserrat M, Ramos SJ, et al. Effect of high pressure and heat treatments on IgA immunoreactivity and lysozyme activity in human milk. Eur Food Res Technol 2016;242:891–8.
77. Viazis S, Farkas BE, Allen JC. Effects of high-pressure processing on immunoglobulin A and lysozyme activity in human milk. J Hum Lact 2007;23:253–61.
78. Braga LP, Palhares DB. Effect of evaporation and pasteurization in the biochemical and immunological composition of human milk. J Pediatr (Rio J) 2007;83:59–63.
79. Chang JC, Chen CH, Fang LJ, et al. Influence of prolonged storage process, pasteurization, and heat treatment on biologically-active human milk proteins. Pediatr Neonatol 2013;54:360–6.
80. Czank C, Prime DK, Hartmann B, et al. Retention of the immunological proteins of pasteurized human milk in relation to pasteurizer design and practice. Pediatr Res 2009;66:374–9.
81. Permanyer M, Castellote C, Ramírez-Santana C, et al. Maintenance of breast milk immunoglobulin A after high-pressure processing. J Dairy Sci 2010;93:877–83.
82. Sousa SG, Delgadillo I, Saraiva JA. Effect of thermal pasteurization and high-pressure processing on immunoglobulin content and lysozyme and lactoperoxidase activity in human colostrum. Food Chem 2014;151:79–85.
83. Evans TJ, Ryley HC, Neale LM, et al. Effect of storage and heat on antimicrobial proteins in human milk. Arch Dis Child 1978;53:239–41.
84. Vieira AA, Soares FV, Pimenta HP, et al. Analysis of the influence of pasteurization, freezing/thawing, and offer processes on human milk's macronutrient concentrations. Early Hum Dev 2011;87:577–80.

85. García-Lara NR, Vieco DE, De la Cruz-Bértolo J, et al. Effect of Holder pasteurization and frozen storage on macronutrients and energy content of breast milk. J Pediatr Gastroenterol Nutr 2013;57:377–82.

86. Silvestre D, Ferrer E, Gaya J, et al. Available lysine content in human milk: stability during manipulation prior to ingestion. Biofactors 2006;26:71–9.

87. Baro C, Giribaldi M, Arslanoglu S, et al. Effect of two pasteurization methods on the protein content of human milk. Front Biosci (Elite Ed) 2011;3:818–29.

88. Carratu B, Ambruzzi AM, Fedele E, et al. Human Milk Banking: influence of different pasteurization temperatures on levels of protein sulphur amino acids and some free amino acids. J Food Sci 2005;70:c373–5.

89. Valentine CJ, Morrow BS, Fernandez S, et al. Docosahexaenoic acid and amino acid contents in pasteurized donor milk are low for preterm infants. J Pediatr 2010;157:906–10.

90. Henderson TR, Fay TN, Hamosh M. Effect of pasteurization on long chain polyunsaturated fatty acid levels and enzyme activities of human milk. J Pediatr 1998;132:876–8.

91. Liebhaber M, Lewiston NJ, Asquith MT, et al. Alterations of lymphocytes and of antibody content of human milk after processing. J Pediatr 1977;91:897–900.

92. Ford JE, Law BA, Marshall VM, et al. Influence of the heat treatment of human milk on some of its protective constituents. J Pediatr 1977;90:29–35.

93. Goldsmith SJ, Dickson JS, Barnhart HM, et al. IgA, IgG, IgM and lactoferrin contents of human milk during early lactation and the effect of processing and storage. J Food Prot 1983;1:4–7.

94. Espinosa-Martos I, Montilla A, de Segura AG, et al. Bacteriological, biochemical, and immunological modifications in human colostrum after Holder pasteurization. J Pediatr Gastroenterol Nutr 2013;56:560–8.

95. Christen L, Lai CT, Hartmann B, et al. The effect of UV-C pasteurization on bacteriostatic properties and immunological proteins of donor human milk. PLoS One 2013;8:e85867.

96. Gibbs JH, Fisher C, Bhattacharya S, et al. Drip breast milk: its composition, collection and pasteurization. Early Hum Dev 1977;1:227–45.

97. Goes HC, Torres AG, Donangelo CM, et al. Nutrient composition of banked human milk in Brazil and influence of processing on zinc distribution in milk fractions. Nutrition 2002;18:590–4.

98. Wardell JM, Hill CM, D'Souza SW. Effect of pasteurization and of freezing and thawing human milk on its triglyceride content. Acta Paediatr Scand 1981;70: 467–71.

99. Romeu-Nadal M, Castellote AI, Gaya A, et al. Effect of pasteurisation on ascorbic acid, dehydroascorbic acid, tocopherols and fatty acids in pooled mature human milk. Food Chem 2008;107:434–8.

100. Ewaschuk JB, Unger S, Harvey S, et al. Effect of pasteurization on immune components of milk: implications for feeding preterm infants. Appl Physiol Nutr Metab 2011;36:175–82.

101. Borgo LA, Coelho Araujo WM, Conceiçao MH, et al. Are fat acids of human milk impacted by pasteurization and freezing? Nutr Hosp 2014;31:1386–93.

102. de Segura AG, Escuder D, Montilla A, et al. Heating-induced bacteriological and biochemical modifications in human donor milk after Holder pasteurization. J Pediatr Gastroenterol Nutr 2012;54:197–203.

103. Bertino E, Coppa GV, Giuliani F, et al. Effects of Holder pasteurization on human milk oligosaccharides. Int J Immunopathol Pharmacol 2008;21:381–5.

104. Coscia A, Peila C, Bertino E, et al. Effect of Holder pasteurization on human milk glycosaminoglycans. J Pediatr Gastroenterol Nutr 2015;60:127–30.
105. Van Zoeren-Grobben D, Schrijver J, Van den Berg H, et al. Human milk vitamin content after pasteurization, storage, or tube feeding. Arch Dis Child 1987;62: 161–5.
106. Gomes FP, Shaw PN, Whitfield K, et al. Effect of pasteurization on the concentrations of vitamin D compounds in donor breastmilk. Int J Food Sci Nutr 2016; 67:16–9.
107. Moltó-Puigmartí C, Permanyer M, Castellote AI, et al. Effects of pasteurization and high pressure processing on vitamin C, tocopherols and fatty acids in mature human milk. Food Chem 2011;124:697–702.
108. Untalan PB, Keeney SE, Palkowetz KH, et al. Heat susceptibility of interleukin-10 and other cytokines in donor human milk. Breastfeed Med 2009;4:137–44.
109. da Costa RS, do Carmo MG, Saunders C, et al. Characterization of iron, copper and zinc levels in the colostrum of mothers of term and pre-term infants before and after pasteurization. Int J Food Sci Nutr 2003;54:111–7.
110. McPherson RJ, Wagner CL. The effect of pasteurization on transforming growth factor alpha and transforming growth factor beta 2 concentrations in human milk. Adv Exp Med Biol 2001;501:559–66.
111. Ley SH, Hanley AJ, Stone D, et al. Effects of pasteurization on adiponectin and insulin concentrations in donor human milk. Pediatr Res 2011;70:278–81.
112. Silvestre D, Miranda M, Muriach M, et al. Antioxidant capacity of human milk: effect of thermal conditions for the pasteurization. Acta Paediatr 2008;97: 1070–4.
113. Silvestre D, Ruiz P, Martínez-Costa C, et al. Effect of pasteurization on the bactericidal capacity of human milk. J Hum Lact 2008;24:371–6.
114. Björkstén B, Burman LG, De Château P, et al. Collecting and banking human milk: to heat or not to heat? Br Med J 1980;281(6243):765–9.
115. Williamson S, Finucane E, Ellis H, et al. Effect of heat treatment of human milk on absorption of nitrogen, fat, sodium, calcium, and phosphorus by preterm infants. Arch Dis Child 1978;53:555–63.
116. Friel JK, Martin SM, Langdon M, et al. Milk from mothers of both premature and full-term infants provides better antioxidant protection than does infant formula. Pediatr Res 2002;51:612–8.
117. Mehta R, Petrova A. Is variation in total antioxidant capacity of human milk associated with levels of bio-active proteins? J Perinatol 2014;34:220–2.
118. Goldblum RM, Dill CW, Albrecht TB, et al. Rapid high-temperature treatment of human milk. J Pediatr 1984;104:380–5.
119. Dhar J, Fichtali J, Skura BJ, et al. Pasteurization efficiency of a HTST system for human milk. J Food Sci 1996;61:569–72.
120. Terpstra FG, Rechtman DJ, Lee ML, et al. Antimicrobial and antiviral effect of high temperature short-time (HTST) pasteurization applied to human milk. Breastfeed Med 2007;2:27–33.
121. Trujillo AJ, Capellas M, Saldo J, et al. Applications of high hydrostatic pressure on milk and dairy products: a review. Innov Food Sci Emerg Technol 2002;3: 295–307.
122. Considine KM, Kelly AL, Fitzgerald GF, et al. High-pressure processing–effects on microbial food safety and food quality. FEMS Microbiol Lett 2008;281:1–9.
123. Mateos-Vivas M, Rodríguez-Gonzalo E, Domínguez-Álvarez J, et al. Analysis of free nucleotide monophosphates in human milk and effect of pasteurisation or

high-pressure processing on their contents by capillary electrophoresis coupled to mass spectrometry. Food Chem 2015;174:348–55.

124. Contador R, Delgado FJ, García-Parra J, et al. Volatile profile of breast milk subjected to high-pressure processing or thermal treatment. Food Chem 2015;180: 17–24.

125. Delgado FJ, Contador R, Álvarez-Barrientos A, et al. Effect of high pressure thermal processing on some essential nutrients and immunological components present in breast milk. Innov Food Sci Emerg Technol 2013;19:50–6.

126. Smelt JM. Recent advances in the microbiology of high pressure processing. Trends Food Sci Technology 1998;9:152–8.

127. Mussa DM, Ramaswamy H. Ultra high pressure pasteurization of milk: kinetics of microbial destruction and changes in physico-chemical characteristics. Lebenson Wiss Technol 1997;30:551–7.

128. Reineke K, Mathys A, Heinz V. Mechanisms of endospore inactivation under high pressure. Trends Microbiol 2013;21:296–304.

129. Demazeau G. A new high hydrostatic pressure treatment of human milk leading both to microbial safety and preservation of the activity of the main components. In: 3rd International Congress of the European Milk Bank Association (EMBA) Abstract book. 2015. Lyon, France. Available at: http://www.biomedia.net/up load/eventoprogramma/1042-programma.pdf. Accessed August 31, 2016.

130. Kingsley DH, Hoover D, Papafragkou E, et al. Inactivation of hepatitis A virus and a calicivirus by high hydrostatic pressure. J Food Prot 2002;65:1605–9.

131. Silva JL, Luan P, Glasser M, et al. Effect of hydrostatic pressure on a membrane-enveloped virus: high immunogenicity of the pressure inactivated virus. J Virol 1992;66:2111–7.

132. Nakagami T, Shigehisa T, Ohmoria T, et al. Inactivation of herpes viruses by high hydrostatic pressure. J Virol Methods 1992;38:255–61.

133. Landolfo S, Gariglio M, Gribaudo G, et al. The human cytomegalovirus. Pharmacol Ther 2003;98:269–97.

134. Nakagami T, Ohno H, Shigehisa T, et al. Inactivation of human immunodeficiency virus by high hydrostatic pressure. Transfusion 1996;36:475–6.

135. Viazis S, Farkas BE, Jaykus LA. Inactivation of bacterial pathogens in human milk by high-pressure processing. J Food Prot 2008;71:109–18.

136. Mayayo C, Montserrat M, Ramos SJ, et al. Kinetic parameters for high-pressure induced denaturation of lactoferrin in human milk. Int Dairy J 2014;39:246–52.

137. Balci AT, Wilbey RA. High pressure processing of milk. The first 100 years in the development of a new technology. Int J Dairy Technol 1999;52:149–55.

138. Moatsou G, Bakopanos C, Katharios D, et al. Effect of high-pressure treatment at various temperatures on indigenous proteolytic enzymes and whey protein denaturation in bovine milk. J Dairy Res 2008;75:262–9.

139. Law AJR, Leaver J, Felipe X, et al. Comparison of the effects of high pressure and thermal treatments on the casein micelles in goat's milk. J Agric Food Chem 1998; 46:2523–30.

140. Russo D, Ortore MG, Spinozzi F, et al. The impact of high hydrostatic pressure on structure and dynamics of β-lactoglobulin. Biochim Biophys Acta 2013;1830: 4974–80.

141. Lopez Fandino R, Carrascosa AV, Olano A. The effects of high pressure on whey protein denaturation and cheese-making properties of raw milk. J Dairy Sci 1996;79:929–1126.

142. Christen L, Lai CT, Hartmann B, et al. Ultraviolet-C irradiation: a novel pasteurization method for donor human milk. PLoS One 2013;8:e68120.

143. Christen L, Lai CT, Hartmann PE. Ultrasonication and the quality of human milk: variation of power and time of exposure. J Dairy Res 2012;79:361–6.
144. Czank C, Simmer K, Hartmann PE. Simultaneous pasteurization and homogenization of human milk by combining heat and ultrasound: effect on milk quality. J Diary Res 2010;77:183–9.
145. Lloyd ML, Hod N, Jayaraman J, et al. Inactivation of cytomegalovirus in breast milk using Ultraviolet-C irradiation: opportunities for a new treatment option in breast milk banking. PLoS One 2016;11:e0161116.
146. Giribaldi M, Coscia A, Peila C, et al. Pasteurization of human milk by a bench top high-temperature short-time device. Innov Food Sci Emerg Technol 2016;36: 228–33.
147. Naicker M, Coutsoudis A, Israel-Ballard K, et al. Demonstrating the efficacy of the FoneAstra pasteurization monitor for human milk pasteurization in resource-limited settings. Breastfeed Med 2015;10:107–12.
148. Coutsoudis I, Adhikari M, Nair N, et al. Feasibility and safety of setting up a donor breastmilk bank in a neonatal prem unit in a resource-limited setting: an observational, longitudinal cohort study. BMC Public Health 2011;11:356.
149. Israel-Ballard K, Coutsoudis A, Chantry CJ, et al. Bacterial safety of flash-heated and unheated expressed breastmilk during storage. J Trop Pediatr 2006;52: 399–405.
150. Chantry CJ, Israel-Ballard K, Moldoveanu Z, et al. Effect of flash-heat treatment on immunoglobulins in breast milk. J Acquir Immune Defic Syndr 2009;51: 264–7.
151. Keim SA, Kulkarni MM, McNamara K, et al. Cow's milk contamination of human milk purchased via the internet. Pediatrics 2015;135:e1157–62.
152. Embleton ND, King C, Jarvis C, et al. Effectiveness of human milk-based fortifiers for preventing necrotizing enterocolitis in preterm infants: case not proven. Breastfeed Med 2013;8:421.
153. Sullivan S, Schanler RJ, Kim JH, et al. An exclusively human milk-based diet is associated with a lower rate of necrotizing enterocolitis than a diet of human milk and bovine milk-based products. J Pediatr 2010;156:562–7.
154. Rochow N, Fusch G, Choi A, et al. Target fortification of breast milk with fat, protein, and carbohydrates for preterm infants. J Pediatr 2013;163:1001–7.
155. Arslanoglu S, Moro GE, Ziegler EE. Adjustable fortification of human milk fed to preterm infants: does it make a difference? J Perinatol 2006;26:614–21.

Postnatal Cytomegalovirus Infection Through Human Milk in Preterm Infants

Transmission, Clinical Presentation, and Prevention

Klaus Hamprecht, MD, PhD[a],*, Rangmar Goelz, MD[b]

KEYWORDS

- Cytomegalovirus • Lactation • Native breast milk • Virus reactivation
- Short- and long-term outcome • Very low birth weight infants (VLBW)
- Virus inactivation • Ganciclovir

KEY POINTS

- Cytomegalovirus (CMV) is reactivated in the lactating breast in up to 96% of CMV sero-positive mothers. The onset, the dynamics, and the end of virus shedding into breast milk are interindividually variable and describe mostly unimodal kinetics.
- As early as on day 3 postpartum infectivity of human breast milk (BM)/colostrum can be detected, and a preterm infant may be infected.
- There is a relevant entity of postnatally acquired symptomatic CMV infection and disease of preterm infants through raw BM.
- Actual data are supporting negative influence on long-term cognitive development.
- Concerning prevention, only heat inactivation eliminates virus infectivity, and short-term heat inactivation is most preservative; this can be applied effectively under routine conditions.
- Short-term heat inactivation for 5 seconds at 62°C maintains the benefits of feeding BM without the disadvantages of CMV transmission.

INTRODUCTION

Besides evident short-term benefits for the baby,[1] breast feeding is associated with improved IQ-scores and increased educational attainment 30 years later.[2] This article will focus on the dynamics of cytomegalovirus (CMV) excretion during lactation, and describe the short- and long-term risks of CMV-infection of small preterm infants, as well as options for prevention.

Both authors contributed equally.
Disclosure statement: The authors state that there is no conflict of interest.
[a] Institute of Medical Virology, University Hospital of Tuebingen, Elfriede-Aulhorn-Str 6, Tuebingen D-72076, Germany; [b] Department of Neonatology, University Children's Hospital, Calwerstr. 7, Tuebingen D-72076, Germany
* Corresponding author.
E-mail address: klaus.hamprecht@med.uni-tuebingen.de

Clin Perinatol 44 (2017) 121–130
http://dx.doi.org/10.1016/j.clp.2016.11.012
0095-5108/17/© 2016 Elsevier Inc. All rights reserved.

In 1967, CMV was first isolated from human breast milk (BM)[3]; thereafter, maternal CMV shedding into milk was related to perinatal infection.[4] A few years later, transmission to term infants fed raw BM was considered to be a form of natural immunization, because there was no or only minimal morbidity.[5] A neonatal exchange transfusion-related CMV infection was reported in 1979.[6] Despite the use of CMV immunoglobulin (IgG)-negative transfusions,[7] postnatal CMV infections, especially in preterm infants, persisted. This observation led the authors to prospectively investigate the role of postnatally acquired CMV infection in preterm infants through raw BM.

CYTOMEGALOVIRUS REACTIVATION DURING LACTATION

CMV, a beta-herpesvirus, persists following primary infection for lifetime in hemato-poetic CD34+ precursor cells and may be reactivated by stress, transient loss of CD4+ and CD8+ T-cell immunity, interleukin (IL)-6 signaling, cell cycle arrest, or DNA-damage.[8] Interestingly, CMV is also reactivated in healthy immunocompetent seropositive women during lactation.[5] The ratio of CMV reactivation at any stage of breastfeeding during the first 3 months after birth is high (>95%) and equals nearly the maternal seroprevalence.[9,10] CMV seroprevalences in Western Europe, the United States, Canada, and Australia range from 40% to 60%, and are above 90% in South Africa, Brazil, India, Japan, and Turkey.[11] The mechanisms leading to viral shedding exclusively into BM are not understood.

DYNAMICS OF CYTOMEGALOVIRUS REACTIVATION

Maternal CMV reactivation of seropositive mothers during lactation with shedding of viral DNA and virolactia[12] can be detected already in colostrum and normally ends after about 3 months after birth. According to the authors' experience with individual kinetics of CMV reactivation in BM of more than 500 healthy breastfeeding mothers of preterm infants, the onset of viral shedding may begin with low viral load (<1000 copies/mL) and low infectivity (without detectable infected fibroblast nuclei in short-term microculture) within 10 days postpartum. Nevertheless, also early onset of viral shedding into colostrum may occur as shown in **Fig. 1** for day 3 postpartum. The onset, dynamics, and the end of virus shedding into milk are interindividually variable and describe mostly unimodal kinetics. Using overnight microculture from cell and fat-free milk whey, peak values of virolactia and viral DNA lactia coincide, varying from 10^3 to 10^6 copies of CMV DNA per milliliter of milk whey.[13]

The study of initiation of viral shedding into colostrum shows divergent results. In a report from Gambia, CMV excretion in colostrum was observed in 100% of congenitally infected infants.[14] A Japanese study of postnatal CMV infection showed, that in 7 cases of very low birthweight (VLBW) infants, the initial viral load in BM in the first week postpartum ranges between 10 and less than 1000 copies/mL CMV DNA.[15] An Italian group detected viral DNA in 31 out of 57 (54%) colostrum samples.[16]

The CMV reactivation of mothers during lactation is a local process without detection of a disseminated or compartmentalized infection in plasma, throat, or cervical swabs.[17–19] Therefore, CMV-DNA, viral late pp67-transcripts and virions can only be detected in BM cells and cell-free milk whey.[12,13,20,21]

SPECTRUM OF CELL TYPES IN BREAST MILK

The BM cells involved in CMV reactivation include CD14+ macrophages.[13] However, CMV-infected milk cells are not essential for virus transmission.[12,19] Milk cells include breast-derived cells like lactocytes, myoepithelial cells, progenitor cells, and stem

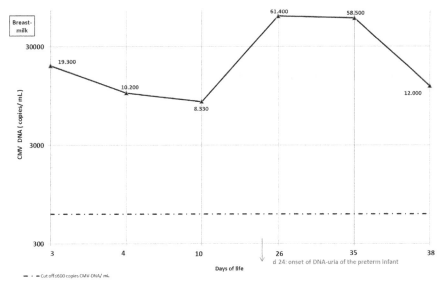

Fig. 1. Early reactivation of CMV in colostrum on day 3 postpartum. Viral DNA lactia was detected using quantitative real-time PCR (CMV R-gene Argene, France) from the milk whey fraction following centrifugation and a 40 μM filtration step.

cells, but also blood-derived cells like immune cells/leukocytes as well as hematopoietic progenitor and stem cells.[22] The nonimmune cells of BM (lactocytes), including luminal epithelial cells express CK18, produce milk proteins and consist of about 30% to 85% of all milk cells.[22]

Several reports found an association between high CMV viral load in BM and risk of transmission.[23,24] However, other observations seem to be important in context of prevention.[15] An inverse correlation between milk CMV-specific IgG avidity and CMV load was also found.[25]

INFLUENCE OF MATERNAL HUMAN IMMUNODEFICIENCY VIRUS/CYTOMEGALOVIRUS COINFECTION

In human immunodeficiency virus (HIV)/CMV coinfected breastfeeding mothers, many of the virological findings in the HIV-negative population are altered. Shedding of CMV and potentially Epstein-Barr virus (EBV) in BM is associated with HIV-1 transmission by breastfeeding.[26] About 5% of HIV-1-positive breastfeeding mothers had detectable CMV DNA perinatally in plasma. There was a strong correlation between cervical CMV DNA detection during pregnancy and later BM CMV levels. Maternal CMV DNA BM levels and CD4 less than 450 cells/mm^3 were determinants of CMV transmission.[27] All HIV-1-infected inocula-like genital secretions, BM, and blood contain cell-free virus and infected cells.[28]

INCIDENCE OF POSTNATAL CYTOMEGALOVIRUS TRANSMISSION THROUGH RAW BREAST MILK

In a prospective study from 1995 to 1998 including all admissions of infants younger than 32 weeks gestational age (GA) or less than 1500 g birthweight (BW), 73 of 76 (96%) CMV seropositive mothers reactivated and shed CMV into BM. Transmission occurred in 33 of 90 (37%) infants by 3 months corrected age; all had been fed with raw, untreated BM.[9] This incidence was subsequently questioned, because lower incidences have been reported.[29] However, in a review summarizing all data published so far, it became clear that transmission rates and clinical presentation of the infected preterm infants were strongly biased by using pretreated BM either by holder pasteurization or cryopreservation, or by shorter observation periods[30] compared with the pilot study. In many studies, the pretreatment procedures were not critically discussed; the high viral reactivation rates detected by CMV DNA from milk whey of up to 96% and the isolation of infectious virus in about 80% of all CMV shedding mothers[9] could be confirmed by other institutions.[10] The main risk factors for symptomatic disease are extremely low birth weight (ELBW), early transmission, low GA, and low infantile IgG titers.[31–33] Sixteen of 33 (48%) infants infected with CMV in the study cited previously[9] had at least 1 symptom; the remaining 17 had none. All symptoms were self-limited.

SYMPTOMATIC POSTNATAL CYTOMEGALOVIRUS INFECTION

Sepsis-like symptoms (SLS) have been introduced as a term to describe symptoms associated with postnatal CMV infection in VLBW preterm infants, comprising apnea and bradycardia, hepatosplenomegaly, hepatitis, gray pallor, distending bowels, thrombocytopenia, neutropenia, and elevated liver enzymes.[34–36] In a controlled study, VLBW-preterm infants had a significantly higher incidence of thrombocytopenia, neutropenia, and mildly increased C-reactive protein (CRP, 10–20 mg/L) than matched controls. For the first time in this study, clinical parameters could be confined to the entity of postnatal CMV infection in preterm infants. All parameters included were self-limited, and there was no impact on neonatal outcomes such as intracranial hemorrhage, periventricular leucomalacia, retinopathy of prematurity, and necrotizing enterocolitis (NEC).[37]

However, several single case reports and case series describe severe illness and even death in VLBW infants, including pneumonia requiring artificial ventilation, hepatitis, and gastrointestinal involvement with necrotizing enterocolitis (NEC), bloody diarrhea, stricture and volvulus. Some infants needed antiviral treatment with (val) ganciclovir.[15,30,32,38–40]

After an initial article reported an association between bronchopulmonary dysplasia (BPD) and postnatal CMV infection,[41] this association was evaluated.[42] In a large propensity-matched retrospective study involving more than 100,000 VLBW infants, BPD and death or BPD had a significantly higher incidence in postnatally CMV infected infants.[42] In an actual case report with lethal neonatal outcome and a complete autopsy, a generalized CMV infection comprising all organs including lungs and brain has been described.[43]

Summarizing these data, it is clear that there is a definite clinical entity of postnatally aquired (through raw BM) symptomatic CMV infection of preterm infants. Symptoms are mostly self-limiting, but these infants might be at increased risk for BPD. Moreover, some infants may become seriously ill and even die, particularly those born at less than 32 weeks GA.

CASE REPORT: SYMPTOMATIC POSTNATAL CYTOMEGALOVIRUS INFECTION AND ANTIVIRAL THERAPY

The authors describe an infant (**Figs. 1–3**) summarizing nearly all findings of postnatal CMV infection: extremely preterm (25 weeks GA) and extremely low BW (350 g), with early onset of CMV reactivation in colostrum on day 3 postpartum containing 19,300 copies CMV DNA per milliliter in milk whey and 8 infected fibroblast nuclei per milliliter milk whey (see **Fig. 1**). Inactivation of BM started at day 4 postpartum. Therefore the infection must have occurred up to this day. Transmission was detected on day 23

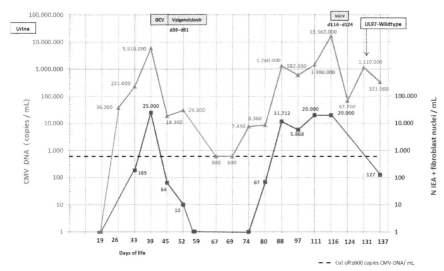

Fig. 2. Quantitative CMV DNA uria and semiquantitative viruria before, during, and after antiviral therapy. CMV detection from urine of the preterm infant was performed by quantitive real-time PCR (CMV R-gene Argene, France) and semiquantitative detection of infectious virus by short-term microculture (18 h) by immunoperoxidase staining of infected fibroblast nuclei using an IE1-specific mAb. The onset of viral DNA uria was defined as the average between the last negative (d19) and the first positive day (d26) of the real-time quantitative PCR assay after birth, in this case day 23 postpartum.

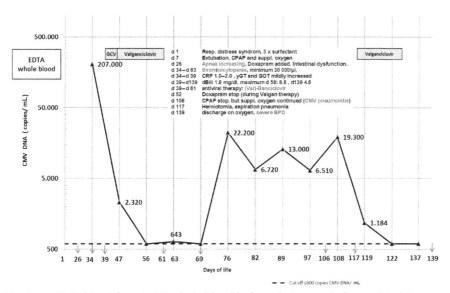

Fig. 3. CMV viral load from EDTA whole blood before, during, and after antiviral therapy. Detection of high viral load in peripheral blood at day 34 postpartum using quantitative real-time PCR (CMV R-gene Argene, France). In contrast to urine, the onset of the presence of the virus in blood cannot be given.

from urine (see **Fig. 2**), followed by detection of viral load with 207,000 copies CMV DNA per milliliter ethylene-diamin-tetra-acidic acid (EDTA) whole blood (see **Fig. 3**). Clinical symptoms included CMV pneumonitis, increasing occurrence of apneas, gastrointestinal malfunction, hepatitis, thrombocytopenia, mildly increased CRP and severe BPD with oxygen requirement during the whole hospital stay and at discharge. During the most critical period, the infant was treated with (val)ganciclovir (21 days, 2×6 mg ganciclovir intravenously or 2×16 mg valganciclovir per day), and before discharge perioperatively because of a herniotomia with orchidopexia complicated by an aspiration pneumonia (9 days). **Fig. 2** depicts the longitudinal course of quantitative viral DNA uria and semiquantitative viruria. The antiviral treatment led to a total loss of infectious virus for a certain period, with decreasing viral DNA uria. This course of intermittent CMV reduction under antiviral therapy for 3 weeks (day 39 to day 61), followed by a strong increase of viral load in blood and urine, is typical for treatment with ganciclovir or its valin ester VGCV. This case demonstrates the value of both detection of CMV via polymerase chain reaction (PCR) and also via semiquantitative short-term culture (18 h) in CMV monitoring for prediction of the efficiency of an antiviral treatment. The rapid effect of the antiviral therapy on CMV detection in blood (see **Fig. 3**) versus urine (see **Fig. 2**) is shown. Interestingly, a complete loss of viral DNA detectable by quantitative real-time PCR in EDTA whole blood can be demonstrated for about 2 weeks (days 56–69) (see **Fig. 3**), while in urine, nearly during the same period (days 59–74) (see **Fig. 2**), infectious virus cannot be detected. Viral DNA-uria lasts only a few days below the cut-off levels of the real-time PCR of 600 copies per milliliter (see **Fig. 2**). In conclusion, PCR from urine may be more sensitive than from blood during antiviral therapy monitoring.

LONG-TERM COGNITIVE OUTCOME OF POSTNATALLY CYTOMEGALOVIRUS INFECTED INFANTS

Long-term outcome has ever been questioned, since the entity of postnatally acquired CMV disease was first observed. In an initial report on a group of 10 children postnatally infected with CMV (GA not given) evaluated at age 9 years, no adverse cognitive, neurologic, auditory, or behavioral sequelae were noted.[44] In contrast, an increased risk of neurologic sequelae and handicap was reported in a group of infants born at less than 2000 g BW with onset of CMV excretion between 3 and 8 weeks after birth and studied at 3 years of age. The CMV excretion starting beyond 8 weeks of age was not associated with an adverse outcome.[45]

In a study from the authors' group, no difference in neurodevelopmental outcome was found between VLBW infants with postnatal CMV infection and a matched control group studied at 2 to 4 years of age using the concept of essential developmental milestones.[46] This is in line with a recent study from Taiwan using Bayley 2 scores for assessment at 2 years.[47] However, this was only true until 5 to 10 years of age. The cognitive outcome of all infants with early postnatal CMV infection at that age was significantly lower than that of matched controls using the Kaufmann-Assessment Battery for Children (ABC) after correction for socioeconomic status. This resembles the result of Paryani 1985.[45] All infants were without audiologic impairment, and the rate of cerebral palsy was not increased.[48,49] At the age of 11 to 16 years, the result was the same assessing neurocognitive outcome with the Wechsler Intelligence Scale, showing a difference of 93 (infected infants) versus 103 (controls, $P<.03$).[50]

It is also noteworthy that imaging by MRI revealed different patterns between CMV-infected and noninfected former preterm infants. A Dutch group of preterm infants with postnatal CMV infection showed a significantly reduced fractional anisotropy in the occipital white matter at term equivalent age compared with controls. The significance of this finding is yet unclear, because neurodevelopment at the age of 16 months was not different.[51] Targeted analyses of participants of the authors' observational study compared with healthy controls using functional MRI revealed significant activation differences in the left hippocampus and in the right anterior cingulate cortex when performing language tasks. Differences in gray matter volume were present in several brain regions, suggesting that long-term neurobiologic consequences of early postnatal CMV infection of preterm infants are detectable even at the age of 14 years, compatible with a higher effort when performing cognitive tasks.[52]

In conclusion, there are now data available supporting the possibility of cognitive long-term consequences of postnatally acquired CMV in preterm infants.

OPTIONS FOR PREVENTION OF VIRUS TRANSMISSION

Effective prevention of CMV transmission is only possible through heat-treatment of BM. Both long-term (30 min, 63°C) and short-term (5 sec, 62°C) pasteurization methods are effective, but short-term pasteurization conserves nutritional and immunologic relevant components in milk like CMV-specific antibodies, enzymes, and hormones, especially growth factors,[53,54] while Holder-pasteurization does not. Recently, in a prospective bicentric intervention study with historical controls, the incidence of CMV transmission was significantly reduced under routine conditions using short-term pasteurization, thus proving effectiveness (Bapistella et al, submitted data). Using this method, the benefits of feeding BM of the own mother can be preserved without the disadvantages of CMV transmission.

Freeze thawing at −20°C for time intervals ranging from 18 hours to 10 days may diminish virus concentrations but is not effective in eliminating the virus.[53,55,56] Two additional techniques have recently been described as capable of eradicating the virus: the first one, microwave irradiation[57] and the second one ultraviolet-C irradiation.[58] These 2 techniques are promising, but until more data are obtained about their efficacy and their potential harmful effects on BM properties, it s not possible to recommend their routine use.

ACKNOWLEDGMENTS

The authors would like to thank all breastfeeding women participating in their studies and Irene Haag for help in generating the figures.

REFERENCES

1. American Academy of Pediatrics. Breast feeding and the use of human milk. Pediatrics 2012;129:e827–41.
2. Victora CG, Horta BL, Loret de Mola C, et al. Association between breastfeeding and intelligence, educational attainment, and income at 30 years of age: a prospective cohort study from Brazil. Lancet Glob Health 2015;3:e199–205.
3. Diosi P, Babusceac L, Nevinglovschi O, et al. Cytomegalovirus infection associated with pregnancy. Lancet 1967;2(7525):1063–6.
4. Reynolds DW, Stagno S, Hosty TS, et al. Maternal cytomegalovirus excretion and perinatal infection. N Engl J Med 1973;289:1–5.
5. Stagno S, Reynolds DW, Pass RF, et al. Breast milk and the risk of cytomegalovirus infection. N Engl J Med 1980;302:1073–6.
6. Benson JW, Bodden SJ, Tobin JO. Cytomegalovirus and blood transfusion in neonates. Arch Dis Child 1979;54(7):538–41.

7. Yeager AS, Grumet FC, Hafleigh EB, et al. Prevention of transfusion acquired cytomegalovirus infections in newborn infants. J Pediatr 1981;98:281–7.
8. Goodrum F, Caviness K, Zagallo P. Human cytomegalovirus persistence. Cell Microbiol 2012;14:644–55.
9. Hamprecht K, Maschmann J, Vochem M, et al. Epidemiology of transmission of cytomegalovirus from mother to preterm infant by breastfeeding. Lancet 2001; 357:513–8.
10. Meier J, Lienicke U, Tschirch E, et al. Human cytomegalovirus reactivation during lactation and mother-to-child transmission in preterm infants. J Clin Microbiol 2005;43:1318–24.
11. Manicklal S, Emery VC, Lazzarotto T, et al. The 'Silent' Global burden of congenital cytomegalovirus. Clin Microbiol Rev 2013;26:86.
12. Hamprecht K, Witzel S, Maschmann J, et al. Rapid detection and quantification of cell free cytomegalovirus by a high-speed centrifugation-based microculture assay: comparison to longitudinally analyzed viral DNA load and pp67 late transcript during lactation. J Clin Virol 2003;28:303–16.
13. Maschmann J, Goelz R, Witzel S, et al. Characterization of human breast milk leukocytes and their potential role in cytomegalovirus transmission to newborns. Neonatology 2015;107:213–9.
14. Kaye S, Miles D, Antoine P, et al. Virological and immunological correlates of mother-to-child transmission of cytomegalovirus in the Gambia. J Infect Dis 2008;197:1307–14.
15. Wakabayashi H, Mizuno K, Kohda C, et al. Low HCMV DNA copies can establish infection and result in significant symptoms in extremely preterm infants: a prospective study. Am J Perinatol 2012;29:377–82.
16. Chiavarini M, Bragetti P, Sensini A, et al. Breastfeeding and transmission of cytomegalovirus to preterm infants. Case report and kinetic of CMV-DNA in breast milk. Ital J Pediatr 2011;37:6.
17. Mosca F, Pugni L, Barbi M, et al. Transmission of cytomegalovirus. Lancet 2001; 357(9270):1800.
18. Numazaki K, Chiba S, Asanuma H. Transmission of cytomegalovirus. Lancet 2001;357(9270):1799.
19. Hamprecht K, Maschmann J, Vochem M, et al. Transmission of cytomegalovirus to preterm infants by breastfeeding. In: Prösch S, Cinatl J, Scholz M, editors. New aspects of CMV-related immunopathology, vol. 24. Basel (Switzerland): Karger; 2003. p. 43–52.
20. Hamprecht K, Vochem M, Baumeister A, et al. Detection of cytomegaloviral DNA in human milk cells and cell free milk whey by nested PCR. J Virol Methods 1998; 70:167–76.
21. Hamprecht K, Witzel S, Maschmann J, et al. Transmission of cytomegalovirus infection through breast milk in term and preterm infants. The role of cell free milk whey and milk cells. Adv Exp Med Biol 2000;478:231–9.
22. Hassiotou F, Hartmann P. At the dawn of a new discovery: the potential of breast milk stem cells. Adv Nutr 2014;5:770–8.
23. van der Strate BW, Harmsen MC, Schäfer P, et al. Viral load in breast milk correlates with transmission of human cytomegalovirus to preterm neonates, but lactoferrin concentrations do not. Clin Diagn Lab Immunol 2001;8:818–21.
24. Jim WT, Shu CH, Chiu NC, et al. High cytomegalovirus load and prolonged virus excretion in breast milk increase risk for viral acquisition by very low birth weight infants. Pediatr Infect Dis J 2009;28:891–4.

25. Ehlinger EP, Webster EM, Kang HH, et al. Maternal cytomegalovirus-specific immune responses and symptomatic postnatal cytomegalovirus transmission in very low-birth-weight preterm infants. J Infect Dis 2011;204:1672–82.
26. Viljoen J, Tuaillon E, Nagot N, et al. Cytomegalovirus, and possibly Epstein–Barr virus, shedding in breast milk is associated with HIV-1 transmission by breastfeeding. AIDS 2015;29:145–53.
27. Slyker J, Farquhar C, Atkinson C, et al. Compartmentalized cytomegalovirus replication and transmission in the setting of maternal HIV-1 infection. Clin Infect Dis 2014;58:564–72.
28. Sagar M. Origin of the transmitted virus in HIV infection: infected cells versus cell-free virus. J Infect Dis 2014;210(Suppl 3):S667–73.
29. Doctor S, Friedman S, Dunn MS, et al. Cytomegalovirus transmission to extremely low-birthweight infants through breast milk. Acta Paediatr 2005;94:53–8.
30. Hamprecht K, Maschmann J, Jahn G, et al. Cytomegalovirus transmission to preterm infants during lactation. J Clin Virol 2008;41(3):198–205.
31. Maschmann J, Hamprecht K, Dietz K, et al. Cytomegalovirus infection of extremely low-birth weight infants via breast milk. Clin Infect Dis 2001;33:1998–2003.
32. Mehler K, Oberthuer A, Lang-Roth R, et al. High rate of symptomatic cytomegalovirus infection in extremely low gestational age preterm infants of 22-24 weeks' gestation after transmission via breast milk. Neonatology 2014;105(1):27–32.
33. Nijman J, van Loon AM, Krediet TG, et al. Maternal and neonatal anti-cytomegalovirus IgG level and risk of postnatal cytomegalovirus transmission in preterm infants. J Med Virol 2013;85:689–95.
34. Ballard RA, Drew WL, Hufnagle KG, et al. Acquired cytomegalovirus infection in preterm infants. Am J Dis Child 1979;133:482–5.
35. Vochem M, Hamprecht K, Jahn G, et al. Transmission of cytomegalovirus to preterm infants through breast milk. Pediatr Infect Dis J 1998;17:53–8.
36. Kurath S, Halwachs-Baumann G, Müller W, et al. Transmission of cytomegalovirus via breast milk to the prematurely born infant: a systematic review. Clin Microbiol Infect 2010;16:1172–8.
37. Neuberger P, Hamprecht K, Vochem M, et al. Case-control study of symptoms and neonatal outcome of human milk-transmitted cytomegalovirus infection in premature infants. J Pediatr 2006;148:326–31.
38. Hamele M, Flanagan R, Loomis CA, et al. Severe morbidity and mortality with breast milk associated cytomegalovirus infection. Pediatr Infect Dis J 2010;29:84–6.
39. Lanzieri TM, Dollard SC, Josephson CD, et al. Breast milk-acquired cytomegalovirus infection and disease in VLBW and premature infants. Pediatrics 2013;131:e1937–45.
40. Goelz R, Hamprecht K, Klingel K, et al. Intestinal manifestations of postnatal and congenital cytomegalovirus infection in term and preterm infants. J Clin Virol 2016;83:29–36.
41. Sawyer MH, Edwards DK, Spector SA. Cytomegalovirus infection and bronchopulmonary dysplasia in premature infants. Am J Dis Child 1987;141:303–5.
42. Kelly MS, Benjamin DK, Puopolo KM, et al. Postnatal cytomegalovirus infection and the risk for bronchopulmonary dysplasia. JAMA Pediatr 2015;169:e153785.
43. Lopes A-A, Belhabri S, Karaoui L. Clinical findings and autopsy of a preterm infant with breast milk-acquired cytomegalovirus infection. AJP Rep 2016;6:e198–202.

44. Kumar ML, Nankervis GA, Jacobs IB, et al. Congenital and postnatally acquired cytomegalovirus infections: long-term follow-up. J Pediatr 1984;104:674–9.
45. Paryani SG, Yeager AS, Hosford-Dunn H, et al. Sequelae of acquired cytomegalovirus infection in premature and sick term infants. J Pediatr 1985;107:451–6.
46. Vollmer B, Seibold-Weiger K, Schmitz-Salue C, et al. Postnatally acquired cytomegalovirus infection via breast milk: effects on hearing and development in preterm infants. Pediatr Infect Dis J 2004;23:322–7.
47. Jim WT, Chiu NC, Ho CS, et al. Outcome of preterm infants with postnatal cytomegalovirus infection via breast milk: a two-year prospective follow-up study. Medicine (Baltimore) 2015;94:e1835.
48. Goelz R, Meisner C, Bevot A, et al. Long-term cognitive and neurological outcome of preterm infants with postnatally acquired CMV infection through breast milk. Arch Dis Child Fetal Neonatal Ed 2013;98:F430–3.
49. Bevot A, Hamprecht K, Krägeloh-Mann I, et al. Long-term outcome in preterm children with human cytomegalovirus infection transmitted via breast milk. Acta Paediatr 2012;101:e167–72.
50. Brecht KF, Goelz R, Bevot A, et al. Postnatal human cytomegalovirus infection in preterm infants has long-term neuropsychological sequelae. J Pediatr 2015;166:834–9.
51. Nijman J, Gunkel J, de Vries LS, et al. Reduced occipital fractional anisotropy on cerebral diffusion tensor imaging in preterm infants with postnatally acquired cytomegalovirus infection. Neonatology 2013;104:143–50.
52. Dorn M, Lidzba K, Bevot A, et al. Long-term neurobiological consequences of early postnatal hCMV-infection in former preterms: a functional MRI study. Hum Brain Mapp 2014;35:2594–606.
53. Hamprecht K, Maschmann J, Müller D, et al. Cytomegalovirus (CMV) inactivation in breast milk: reassessment of pasteurization and freeze-thawing. Pediatr Res 2004;56:529–35.
54. Goelz R, Hihn E, Hamprecht K, et al. Effects of different CMV-heat-inactivation-methods on growth factors in human breast milk. Pediatr Res 2009;65:458–61.
55. Maschmann J, Hamprecht K, Weissbrich B, et al. Freeze-thawing of breast milk does not prevent cytomegalovirus transmission to a preterm infant. Arch Dis Child Fetal Neonatal Ed 2006;91:F288–90.
56. Curtis N, Chau L, Garland S, et al. Cytomegalovirus remains viable in naturally infected breast milk despite being frozen for 10 days. Arch Dis Child Fetal Neonatal Ed 2005;90:F529–30.
57. Ben-Shoshan M, Mandel D, Lubetzky R, et al. Eradication of cytomegalovirus from human milk by microwave irradiation: a pilot study. Breastfeed Med 2016;11:186–7.
58. Lloyd ML, Hod N, Jayaraman J, et al. Inactivation of cytomegalovirus in breast milk using ultraviolet-C irradiation: opportunities for a new treatment option in breast milk banking. PLoS One 2016;11(8):e0161116.

Ensuring Safety in Donor Human Milk Banking in Neonatal Intensive Care

Ben T. Hartmann, PhD[a,b],*

KEYWORDS

- Donor human milk banking • Guidelines • Best practice

KEY POINTS

- There is a significant variation in practice in human milk banking across jurisdictions.
- A single international standard of practice is not possible and there are currently few methods to assess appropriate milk-banking practice.
- Milk banks must assess both clinical responsibility and social responsibility to both their donors and recipients.
- Universal hazards and benefits should be defined by donor human milk-banking services using a systematic method.
- Local jurisdictions will need to assess these benefits and hazards using existing and internationally recognized hazard assessment tools.

INTRODUCTION

At its most basic definition, a donor human milk bank can be considered to be "a store of donated human milk for later use when required." This definition is simplistic but useful, as it is one of the few available that covers the diverse range of milk-banking practices. It implies that any donor human milk-banking service (DHMBS) will engage in a process of selection of donors, storage, and/or processing of product and will then dispense that product to appropriate recipients. Within each of

Disclosure Statement: The author has accepted travel funding to attend scientific meetings as an invited speaker from Medela AG, and travel funding to attend a conference from the conference sponsor Prolacta Bioscience. The author has undertaken professional consultancy for the Australian Red Cross Blood Service.
[a] Perron Rotary Express Mothers (PREM) Milk Bank, Neonatology Clinical Care Unit, King Edward Memorial Hospital, 1st Floor Block A, 374 Bagot Road, Subiaco, Western Australia 6008, Australia; [b] Centre for Neonatal Research and Education, The University of Western Australia (M550), 35 Stirling Highway Crawley, Perth, Western Australia 6009, Australia
* Perron Rotary Express Mothers (PREM) Milk Bank, Neonatology Clinical Care Unit, King Edward Memorial Hospital, 1st Floor Block A, 374 Bagot Road, Subiaco, Western Australia 6008, Australia.
E-mail address: ben.hartmann@health.wa.gov.au

these basic functions, practice in milk banking varies across and even within jurisdictions.[1] The result is that there are now various definitions of an appropriate donor; a range of collection, storage, and processing practices; and a range of recipients of donor milk products.[1–6] This presents a difficulty for new human milk-banking projects and when assessing appropriate DHMBS practice. There is growing availability of donor milk in the neonatal intensive care unit (NICU) and for the vulnerable patient it is desirable to standardize practice to ensure DHMBSs are providing a safe and credible clinical service. In addition, where donor human milk product itself may cross borders (be that one hospital to another or geographic borders), it is desirable to ensure a uniform standard of safety in donor human milks. The recent development of an ISBT128 standard for donor human milk labeling has been an important step in this process.[7] Recent editorials[8] rightly question the unregulated expansion of donor human milk banking with limited evidence for the benefit of donor milk in NICU. DHMBSs must adequately respond to these concerns. There is also a growing interest in the community toward informal sharing of breast milk.[9] This practice is often confused with formal human milk banking in the NICU, whereas it is clear they are very different public health issues and should be considered separately. However, DHMBSs in some jurisdictions do provide a service to both NICU patients and the general community.[9] A clear description of the wide range of considerations for safe and ethical milk-banking practice in the NICU may assist parents, policy makers, and clinicians requiring an objective measure of a minimum acceptable standard of safety when sharing breast milk.

This article aims to develop a potential framework to design and assess appropriate milk-banking practice to ensure safety. The principles that were used to establish safe donor human milk banking in Perth, Western Australia, where contemporary human milk banking began in 2006,[3] are defined. Although discussion focuses on the activity of a DHMBS in an Australian NICU, these general principles may serve as a foundation to assess appropriate milk-banking practices in any setting. This article does not recommend a single standard of practice in donor human milk banking or suggest that the practices used at the PREM (Perron Rotary Express Mothers) Milk Bank represent the only safe practice in milk banking. However, the potential hazards and benefits of donor human milk banking are universal and can be defined. By identifying these initial principles of donor human milk-banking practice, DHMBSs can design appropriate processes, or assess and validate existing practice with reference to the intended recipient and with consideration to local issues. The approach outlined in this article is developed with the intention of assessing and validating our own practice, its publication is intended to ensure transparency of our service and provide opportunity for objective criticism. This recognizes an unresolved issue for DHMBS internationally, current services have evolved different practices based on historical experience and local risk factors. This has resulted in significant variation in the practice of human milk banking around the world.

RESPONSIBILITIES OF A DONOR HUMAN MILK-BANKING SERVICE

The guidelines for donor blood services are useful when considering responsibilities for DHMBSs, as there are similarities between these services. The World Health Organization[10] considers the primary responsibility of blood transfusion services "to provide a safe, sufficient and timely supply of blood and blood products." Furthermore, they suggest all prospective blood donors be assessed for their suitability to donate, and that the purpose of this assessment is to

- Protect donor health and safety by collecting blood only from healthy individuals
- Ensure patient safety by collecting blood only from donors whose donations when transfused, will be safe for the recipients
- Identify any factors that might make an individual unsuitable as a donor, either temporarily or permanently
- Reduce the unnecessary deferral of safe and healthy donors
- Ensure the quality of blood products derived from whole blood and apheresis donations
- Minimize the wastage of resources resulting in the collection of unsuitable donations

These appear to be reasonable expectations of a DHMBS. The previously quoted document[10] goes on to state, "In many countries, donor selection criteria are still based on tradition and customary practice rather than evidence" and "criteria from one country are often adopted in other countries without due consideration of the profiles of the general and potential donor populations, the prevailing epidemiology of infectious diseases, local culture and available resources" while concluding that "polices for donor selection should take into account the need for a balance between the safety and sufficiency of the blood supply and availability of resources." It is striking how equally relevant these statements are to current donor human milk-banking practice.

With direct reference to, and adapted from, stated objectives of donor blood services,[10] DHMBSs may commit to the following responsibilities:

The primary responsibility of the DHMBS is to provide a safe, effective, ethical, and sustainable supply of donor human milk products. DHMBSs should ensure that the act of donation is safe and causes no harm to the donor or the infant/family. They should maintain a pool of safe, voluntary nonremunerated donors and take all necessary steps to ensure that donor human milk products are efficacious for the recipient, with minimal risk of infection or harm. This includes harm resulting from detrimental breastfeeding outcomes in recipient populations.

- The safety of human milk donors must be protected by ensuring confidentiality, privacy, self-determination, and nondiscrimination.
- The safety of the recipients of donor human milk products must be protected by ensuring the safety, quality, and availability of donor human milk products.
- Human milk donors have a responsibility to self-defer if they are aware of any concern that may influence their suitability to donate. Donors have the right to withdraw at any stage of the donation process.
- Recipients have the right to be protected from avoidable adverse events associated with donor human milk products.
- Although anyone may offer to become a milk donor, there is no intrinsic right to donate milk. Where self-determination conflicts with safety of donor or recipient, safety considerations will decide acceptability of donation.

The question for DHMBSs, such as the PREM Milk Bank, now becomes how to transparently achieve these objectives? Additionally, the lack of national and international regulatory bodies governing DHMBSs increases the need for donor human milk banks to be transparent in the decisions made during the course of their operation. There may be wider value in the development of systematic approaches to assess DHMBSs.

A first step in our reassessment of our own milk-banking practice against the previously stated principle has been to review a clear description of the intended outcomes of our service. We also seek to review all potential positive and negative impacts of our service. Our risk/benefit model is diagrammatically represented in **Fig. 1**.

When conceiving or assessing the scope of practice of a donor human milk bank, **Fig. 1** may provide a useful starting point to ensure all potential positive and negative impacts of a project are considered. Each segment of the Venn diagram represents an area of impact to be considered by a donor human milk bank. The potential risk or benefits may vary in nature. For example, at the PREM Milk Bank we consider the primary clinical benefit of our donor human milk bank to deliver a reduction in the risk of necrotizing enterocolitis (NEC) in very low birthweight (VLBW) preterm infants.[3] This is based on the available systematic reviews of the literature.[11] We have also considered the potential clinical risk to our recipients of donor milk in Perth, based on well-established hazards in donor human milk.[3] We have endeavored to measure and manage the risks of these hazards in our local population of donors and recipients using methods such as HACCP (Hazard Analysis Critical Control Point).[3] These risk management tools are now required by many DHMBS guidelines.[3–5,12] However, it is clear that the clinical risks and benefits are not the only responsibilities of a milk bank. Similar to concepts established for blood banks,[10] the health and safety of the milk donor is also important and clearly there are wider considerations to ensuring milk banking is not disruptive to breastfeeding outcomes of our donors and recipients. These "social responsibilities" are important considerations for the design and assessment of milk-banking practice. From **Fig. 1** it is then possible to formulate an overview (**Table 1**) of the range of implications and considerations for a milk-banking service. In Perth, we have focused much of our early practice on ensuring 2 key outcomes: that our service is safe and that it provides an intervention beneficial to recipients.[3] However, our practice has always had the key goal of promoting and supporting breastfeeding outcomes in both the donor or recipient population.

We have previously published descriptions of formal "quantifiable" risk assessment methods that can be applied to the clinical hazards identified in milk banking,[3,9] and these methods have also been developed by other DHMBSs.[4,5,12] However, benefit assessment methods are less well established. For the purposes of determining the

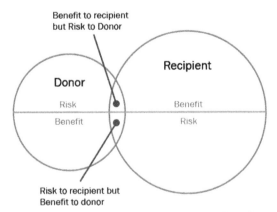

Fig. 1. A risk/benefit model of donor human milk banking. Although removed for simplification, any impact must consider both a donor and her infant or a recipient and her mother. For each segment of the Venn diagram, both clinical and social responsibilities of a DHMBS can be identified.

Table 1
The range of clinical and social responsibilities for a DHMBS to ensure *safety, efficacy, ethical practice*, and *sustainability*

Stakeholder	Type	Risk/Benefit	Example (Potential Hazard or Potential Benefit)	Method of Assessment	Quality	Resulting DHMBS Program/Process
Recipient	Clinical responsibility	Risk	Disease transmission (HIV) (Can be defined by literature review and hazard identification)	Risk assessment	Quantifiable (eg, HACCP)	Process development, donor screening, outcomes tracking, adverse events
	Clinical responsibility	Benefit	Reduce NEC	Benefit assessment	Ranked, quantifiable by outcomes tracking	Outcomes tracking
Recipient	Social responsibility	Risk	Reduce breastfeeding in NICU	Risk assessment	Semi quantifiable	Outcomes tracking
	Social responsibility	Benefit	Increase breastfeeding success in NICU	Benefit assessment	Ranked	Outcomes tracking
Donor	Clinical responsibility	Risk	Injury from breast pump	Risk assessment	Quantifiable	Donor management
	Clinical responsibility	Benefit	Sustained breastfeeding where excessive maternal oversupply; reduced mastitis	Benefit assessment	Ranked	Outcomes tracking, marketing/communications plan
Donor	Social responsibility	Risk	Donation negatively impacts donors breastfeeding	Risk assessment	Semi-quantifiable/ranked	Donor management, screening, outcomes tracking
	Social responsibility	Benefit	Positive donor experience (altruism)	Benefit assessment	Ranked	Marketing/communications, outcomes tracking

The green section indicates issues that are common considerations for all DHMBS. The red section denotes a process that must be undertaken by individual DHMBS following a common methodology.

Abbreviations: DHMBS, donor human milk bank services; HACCP, Hazard Analysis Critical Control Point; HIV, human immunodeficiency virus; NEC, necrotizing enterocolitis; NICU, neonatal intensive care unit.

appropriate practice in a DHMBS it is probably sufficient for a service to identify the intended benefits and rank them in terms of the importance to the project. For example, we consider the primary clinical benefit of the PREM Milk Bank to be in the reduction of the incidence of NEC in VLBW preterm infants by avoiding early formula feeding of infants less than 32 weeks' gestation and/or less than 1500 g birth weight.[3] However, we also intend the operation of our DHMBS to improve (or at least not be detrimental to) breastfeeding outcomes at discharge. Clearly, if these are the stated aims of our project, they are outcome measures that we should commit to tracking. To achieve a sustainable business model for our DHMBS the PREM Milk Bank must demonstrate that we are achieving the clinical aims of the service.

DHMBSs in other jurisdictions may value these intended benefits differently. However, identification of the intended benefit will also identify the outcome measures that it is necessary to track. This begins to demonstrate the value of this type of assessment of a DHMBS during the design of the service. The final column of **Table 1** shows the operational program of the donor human milk bank that will be the direct outcome of the decisions and assessment made during this process.

There are 2 key questions we ask with regard to an assessment of our practice:

1. What are the known hazards and intended benefits of the proposed service (see **Table 1** in green)?
2. What are the risks presented by these hazards for our intended recipient or donor and how do we maximize and measure the proposed benefits (see **Table 1** in red)?

The answers to question 1 (those shown in green in **Table 1**) are universal considerations that can be established by existing DHMBSs, whereas question 2 (shown in red in **Table 1**) will be a process undertaken by local jurisdictions and projects. This will allow a clear statement of the goals and responsibilities of a service and ensure they are achieved. An additional benefit for milk banks under development is that a clear description of the recipient and donor and the intended outcomes of the service will allow projects to better model the size and scope of the clinical demand and better develop resources to meet these expected demands.

There is clear distinction between the identification of any potential hazard present in donor human milk (anything that may cause harm) and the associated risk to a recipient (a measure of the chance that the hazard will cause harm). The rest of this discussion will be limited to the identification of the potential hazards and intended benefits of donor milk banking (green section of **Table 1**) from our experience in Perth. These were either identified during the establishment of the PREM Milk Bank, or include issues that have become apparent during the 10 years of operation of our service. It also seeks to identify additional issues based on recommendations in similar industries or from examination of the literature. They are grouped as either clinical responsibilities or social responsibilities. These require assessment with regard to the risk they present to the intended recipient. Not every potential hazard identified will present an unacceptable risk to a recipient or donor, and the social benefits and hazards are not the sole responsibility of DHMBSs, but they are all relevant considerations that require assessment by a DHMBS.

CLINICAL RESPONSIBILITIES OF A DHMBS
Recipient

Potential clinical hazards of donor human milk
General donor assessment As in blood donation, an initial assessment of the donor may identify issues that impact the safety and quality of a donation. This may include occupational exposure to chemicals that can be transferred to breast milk and present a potential hazard to a preterm infant. As the recipient infant may not have been exposed to these hazards in utero, a milk bank may assess these issues differently to recommendations for mothers feeding their own infant. There are more similarities in the composition of human milk from women of different geographic, ethnic, and socioeconomic backgrounds than there are differences.[13] Many studies show that breast milk quality is conserved in mothers living in impoverished circumstances.[13] Diets low in B12 (vegan or vegetarian without supplementation) may result in low breast milk B12 and insufficiency in infants.[14] There are significant differences in the macronutrient composition in individual women across stages of lactation (colostrum, transitional milk, mature milk, and involution) and significant differences in macronutrient composition among individual women.[13] Milk quality may be related to parity with evidence of "reduced quality" from mothers of very high parity (>9).[13] Decisions regarding general donor suitability with regard to stage of lactation should be made

with respect to the clinical relevance of this variation considering how preterm infant growth is managed in a neonatal unit (growth monitoring and fortification regimes should be considered) (**Table 2**).

Donor medical history: noncommunicable disease Some illnesses alter components in maternal milk, assessment of the risk these present to the intended recipient should be undertaken. Recommendations for blood donors[10] suggest acceptance of individual donors with a past history of mental health problems depends on their ability to fully answer the donor questionnaire and give informed consent. Milk banks may consider similar assessments necessary. In general, donors with chronic or ongoing illness that does not affect their milk supply or composition may donate subject to the assessment of the safety of any maternal medications. Donors should not be unnecessarily excluded from donation (**Table 3**).

Donor medical history: medical and surgical interventions Any relevant medical or surgical history that may affect the safety or quality of donated human milk for the intended recipient should be considered by a DHMBS. Any donor medications should be reviewed with respect to the underlying condition for which they are taken (compare with Ref.[10]) their transfer to breast milk and their risk to a recipient infant. All medication ingested by a mother enters the breast milk compartment, but the vast majority do so in such small concentrations that the amount is clinically irrelevant.[22] An appropriately qualified individual should undertake individual review of donor medications, their transfer to breast milk, their oral availability to the recipient, and interactions with common medications in the NICU. General recommendations for common medications could be developed by existing DHMBSs and do appear in various milk-banking guidelines.[6] We encounter milk donors who use alternative

Table 2 General donor assessments		
Potential Hazard	**Comment**	**Reference**
Age	Maternal age may have minor influence on milk composition, unlikely to be clinically significant for NICU patient, but review required	Kedem et al,[15] 2013; Argov-Argaman et al,[16] 2016
General Health	Weight (BMI)*, diet (low B-12, high iodine)**	*Grote et al,[17] 2016 **Specker et al,[14] 1990; Shumer et al,[18] 2013
Occupation	Exposure to environmental toxin, chemical	Picone & Paolillo,[19] 2013
Country of residence	Exposure to pesticide, accumulation in donor's milk	Tai et al,[20] 2013
Smoking	Transfer of nicotine and metabolites to breast milk	Dahlstrom et al,[21] 2008
Alcohol consumption	Transfer to breast milk	Hale,[22] 2003
Caffeine consumption	Transfer to breast milk*, use of caffeine as medication in NICU	Escuder-Vieco et al,[23] 2016
Stage of lactation	Milk composition (suitability to support growth in preterm infants)	Prentice,[13] 1995

Abbreviations: BMI, body mass index; NICU, neonatal intensive care unit.

Table 3
Donor noncommunicable disease

Potential Hazard	Comment	Reference
Psychiatric disorders	Consider with reference to recommendations for blood donors* and the principle of self-determination of the donor.	World Health Organisation,[10] 2012
Other illness	If no risk to donor's milk supply, major compositional change and if medications are assessed as safe, minor illness does not preclude donation. Acute febrile illness does not affect major macronutrients in breast milk.*	*Zavaleta et al,[24] 1995

medicines, complementary therapy, and herbal preparations. It may be difficult to distinguish between herbal "medication" and a food ingredient. Postnatal cultural practices may require assessment for their safety with regard to milk donation. Consumption of traditional "soups" to improve a mother's milk production and that contain seaweed may result in high levels of iodine and these have been associated with acquired hypothyroidism in an infant.[18] Potential causes for excessive iodine in the maternal diet may require identification.

There is little evidence that previous breast surgery or breast implants (saline or silicone) affect milk quality or safety.[25] We have experienced donor self-disclosure of this history due to their concern to ensure the safety of their donation; formal review of the issue should allow a milk bank to form an appropriate policy. Breast reduction and augmentation may not reduce a mother's milk supply when glandular tissue is not removed or when scar tissue does not disrupt milk ducts.[26] A history of breast surgery may prompt caution to ensure donor has oversupply (**Table 4**).

Table 4
Donor medical and surgical interventions

Potential Hazard	Comment	Reference
Immunizations and vaccinations	Assess maternal vaccination with live attenuated virus vaccines (eg, measles mumps, rubella, smallpox).	HMBANA,[6] 2015
Medications	Exclusion or temporary deferral periods can be developed where appropriate. When a voluntary donor has a true oversupply and illness and/or medication does not present a risk to the recipient population, it seems reasonable to allow donation.	
Blood transfusion or transplantation	Transfusion Transmitted Infection risk after blood transfusion (country of transfusion).	
Diagnostic and surgical procedures	Safety of donation after silicone or saline implant may need to be assessed. Unlikely to present a hazard to recipient.	Semple et al,[25] 1998
Alternative and complementary medicines	Pharmacologic effects often poorly researched, questions remain about purity of preparations. Caution seems appropriate in most cases. Can be difficult to distinguish during screening between food ingredient and herbal "medicine."	

Donor human milk transmissible infections Infections potentially transmitted via human milk present the most clinically relevant risk to preterm recipients of donor human milk, although the likelihood of transmission via human milk is in most cases quite low.[9] Transmission of infection is the most well understood risk and of most concern to the parents of recipients. Strategies can be developed to appropriately mitigate the hazard. Local assessments of these risks will be required, as geographic variation in the incidence of viruses must be considered (**Table 5**).

Hazards resulting from uncontrolled collection In most DHMBSs, the collection of milk and its initial storage may be uncontrolled by the DHMBS and occur in the donor's home. Time and temperature of storage and during transport impact milk quality and safety.[29] Control measures may be developed to ensure compositional and bacterial content of donated milk is safe. Collection method may also affect bacterial content and shared pumping equipment could result in cross-contamination with unknown/unscreened milk. Where collection is uncontrolled, there is a possibility of the substitution of another's milk and DHMBS may manage this by a range of methods from signed declaration by the donor through to DNA testing (**Table 6**).

Hazards of storage method Human milk banks should consider the potential hazards associated with the intended storage method. Both the duration of storage and the temperature of storage have been shown to alter the bacterial content of human milk and composition[29] (**Table 7**).

Table 5
Human milk transmissible infections

Potential Hazard	Comment	Reference
Viral infections	HIV, HTLV, CMV HCV, HBV other enveloped viruses Nonenveloped viruses	Landers & Hartmann,[9] 2013
Bacterial infections (of breast)	Although processing methods, such as pasteurization, kill most bacteria, high levels of bacteria may not be removed by processing method or some processing methods germinate bacteria endospores.	Landers & Updegrove,[27] 2010
Fungal infections (of breast)	Usually removed by processing methods (pasteurization) but may indicate donor (mammary gland) is not healthy. Fungal transmission may also be reduced by freezing milk.*	*Omarsdottir et al,[28] 2015
Protozoal infections	Requires assessment	
Prion disease (CJD, vCJD)	Unknown transmission risk in breast milk. Excluded as donors in some countries.	Hartmann et al,[3] 2007; HMBANA,[6] 2015
High-risk behaviors	High-risk sexual behavior, IV drug use, prison, occupation (eg, needle stick), cosmetic treatments (including acupuncture or tattoo).	World Health Organisation,[10] 2012
Country of residence and travel	As geographic prevalence of disease varies so does the assessment of the risk.	World Health Organisation,[10] 2012

Abbreviations: CJD, Creutzfeldt-Jakob disease; CMV, cytomegalovirus; DHMBS, donor human milk bank services; HBV, hepatitis B virus; HCV, hepatitis C virus; HIV, human immunodeficiency virus; HTLV, human T-Cell lymphotropic virus; IV, intravenous; vCJD, variant Creutzfeldt-Jakob disease.

Table 6
Hazards from uncontrolled collection

Potential Hazard	Comment	Reference
Hygienic collection and storage	Bacterial contamination risk. Composition changes with storage.	Hartmann & Christen,[29] 2013
Positive identification of donor	A hazard only when collection is uncontrolled.	
Adulteration	A hazard only when collection is uncontrolled.	Keim et al,[30] 2015
Contamination	Accidental or deliberate*, by donor or milk bank staff or volunteers.	*Keim et al,[31] 2013
Allergens	Occasional concern is expressed about cow's milk protein in human milk in the neonatal intensive care unit but this appears to be based on sparse evidence. It does not appear necessary to require donors to exclude dairy products from their diet.	

Hazards specific to processing method Jean-Charles Picaud and Rachel Buffin discuss the effect of various processing methods on donor milk quality (see, "Human Milk—Treatment and Quality of Banked Human Milk," in this issue). Any assessment of the safety of a DHMBS must review the entire process, as different processing methods may exhibit different efficacy against identified hazards and the treatment method itself may introduce specific hazards. For example, it is well established in the food safety literature and milk-banking literature that Holder pasteurization (62.5°C for 30 minutes) germinates *Bacillus cereus* endospores if present in a donated sample.[27] Thermal treatments kill most bacteria in human milk but may not remove heat-stable bacterial enterotoxin, this is established in the food literature for organisms such as *Staphylococcus aureus*.[32] There also may be different considerations with regard to the safety of live versus dead bacteria. Killing bacteria in donor milk may introduce an additional hazard. Gram-negative bacteria may release heat-

Table 7
Potential hazards related to storage method

Potential Hazard	Comment	Reference
Time and temperature of storage	Where donation is stored outside milk bank control, consideration may be given to methods to identify appropriate storage has occurred.	Hartmann & Christen,[29] 2013
Collection container	Material of collection container (stainless steel, glass, plastic) has been demonstrated to affect composition of breast milk due to adherence of components to container wall. There may be intrinsic food safety risks associated with particular containers (glass subject to chipping). Container material itself may leach chemicals into stored product (eg, BPA [Bisphenol-A]). Reprocessed containers may contribute bacterial contamination or cleaning chemical to product.	Hartmann & Christen,[29] 2013

stable endotoxin (lipopolysaccharide) after they die.[32] These bacterial toxins have been associated with NEC in preterm infants.[33] Risk assessments need to consider not only the likelihood and significance of adverse events associated with these hazards but the degree to which adverse events could be identified and attributed to these hazards. As potential adverse events associated with the presence of bacterial toxins in pasteurized donor human milk in a preterm infant (ranging from feed intolerance to NEC) are regular events associated with all feeding types in preterm infants, the ability to attribute these outcomes to PDHM (pasteurised donor human milk) would appear low. It appears unlikely that a universal "bacterial standard" can be developed for all DHMBSs; however, identification of all potential hazards associated with bacterial content of donor human milk will allow local guideline development.

All processing methods designed to remove bacterial or viral hazards will impact the quality of donor human milk. Although direct association with the amount of bioactive protein content in human milk and the clinical outcome in a preterm infant have rarely been established it is hypothesized that maximizing the retention of these components in donor milk may be beneficial to the recipient. Processing methods have varying effects on the retention of bioactive components; excessive damage to these components may reduce the clinical efficacy of the product and increase the risk of adverse events in the recipient.

Research has also suggested that preterm infants fed pasteurized donor human milk exhibit suboptimal growth.[11] Recent research suggests adequate preterm infant growth rates can be achieved on a full human milk and donor human milk diet[34] (**Table 8**).

Potential clinical benefits of donor milk

The clinical benefit of pasteurized donor human milk for the recipient is under continual review by the available literature. This is not intended to constitute a critical review. However, there are beneficial outcomes associated with PDHM use that have a higher quality of evidence than others. These have been discussed elsewhere.[29,37] **Table 9** also considers benefits that are less well established and may be suited to additional research by DHMB. Although milk banks in low-income and middle-income countries may provide product to NICU with the goal of reducing the risk of NEC, product may be provided to other patient groups. These beneficial clinical outcomes for the recipient usually constitute the business case for the cost of a DHMBS. As such, they should be outcomes that are measured.

Table 8
Potential hazards specific to intended processing method

Potential Hazard	Comment	Reference
Bacillus endospore germination	Holder pasteurization.	Landers & Updegrove,[27] 2010
Heat-stable bacterial toxin	Not affected by pasteurization.	Balmer & Wharton,[32] 1992
Bacterial toxin release after death	Identification of bacteria present in donation may be required.	Balmer & Wharton,[32] 1992
Differential effect of processing on viruses	For example, UVC less effective against human immunodeficiency virus.	Christen,[35] 2014
Processing-induced hazards	Reactive oxygen species production by UVC. May not be clinically relevant but requires assessment.	Christen et al,[36] 2013

Table 9
Potential clinical benefits of donor milk banking

Potential Benefit	Comment	Reference
NEC, feed intolerance, postsurgical bowel anomalies, and so forth	Only beneficial in absence of maternal breast milk	Landers & Hartmann,[9] 2013
Increased thymus size in HIV exposed uninfected infants	More research required	Jeppesen et al,[38] 2013
Potential use in pediatric bone marrow transplant recipients	More research required	Davies,[39] 2015

Abbreviations: HIV, human immunodeficiency virus; NEC, necrotizing enterocolitis.

For Donor

Potential clinical hazards of milk donation
There is very little published information regarding the potential clinical risk to a donor from milk donation. **Table 10** was generated from our experience over 10 years and highlights that this is an area that could be subject to additional research.

Potential clinical benefits of milk donation
There may be some clinical benefits of donation for the donor. **Table 11** was generated from our experience of milk banking in Perth.

SOCIAL RESPONSIBILITY OF DONOR HUMAN MILK-BANKING SERVICES

A major goal of this current reassessment of our practice is to ensure that equal attention is given to the social responsibilities of our service, as these have received less attention in the available literature. Recent publications exploring the ethics of donor milk focus mostly on the ethical use of a scarce resource[40] or narrow discussion regarding the ethics of for-profit DHMBS.[41] With the current expansion of milk-banking practice worldwide and the operation of for-profit milk banks it is timely to address the social responsibility of a donor human milk bank. This is done with reference to the previously stated principle that DHMBSs should provide evidence of benefit for recipients and should cause no harm to donors or recipients and with reference to the risk/benefit model for donors and recipients shown in **Fig. 1**.

Table 10
Potential clinical hazards for donor

Potential Hazard	Comment
Nipple trauma from breast pump	Requires suitably qualified staff to assess collection equipment and instruction.
Own infant breastfeeding	Requires development of appropriate screening assessment to ensure excess milk donated and that donor infant's health is protected.
Medications	An individual's desire to donate may influence her decision to start or resume a required medication (depression) and avoid deferral from donation for this reason.
Hazards of collection	Cleaning and sterilization instructions for hygienic collection of donor milk may include hazards (steam burns associated with thermal disinfection of collection bottles).

Table 11	
Potential benefits of milk donation for donor	
Potential Benefit	**Comment**
Sustained lactation	Donors experiencing very large oversupply (2–3 L per day) report being overwhelmed by amount of their milk production. Anecdotally, some of these mothers report before donation they considered ceasing breastfeeding but the "value" of their donation allowed them to continue feeding their own infant.
Reduced mastitis, blocked ducts due to oversupply	Anecdotal reports may be interesting subject for research.
Altruism of donation positively affects postnatal depression	Anecdotally, donors with a history of postnatal depression have reported the value (altruism) associated with donation helped cope with this issue better than after previous childbirth. Research may address this question.

For Recipient

Hazards of donor human milk banking (social responsibility)

In any jurisdiction, DHMBSs should be used only in the absence of a sufficient supply of maternal breast milk. The current recommendation of the American Academy of Pediatrics is as follows:

1. The potential benefits of human milk are such that all preterm infants should receive human milk. Mother's own, fresh or frozen, should be the primary diet for preterm infants, and it should be fortified appropriately for the infant born weighing less than 1500 g.
2. If a mother's own milk is unavailable despite significant lactation support, pasteurized donor milk should be used.[9]

Thus, DHMBS should ensure provision of PDHM does not negatively impact maternal breastfeeding success in the NICU. Practices that may reduce emphasis and support for maternal lactation success should be identified. Williams and colleagues[42] conclude that there is evidence of mainly positive but in some settings, negative effects on maternal breastfeeding when donor human milk is introduced to a neonatal unit. This may indicate that local DHMBS practice influences maternal breastfeeding success.

DHMBSs should also assess the cultural appropriateness of donor human milk-banking practices. The literature reports some milk-banking practices may be a barrier to use by Muslim parents.[43] In principle, DHMBS should provide a service to all patients identified by research as at risk of fed infant formula. A religious belief may a valid reason for parents to not give consent for their infant to receive donor milk. However, recent research suggests milk kinship beliefs for Muslim parents need not be a barrier for donor milk use if strict conditions are met in milk bank practice[43] (**Table 12**).

Benefits of donor human milk banking

An aim of our service is to increase breastfeeding success in the NICU and not decrease maternal breastfeeding at discharge. Audit results suggest we are meeting this aim.[29,42] It must also be shown to be an effective intervention reducing NEC in patients otherwise receiving formula.

Table 12
Potential hazards for recipient/mother

Potential Hazard	Comment	Reference
Donor human milk negatively impacts breastfeeding success in NICU	Possible reduced emphasis on early maternal milk supply.	Williams et al,[42] 2016
Maternal perceptions/expectations of breastfeeding	Research required to better understand interaction between donor milk use and recipient mother's breastfeeding experience.	
Cultural appropriateness of donor milk	Cultural implications for receiving population should be assessed. Milk kinship for Muslim parents is reported in literature*; other cultural beliefs may impact the acceptability of a DHMBS.	*Khalil et al,[43] 2016

Abbreviations: DHMBS, donor human milk bank services; NICU, neonatal intensive care unit.

For Donor

Hazards of human milk banking

In general terms, it is a responsibility of the DHMBS to ensure a donor's own breastfeeding is not affected by the act of donating. The PREM Milk Bank has intermittently received offers of donation from mothers who have self-diagnosed "lactose intolerance" in their breastfed infant. During the assessment of their breastfeeding, it has become evident that they have chosen to formula feed their infant but sustain lactation so as to donate to the PREM Milk Bank. There are ethical concerns about receiving such donations. Some medications are known to decrease milk production.[22] These may be revealed during the course of a milk donor screen. It is a responsibility of the DHMBS to inform the donor of this risk and manage or defer the donor as appropriate to ensure her milk supply is protected for her own infant. Estrogens, progestins (early in lactation), ergot alkaloids, and pseudoephedrine have been shown to decrease milk supply.[22]

Prolonged donation after neonatal death is an area requiring more research. Although in some cases it may be of high value, these studies may exclude participants who did not benefit from bereaved donation.[44] Research is required to ensure it is not harmful to either parent (**Table 13**).

Table 13
Hazards for donor of milk banking

Potential Hazard	Comment
Age (lower limit)	Local legal requirements for informed consent (blood test and donation).
Own infant breastfeeding	Infant must be fully breastfed, not substituting formula so she has excess breast milk.
Stage of lactation	Are donations of colostrum ethical?
Privacy of donor	Should be maintained.
Ethical use of data	Policy should be developed consistent with local requirement.
Sustained donation after neonatal death	Research required to demonstrate no harm for either parent.
Cultural appropriateness	For example, Muslim parents.

Benefits of human milk banking
The establishment of a DHMBS in Perth has increased community engagement with our NICU. We have established a policy supporting donations after neonatal death, where these are of previously expressed milk or made as a mother progresses naturally toward involution. Until research confirms prolonged donation after neonatal death benefits all parents, we are cautious about encouraging this activity (**Table 14**).

COMPLEX ISSUES FOR MILK BANKS

With reference to the risk-benefit model proposed in **Fig. 1**, the previous discussion has not addressed the intersection between risks/benefits for the donor and the risks/benefits for the recipient. This is one of the strengths of this model. It highlights areas of practice in which clinical and social responsibilities of milk banking may conflict, and as such it is an important consideration for milk bank design. It is important for DHMBS to assess practices that may seek to maximize clinical benefit for recipients at the expense of increased risks to the donor. Likewise, there may be practices that benefit the donor and increase the availability and quantity of donation but at the expense of increasing the risk of harm to the recipient. DHMBS must determine appropriate practices that balance these concerns. The most obvious example of such an issue is remuneration of the donor. One hundred percent nonremunerated blood donation is a stated goal of organizations such as the World Health Organization,[45] acknowledging it is the foundation of a safe sustainable blood supply. Although it could be considered a social responsibility (ethical) to financially compensate a mother for her milk,[41] this practice may increase the risk of harm to both recipients and donors. This is of course no longer "donor" human milk banking. Payment may encourage mothers to sell their breast milk and formula feed their own infant, as occurred in Brazil until the 1990s.[46] Or it may incentivize participants to nondisclose potential risks (lifestyle, medication, and illness) that would exclude the sale of their milk. Nondisclosure increases risk of harm to the recipient. Other complex issues appear in **Table 15** .

In addition to the concerns raised in **Table 15** regarding "donor" payments, recent business models encouraging the globalization and commercialization of human milk markets[41] raise the disturbing prospect of commercial milk banks sourcing human milk in low-income and middle-income countries and exporting product for profit to high-income countries. These services cannot use the history of safe donor human milk-banking practice to promote the safety of their service, as the risk profile of the associated product and the potential harm to women selling their milk is very different from the altruistic model. The prior experience in Brazil, where significant harm to breastfeeding outcomes and resulting infant mortality has now been recognized and addressed by milk banks,[46] may be a better model of what to expect from these commercial services.

Table 14	
Potential benefits of human milk banking for donors	
Potential Benefit	**Comment**
Donation after neonatal death	May be high value to donor
Altruism	
Community engagement with neonatal intensive care unit	

Table 15
Benefit to one party, hazard to the other

Benefit or Hazard	Comment
Increased availability of product by payment for milk	Increases clinical hazards to recipient by incentivizing nondisclosure, adulteration, or substitution.[30,31]
Payment for milk benefits "donor"	As above.
Free blood testing service for informal milk sharing	The PREM Milk Bank observes online posts from mothers "advertising" their screening at our bank to others seeking to informally share. Uses milk bank resources and reduces available milk to intended recipient.
Altruism more than oversupply	Screened donors whose desire to help leads to "overestimating" their oversupply. Reduces availability of product to intended recipient.

The PREM Milk Bank is a government-funded public health service. Our goals are similar to not-for-profit services elsewhere. Ironically, the measure of success of the PREM Milk Bank may be how little donor milk product we use, as we seek to maximize maternal breastfeeding success. This meets our social responsibility to support desirable public health outcomes and support breastfeeding and our clinical responsibility to ensure optimal clinical outcomes for preterm infants. This measure of success appears in direct contrast to a commercial service in which profit lies in maximizing the market for a product that is a less desirable outcome to maternal lactation success. We must focus equal research attention on understanding the physiologic barriers to successful lactation after preterm birth.

SUMMARY

The statement "human milk for human babies" is not sufficient justification for the existence of DHMBSs. Evidence of benefit and absence of harm must be continually established by these services. This is particularly the case in which the raw material required by this process is provided by the generosity of individual mothers whose most important role is providing this biological necessity for their own infant. The approach described in this article is considered a starting point for the reassessment of 10 years of safe milk-banking practice in our NICU. By clearly examining the intended benefits and potential hazards of our service, we can improve future practice and inform the development of DHMBSs. The identification of potential hazards undertaken in the preceding sections of this article may serve to highlight the significant differences between donor human milk banking, commercial milk banking, and uncontrolled informal sharing of human milk. Using this assessment as a template, DHMBSs can develop their own recommendations for managing each benefit or hazard identified. This may be the only way to define minimum standards for all forms of milk sharing. Each issue will require local or jurisdictional assessment with regard to the intended service outcomes.

The growth of commercial milk banking and informal sharing bring concerns regarding effective interventions, ethical practice, and safety. With little regulation of milk bank practice, this is unavoidable. Parents, clinicians, communities, and governments will decide acceptable principles; however, we hope that the preceding discussion and systematic approach to describing donor human milk-banking practice informs this discussion and allows objective assessment of the role DHMBS in neonatal intensive care.

Best practices

What is the current practice?

Donor human milk banking is currently informed by historical practice and experience. Evidence-based practice suggests value in the use of pasteurized donor human milk to avoid early formula feeding in VLBW preterm infants. However, DHMBSs provide a wider service with varying levels of evidence of benefit. The expansion of for-profit milk banking risks harm when payment to donor occurs and when profit lies in maximizing use of product in the NICU.

What changes in practice are likely to improve outcome?

The clear and systematic approach outlined in this article to assess both clinical and social responsibility in DHMBS, identifying risks and benefits for both donors and recipients, will define the minimum acceptable standard to practice safe, effective, ethical, and sustainable donor human milk banking.

ACKNOWLEDGMENT

The author acknowledges Tracey Sedgwick and Professor Karen Simmer, who contributed experience and critical review during the preparation of this article.

REFERENCES

1. Omarsdottir S, Casper C, Åkerman A, et al. Breastmilk handling routines for preterm infants in Sweden: a national cross-sectional study. Breastfeed Med 2008; 3(3):165–70.
2. Grøvslien AH, Grønn M. Donor milk banking and breastfeeding in Norway. J Hum Lact 2009;25(2):206–10.
3. Hartmann BT, Pang WW, Keil AD, et al. Best practice guidelines for the operation of a donor human milk bank in an Australian NICU. Early Hum Dev 2007;83:667–73.
4. National Institute for Health and Clinical Excellence. Donor breast milk banks: the operation of donor milk bank services. London: Clinical Guideline (CG) 93, National Institute for Health and Clinical Excellence; 2010.
5. PATH. Strengthening human milk banking: a global implementation framework. Seattle, Washington: PATH, Bill & Melinda Gates Foundation Grand Challenges Initiative; 2013.
6. HMBANA. Guidelines for the establishment and operation of a donor human milk bank. Fort Worth (TX): Human Milk Banking Association of North America; 2015.
7. ICCBBA. ISBT 128 Standard: labelling of human milk banking products. San Bernadino (CA): ICCBBA; 2016.
8. Modi N. Donor breast milk banking: unregulated expansion requires evidence of benefit. BMJ 2006;333:1133–4.
9. Landers S, Hartmann BT. Donor human milk banking and the emergence of milk sharing. Pediatr Clin North Am 2013;60:247–60.
10. World Health Organisation. Blood donor selection: guidelines on assessing donor suitability for blood donation. Geneva (Switzerland): World Health Organisation; 2012. Contract No.: ISBN 978 92 4 154851 9.
11. Quigley MA, Henderson G, Anthony MY, et al. Formula milk versus donor breast milk for feeding preterm or low birthweight infants. Cochrane Database Syst Rev 2007;(4):CD002971.

12. Arslanoglu S, Bertino E, Tonetto P, et al. Guidelines for the Establishment and Operation of a Donor Human Milk Bank. J Matern Fetal Neonatal Med 2010; 23(S2):1–20.
13. Prentice A. Regional variations in the composition of human milk. In: Jensen RG, editor. Handbook of milk composition. Food science and technology. CT: Academic Press; 1995. p. 115–221.
14. Specker BL, Black A, Allen L, et al. Vitamin B-12: low milk concentrations are related to low serum concentrations in vegetarian women and to methylmalonic aciduria in their infants. Am J Clin Nutr 1990;52(6):1073–6.
15. Kedem MH, Mandel D, Domani KA, et al. The effect of advanced maternal age upon human milk fat content. Breastfeed Med 2013;8(1):116–9.
16. Argov-Argaman N, Mandel D, Lubetzky R, et al. Human milk fatty acids composition is affected by maternal age. J Matern Fetal Neonatal Med 2016;1–4 [Epub ahead of print].
17. Grote V, Verduci E, Scaglioni S, et al. Breast milk composition and infant nutrition intakes during the first 12 months of life. Eur J Clin Nutr 2016;70:250–6.
18. Shumer DE, Mehringer JE, Braverman L, et al. Acquired hypothyroidism in an infant related to excessive maternal iodine intake: food for thought. Endocr Pract 2013;19(4):729–31.
19. Picone S, Paolillo P. Chemical contaminants in breast milk. Early Hum Dev 2013; 89:S117–8.
20. Tai PT, Nishijo M, Ahn NTN, et al. Dioxin exposure in breast milk and infant neurodevelopment in Vietnam. Occup Environ Med 2013;70:656–62.
21. Dahlstrom A, Ebersjo C, Lundell B. Nicotine in breast milk influences heart rate variability in the infant. Acta Paediatr 2008;97:1075–9.
22. Hale TW. Medications in breastfeeding mothers of preterm infants. Pediatr Ann 2003;32(5):337–47.
23. Escuder-Vieco D, Garcia-Algar Ó, Joya X, et al. Breast milk and hair testing to detect illegal drugs, nicotine and caffeine in donors to a human milk bank. J Hum Lact 2016;32(3):542–5.
24. Zavaleta N, Lanata C, Butron B, et al. Effect of acute maternal infection on quantity and composition of breast milk. Am J Clin Nutr 1995;62:559–63.
25. Semple JL, Lugowski SJ, Baines CJ, et al. Breast milk contamination and silicone implants: preliminary results using silicon as a proxy measurement for silicone. Plast Reconstr Surg 1998;102(2):528–33.
26. Lawrence RA, Lawrence RM. Breastfeeding: a guide for the medical professional. 6th edition. Elsevier; 2005. p. 1152.
27. Landers S, Updegrove K. Bacteriological screening of donor human milk before and after Holder pasteurisation. Breastfeed Med 2010;5(3):117–21.
28. Omarsdottir S, Casper C, Navér L, et al. Cytomegalovirus infection and neonatal outcome in extremely preterm infants after freezing of maternal milk. Pediatr Infect Dis J 2015;34:482–9.
29. Hartmann BT, Christen L. Donor human milk banking in neonatal intensive care. In: Patole S, editor. Nutrition for the preterm neonate: a clinical perspective. New York: Springer; 2013. p. 367–87.
30. Keim SA, Kulkarni MM, McNamara K, et al. Cow's milk contamination of human milk purchased via the Internet. Pediatrics 2015;135(5):1–5.
31. Keim SA, Hogan JS, McNamara K, et al. Microbial contamination of human milk purchased via the internet. Pediatrics 2013;132(5):e1227–35.
32. Balmer SE, Wharton BA. Human milk banking at a Sorrento maternity hospital, Birmingham. Arch Dis Child 1992;67:556–9.

33. Duffy LC, Zielezny MA, Carrion V, et al. Bacterial toxins and enteral feeding of premature infants at risk for necrotizing enterocolitis. Am J Hum Biol 1998;10:211–9.
34. Hair AB, Hawthorne KM, Chetta KE, et al. Human milk feeding supports adequate growth in infants 1250 grams birth weight. BMC Res Notes 2013;6:459.
35. Christen L. Pasteurization of donor human milk for the use in the neonatal intensive care unit. Crawley: The University of Western Australia; 2014.
36. Christen L, Lai CT, Hartmann BT, et al. The effect of UV-C pasteurisation on bacteriostatic properties and immunological proteins of donor human milk. PLoS One 2013;8(12):e85867.
37. Simmer K, Hartmann BT. The knowns and unknowns of human milk banking. Early Hum Dev 2009;85:701–4.
38. Jeppesen DL, Ersbøll AK, Hoppe TU, et al. Normal thymic size and low rate of infections in human donor milk fed HIV-exposed uninfected infants from birth to 18 months of age. Int J Pediatr 2013;2013:8.
39. Davies S, editor. The potential use of donor milk in young bone marrow transplant recipients. 3rd Annual International Conference on Human Milk Science and Innovation held at Pasadena (CA). September 9–11, 2015.
40. Miracle DJ, Szucs KA, Torke AM, et al. Contemporary ethical issues in human milk banking in the United States. Pediatrics 2011;128:1–6.
41. Medo ET. Increasing the global supply and affordability of donor milk. Breastfeed Med 2013;8(5):438–41.
42. Williams T, Nair H, Simpson J, et al. Use of donor human milk and maternal breasfeeding rates: a systematic review. J Hum Lact 2016;32(2):212–20.
43. Khalil A, Buffin R, Sanlaville D, et al. Milk kinship is not an obstacle to using donor human milk to feed preterm infants in Muslim countries. Acta Paediatr 2016;105:462–7.
44. Welborn J. The experience of expressing and donating breast milk following a perinatal loss. J Hum Lact 2012;28(4):506–10.
45. World Health Organisation. Towards 100% voluntary blood donation. Geneva (Switzerland): World Health Organisation International Federation of Red Cross and Red Crescent Societies; 2010.
46. Arnold LDW. Donor human milk banking: creating public health policy in the 21st century. Cincinnati (OH): Union Institute and University of Cincinnati; 2005.

Variation of Metabolite and Hormone Contents in Human Milk

Hans Demmelmair, PhD*, Berthold Koletzko, MD, PhD

KEYWORDS

- Metabolite • Amino acid • Leptin • Insulin • Body mass index • Human milk

KEY POINTS

- Animal studies show that the lactation period contributes to metabolic programming of offspring health and bioactivity of orally ingested leptin and insulin.
- Levels of many small molecules in human milk are influenced by stage of lactation.
- Variability of small molecule concentrations seems higher in preterm milk than in term milk.
- Maternal body mass index influences milk leptin levels.

Human milk (HM) is the optimal nutrition for infants born at term during the first months of life by itself and thereafter in combination with complementary feeding[1] and for preterm infants if fortified with protein and other nutrients.[2,3] HM is a complex mixture of nutrients with variable composition. The energy content shows large interindividual variation from 50 to 86 kcal/100 mL (mean [M] $\pm$ 2 standard deviation [SD]), as determined in a recent meta-analysis.[4] The variance of the energy content primarily reflects high variation of the fat content but also protein and, to a lesser extent, lactose contents as shown in the analysis of 2554 expressed HM samples in Denmark (**Table 1**).[5] Milk changes with duration of lactation, in particular protein content decreases (**Fig. 1**) whereas fat content increases.[6] Other factors associated with variation in milk composition include duration of gestation, maternal diseases such as diabetes mellitus or malnutrition, genotype, and maternal diet.[7] Energy and macronutrient supply to the breastfed term infant may modulate growth and body composition. For example, higher contribution of protein to total milk energy content at 4 to 8 weeks of lactation has recently been found to predict a higher body mass index at the age of 1 year (**Fig. 2**).[8]

Disclosure Statement: The authors have nothing to disclose.
Division of Metabolism and Nutritional Medicine, Dr. von Hauner Childrens Hospital, University of Munich Medical Center, Lindwurmstrasse 4, 80337 München, Germany
* Corresponding author.
E-mail address: hans.demmelmair@med.uni-muenchen.de

Table 1
Variation of macronutrient and energy content in 2554 human milk samples collected from 224 mothers

Percentiles (%)	2.5	10	50	90	97.5	Ratio 97.5/2.5
Protein (g/L)	6.3	6.9	8.6	11.4	14.3	2.3
Fat (g/L)	18.4	23.8	36.1	54.6	89.0	4.8
Lactose (g/L)	64.2	68.4	72.4	75.2	76.5	1.2
Energy (kcal/L)	500	557	668	840	1115	2.3

Modified from Michaelsen KF, Skafte L, Badsberg JH, et al. Variation in macronutrients in human bank milk: influencing factors and implications for human milk banking. J Pediatr Gastroenterol Nutr 1990;11(2):229–39.

More information has become available in recent years on the concentrations of small molecules and hormones in HM and their variability. This article aims to identify recent information obtained on a broader spectrum of the small molecules in milk by searching the Web site *"Web of Science"* (Available at: http://www.ipscience. thomsonreuters.com/product/web-of-science/. Accessed September 15, 2016) for articles identified by the keywords "metabolomics" and "human milk OR breast milk" (45 articles) and the references in the articles deemed relevant. The discussion of hormones in milk is limited to leptin and insulin, although the presence of a series of further hormones and their potential relevance for the infant has been described. The studies mentioned were identified from the review by Andreas and colleagues[9] or from a *"Web of Science"* search for articles published after 2014 matching the search terms (human milk OR breast milk) and (insulin OR leptin).

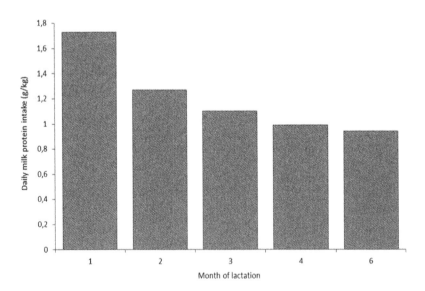

Fig. 1. During the first 6 months of lactation, the protein supply to an exclusively breastfed infant decreases to about 55% of the initial values due to decreasing milk protein concentration. Milk protein intake is calculated as 75% of crude protein intake. (*Data from* World Health Organization. Protein and amino acid requirements in human nutrition. World Health Organ Tech Rep Ser 2002;935:265.)

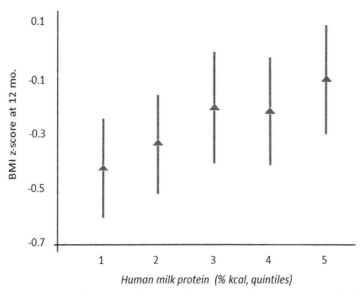

Fig. 2. Protein content of human milk protein from 614 mothers at 4 to 8 weeks of lactation is positively associated with infant BMI z-score at 12 months of age. (*Data from* Prentice P, Ong KK, Schoemaker MH, et al. Breast milk nutrient content and infancy growth. Acta Paediatr 2016;105(6):641–7.)

SMALL MOLECULES AND HORMONES IN HUMAN MILK

In animal studies exploring the impact of lactation on early metabolic programming of the offspring, milk leptin and insulin were reported to induce long-term effects on body weight homeostasis and insulin sensitivity.[10,11] Considerable variability has been described for the concentrations of small molecules in milk found in milk fat globules (eg, triacylglycerol species, glycerophospholipid species, sphingomyelin species, cholesterol), as well as proteins and peptides (proteinogenic amino acids), disaccharides and oligosaccharides (eg, glucose, galactose, fucose), and other components dissolved in HM (eg, amino acids, urea, citrate, 2-ketoglutarate, choline, nucleotides).[12] HM oligosaccharides are not absorbed by the infant to an appreciable extent but bind to endothelial receptors and act as prebiotics with modulating effects on the infant gut microbiome, whereas many of the proteins and peptides seem to have bioactive functions.[6] Among the peptides in HM are peptide hormones (ie, insulin, insulin-like growth factors, leptin, adiponectin, ghrelin) that may contribute to the effects of breastfeeding, such as the lower risk of later obesity, compared with infant formula feeding.[13]

Metabolite, insulin, and leptin levels in the circulation have been studied in relation to infant growth and the risk of obesity, suggesting associations between branched-chain amino acids, hormones, and body weight.[14,15] Investigation of effects of HM metabolite and hormone levels on infant development requires identification and consideration of maternal factors associated with the HM levels to enable interpretation of findings. This article aims at identifying some relevant aspects of HM metabolites, insulin, and leptin, as well as their potential effects on the infant.

The small molecules contained in HM have only recently been in the focus of research. Although they hardly contribute to the total amount of nutrients delivered to the baby, they may have effects on infant growth as well as the development of the gut, the immune system, the nervous system, and other tissues. The concentration of such molecules may reflect maternal metabolism because it is likely that the concentrations of small water-soluble molecules in HM are related to their concentrations in the maternal circulation. Small molecules up to a molecular size of about 1500 d can be studied by metabolomics methodology (ie, the qualitative and quantitative characterization of a large variety of small molecules in biological samples). Several studies have been published applying metabolomics methodology to HM, which have used different analytical techniques (see **Table 1**). Metabolomic analyses allow assessment of a large number of compounds in milk samples, which necessitates the application of sophisticated statistical tools for data analysis. Most HM metabolome studies applied nuclear magnetic resonance (NMR) as the analytical technique (see **Table 1**). NMR covers a wide range of small molecules, and the currently applied technology is suitable to determine concentrations of about 1 μmol/L or higher.[12]

Using a combination of different techniques, Andreas and colleagues[16] detected 710 metabolites in HM with suitable reproducibility using modifications of established procedures for plasma analyses, including Folch extraction, protein elimination by ultrafiltration, and sample preparation with a mixture of methanol and tertiary-butyl-methylether, combined with analyses by NMR, capillary electrophoresis (CE)-mass spectrometry (MS), liquid chromatography (LC)-MS, and gas chromatography (GC)-MS.[16] Villasenor and colleagues[17] described the single-phase extraction of HM with tertiary-butyl-methylether/methanol (1/1), which avoids the distribution of components between a polar and an unpolar phase, and provides an extract suitable for LC analyses and, after derivatization, for GC analyses. The single-phase extraction enables the quantification of polar amino, unpolar diacylglycerols, and many molecules of intermediate polarity from 1 sample extract. In combination with sensitive MS, a 10 to 100 times higher sensitivity compared with NMR can be achieved.[17] Single-phase extraction is also suitable for the quantification of triglyceride-bound fatty acids after their transesterification into methyl esters (Hans Demmelmair, PhD, 2016, unpublished work). The available metabolomics studies (see **Table 1**) have focused on investigating differences between preterm and term milk, and looked at the dependence of metabolite concentrations on the time since delivery. The change of milk composition with lactational stage is relevant for macronutrients[4] because infant dietary requirements change with age, especially protein needs (see **Fig. 1**).[18,19] Six of the 9 identified metabolomics studies reported changes of small molecule concentrations with the duration of lactation (**Table 2**). Changes during the first month of lactation have been reported for carbohydrates but also changes of amino acids have been identified. Thus, for the identification of further factors influencing the small molecules in HM, the day of lactation when the sample is obtained needs to be taken into account, either by collection standardized for duration of lactation, or by corresponding statistical adjustments. Moreover, preterm birth seems to influence metabolites primarily in milk samples collected during early phase of lactation, which corresponds to the finding of attenuated differences of macronutrient contents between term and preterm milk from the third month of lactation onward.[4]

LIPIDS

Regarding HM lipids, metabolomic analyses indicate some influence of gestational and lactational age on short-chain and medium-chain fatty acids, and on triacylglycerol molecular species. Metabolomic studies based on MS can be complemented by the analysis of milk fatty acid composition by transferring esterified fatty acids into methyl esters and subsequent gas liquid chromatographic analyses. Such studies have identified associations of lactation duration, maternal diet,[20] and maternal body mass index (BMI) with milk fatty acid composition.[21]

Table 2
Metabolomics studies of human milk collected during the first 3 months of lactation

Author	Techniques Applied	Focus	Number of Metabolites Detected	Main Findings
Marincola et al,[68] 2012	NMR, GC-MS	Proof of principle	—	PCA differentiates milk metabolome according to lactational week, differences between human milk and formula
Smilowitz et al,[12] 2013	NMR	Analytical and biological variance at day 90 of lactation	65 (including sugars, amino acids, fatty acids, nucleotides)	Relative biological variance only 4% for lactose, <25% for urea, creatinine, glutamate, myo-inositol, valine, citrate, up to 120% for other metabolites alanine and galactose depend on postprandial state
Pratico et al,[69] 2014	NMR	Methodological	43 identified	PCA differentiates samples according to maternal secretor status
Longini et al,[70] 2014	NMR	Influence of gestational and lactational age	—	Only very preterm birth can be identified in the milk metabolome
Villasenor et al,[17] 2014	Single-phase extraction, LC-MS, GC-MS	Methodological	1146	Single-phase extraction is suitable for GC and LC analyses, PCA based on LC-MS data shows differences due to week of collection (week 1 vs week 4)
Andreas et al,[16] 2015	LC-MS, GC-MS, CE-MS, NMR	Methodological	710	Changing metabolite concentrations during the first 10 d of lactation
Spevacek et al,[71] 2015	NMR	Influence of gestational and lactational age	69 (including sugars, amino acids, fatty acids, nucleotides)	Most metabolites changes between day 0–5, day 14, and day 28 of lactation change over time seem different between term and preterm milk
Wu et al,[72] 2016	NMR	Influence of lactational age (day 9–87) in 1 subject	36	PCA differentiates early (until day 24) and late samples
Sundekilde et al,[73] 2016	NMR	Influence of gestational and lactational age	51 identified	Metabolites different between term and preterm infants include: lactose, carnitine, citrate, oligosaccharides after 5–7 wk of lactation milk metabolome is independent of length of gestation

Abbreviation: PCA, Principal Component Analysis.

Observational studies indicate that the influence of the dietary intake on the total content of HM macronutrients, including fat, lactose, and protein, is modest.[22–25] In contrast, dietary fatty acid intake modifies milk fatty acid composition, although body fat stores contribute significantly to milk fatty acid content.[26] As for other lipid compartments, an effect of genetic variation of the enzymes desaturating and elongating essential fatty acids to long-chain polyunsaturated fatty acids has been shown for HM fat.[27] This agrees with the concept that maternal metabolism buffers a wide range of variations of dietary intake ensuring a stable HM macronutrient content. However, variable dietary intake in time or between subject differences of diet or genotype result in different compositions of milk fat and, potentially, in the concentration of dissolved small molecules.

AMINO ACIDS

The influence of maternal body weight on HM macronutrient content has generally been found low in observational studies, with the strongest associations observed for milk protein.[22,28] In infants, higher protein intake has been associated with higher serum amino acid concentrations,[15] higher early weight gain,[8,29,30] and markedly increased obesity risk in later childhood.[31] This agrees with a possible influence of protein content on infant weight gain, observed as unremarkable levels of hormones, lipid species, and carnitine, in a sample of HM consumed by an infant with excessive weight gain (>97. percentile) but with a 1.7-fold higher protein content than expected.[30] If maternal BMI significantly influences free and total milk amino acids, this might contribute to modulating the risk of later offspring obesity. Although several studies have looked at the concentration of free amino acids in breast milk,[32] so far only 1 study has compared the concentrations of free amino acids between lean and obese mothers.[33] In this study, milk samples were collected after 1 month of lactation from 2 groups of 45 women each with a BMI of 21.6 ± 1.4 kg/m^2 (M ± SD) and 34.3 ± 3.9 kg/m^2, respectively. Measured amino acid concentrations were generally similar to previous reports and concentrations of most amino acids did not differ between the groups but there were significantly higher concentrations of branched-chain amino acids (20%), tyrosine (30%), and alanine (12%) in the milk of obese women. Plasma concentrations of these amino acids have been found related to obesity in metabolomics studies.[34] It is assumed that leucine, as a major representative of the branched-chain amino acids, increases anabolism, including protein and lipid synthesis via the mechanistic target of rapamycin (mTOR) pathway.[35] Tyrosine is related to insulin sensitivity.[36] Given that plasma concentrations of these amino acids have been found increased in obese children and nonlactating adults,[34] such increased plasma concentrations might lead to increased milk content. Whether such concentration differences are of relevance for the breastfed baby needs to be clarified because, for most amino acids, the contribution of free amino acids to total amino acid intake is small. The average total branched-chain amino acid content of HM combining free and protein-bound amino acids has been estimated to be around 20 mmol/L, whereas free branched-chain amino acids contribute less than 1% to this amount.[32] Consequently, a 20% relative difference in free amino acids only marginally affects total intake. Nevertheless, free amino acids might have other effects beyond their nutritive value because they may affect gut function via interaction with the G protein-coupled receptor[37] and they enter the circulation more rapidly than protein-bound amino acids.[38]

BIOLOGICAL ROLES OF SMALL MOLECULES IN MILK

The results of animal studies provide further support for the potential importance of small molecules in milk. A series of recent studies in rodents showed that maternal obesity achieved by ad libitum feeding of high-fat diets leads to higher offspring body weight, body fat percentage, and blood pressure in early adulthood, compared with offspring of lean control dams.[39,40] Cross-fostering of the offspring between obese and control dams demonstrated that adverse effects are observed in offspring exposed to overnutrition either during pregnancy or during the lactation period only, or during both periods, demonstrating both prenatal and postnatal metabolic programming in rodents. A protein-reduced ad libitum diet of the dams did not induce changes of protein and lactose content of the milk but fat content decreased. Principal component analysis revealed differences of the concentrations of small molecules analyzed by LC–time-of-flight MS.[41] Further targeted analyses revealed significant differences of the concentrations of free amino acids, which could explain altered metabolic status later in life. The important impact of milk composition is demonstrated by the observation that male rats born after a pregnancy with normal protein supply and switched to milk feeding by dams with a reduced protein diet during lactation showed a slower postnatal growth rate and were protected later in life against fat accretion or insulin-sensitivity loss when exposed to a western diet.[42]

HUMAN MILK HORMONES

The investigation of peptide hormones in HM has received considerable attention. Human studies aim at identifying the maternal predictors of hormone concentrations and their consequences for the infant. The studies in humans are complemented by mechanistic studies in animals. Peptide hormones are a further class of compounds that differentiate HM from infant formula, and they might contribute to the lower obesity risk in breastfed compared with formula-fed infants.[43]

The interest in HM leptin has been stimulated by the finding that gastric cells produce leptin, which is mostly secreted into the gastric lumen and interacts with leptin receptors in the intestine to influence satiety.[44] Thus, milk leptin jointly with stomach-derived leptin may affect dietary intake and infant growth. This points toward a possible important role of HM leptin during the first postnatal weeks, when digestive activity is not yet fully developed and gastric leptin production is still limited, as documented in rats.[45] In fact, infant studies reported inverse relationships between leptin levels in HM collected at the ages of 1, 2, and 4 weeks and later body weight, whereas leptin in milk collected at later ages showed no such relationship.[46–48] A prerequisite for biological activity of HM leptin is that it is not fully denatured in the digestive tract. This can be achieved by a relatively high pH in the stomach of newborn infants but might also be facilitated by binding of leptin to the leptin-binding protein (ie, the soluble form of the leptin receptor).[49] Therefore, not only milk leptin but also the milk concentration of leptin-binding protein should be considered in investigations of the effects on infant development.[50]

The establishment of the maternal BMI as a significant determinant of HM leptin suggests that milk leptin is a component that differentiates milk of obese women from milk of lean women.[9] However, this complicates the investigation of leptin effects on infant growth and adiposity because anthropometric outcomes in infants are also predicted by maternal body weight and body composition.[51] Maternal BMI as a determinant of both HM leptin and infant BMI might establish a correlation between HM leptin and infant fat mass without a direct relevance of HM leptin for infant growth.

Other factors have also been associated with HM leptin (**Table 3**) and, in some cases (eg, years of education, preterm birth), these associations might be partly due to linkage of these factors with maternal BMI. Only 1 study reported a dependence

Table 3
Reported factors associated with human milk leptin concentrations other than maternal body mass index in studies included in the systematic review by Andreas et al[9] and further studies published after 2014

	Maternal BMI	Relationship of Other Factors with HM Leptin Level Reported
Houseknecht et al,[74] 1997	Yes	None reported
Ucar et al,[75] 2000	No	Negative association with maternal high-density lipoprotein cholesterol
Uysal et al,[76] 2002	Yes	None reported
Bielicki et al,[77] 2004	Yes or No	Lower in preterm than in term infants
Dundar et al,[48] 2005	No	Negative association with infant birthweight
Bronsky et al,[78] 2006	Yes	Lower in preterm than in term infants, no effect of infant sex, no effect of cesarean section, no correlation with maternal age
Miralles et al,[47] 2006	Yes	None reported
Weyermann et al,[52] 2007	Yes	Infant sex (lower with male infants), higher in Turkish than in German mothers, higher in mothers with less years of education
Bronsky et al,[79] 2011	No	Month of lactation (colostrum shows highest values, decrease until month 6 of lactation and subsequent increase until month 12)
Eilers et al,[80] 2011	Yes	No difference between term and preterm infants, no association with milk fat content
Schuster et al,[46] 2011	Yes	No association with duration of gestation, birthweight, birth length, infant sex
Fields & Demerath,[81] 2012	Yes	None reported
Savino et al,[82] 2012	No	None reported
Schueler et al,[83] 2013	Yes	No relation to fat content
Brunner et al,[84] 2015	Yes	No effect of n-6 and n-3 fatty acid status
Quinn et al,[85] 2015	Yes	No effect of daily breastfeeding frequency, energy intake, percentage calories from fat in the diet, parity, household wealth, mother's education
Savino et al,[86] 2016	Yes	No effect of infant sex, no influence of duration of lactation
Lemas et al,[60] 2016	Yes	Association between leptin and infant microbiome
Andreas et al,[61] 2016	Yes (foremilk)	Positive association with fat content at lactation day 7, no difference between exclusive and partial breastfeeding

of HM leptin on infant sex, with lower HM leptin in male than in female infants,[52] whereas 3 studies reported no effect of infant sex (see **Table 3**). On the other hand, circulating leptin seems to be lower in male infants than in female infants,[53,54] reflecting higher body fat percentage in female infants at this age.[55] It seems possible that HM leptin might affect growth and body composition differently in male and female infants because the importance of dietary leptin in relation to less endogenously produced leptin could be higher in boys.

The identification of the sources of milk hormones is a further research objective. Milk hormones may be transferred from the maternal circulation into breast milk or synthesized by mammary gland cells and subsequently secreted into milk.[56,57] HM leptin was found to depend on maternal BMI.[9] This suggests that HM leptin reflects maternal leptin synthesis in adipose tissue and/or an increased leptin synthesis in the mammary gland in obese women, as suggested by studies in mice.[58]

Milk insulin is bioactive and can influence offspring growth in animals.[59] Clearly higher HM insulin concentrations have been reported in obese than in lean mothers[60]; however, only 2 of the 4 studies included in the systematic review by Andreas and colleagues[61] showed a significant positive correlation between BMI and HM insulin, whereas 2 other studies reported no correlation. This is unexpected because serum insulin increases with higher BMI.[62] Whether an influence of lactational stage on HM insulin complicates the identification of an association between maternal BMI and HM concentrations of insulin is controversial because not all studies report a change of concentrations between the first week and month 3 of lactation.[13,63] In studies enrolling lean and obese women, Ley and colleagues[64] reported a more than 50% decrease of HM insulin from lactation day 2 (0–7 days) to day 95 (170 pmol/L vs 52 pmol/L, median, n = 117), whereas Andreas and colleagues[61] observed almost identical values for samples from week 1 and month 3 (fore milk: 515 ng/mL vs 525 ng/mL, hind milk: 440 ng/mL vs 457 ng/mL, M, n ≥ 81). The discrepancy may be explained by high variation of the concentration during the first week and slightly later collection of the samples by Andreas and colleagues.[61] Interestingly, Ley and colleagues[64] did not find associations of the HM insulin level with maternal metabolic parameters for early milk samples; however, HM insulin in samples of day 95 was related to prepregnancy BMI, Homeostasis Model Assessment (HOMA) index (week 30 of gestation), and insulin sensitivity (week 30 of gestation).[64] During the first lactation week, HM insulin seems highly variable with time and single measurements might not be sufficient to detect influencing factors and associations with offspring outcome.

HM insulin concentrations have been found similar to plasma concentrations and an active transfer of pancreas-derived insulin into milk has been proposed.[65] This is in contrast to leptin, which shows much lower concentrations in HM than in plasma, although synthesis activity in the mammary gland has been shown.[56] This could suggest that unidentified factors influence the insulin transfer into HM and attenuate the association between maternal BMI and HM insulin concentration.

In addition to confounding factors, covariance of peptide hormones and other components of milk might have to be considered in investigations of the influence of HM hormone concentrations on infant growth and other outcomes. Although this is not obvious for some hormones, in other cases this could be of relevance. Because leptin has been found related to maternal adiposity,[9] this could be related with higher availability of lipid precursors in the circulation, stimulating mammary gland lipid synthesis from long-chain fatty acids and leading finally to milk with a higher fat content or an altered fatty acid composition. Two studies have reported no association of HM leptin and fat content but 1 study found a positive correlation (see **Table 3**).

PERSPECTIVE

Although the number of studies looking at the determinants and effects of small molecules and hormones in HM is still limited, the potential and applicability of such investigations is most promising. Dissolved small molecules in HM might well reflect maternal metabolism but most of the metabolites contribute to the infant diet as components of the macronutrients. There are indications that HM macronutrient composition[8] and hormones influence infant growth, and identification of effects specific for a metabolite or hormone may depend on corresponding adjustments in the data evaluation. Surprisingly, there are very limited data only comparing milk of preterm and term infants, even though the biological relevance of small molecules and hormones provided with milk might be even greater for preterm infants. Lactational stage influences the milk content of many small molecules and maternal BMI modulates free amino acid concentrations[33] and fatty acid composition.[21] Also, maternal obesity, gestational diabetes, and high gestational weight gain, as well as fetal intrauterine growth restriction, may well be related to milk metabolite concentrations.[66,67] Further investigation of determinants of the concentrations of metabolites in HM are warranted, given that milk metabolites must be expected to contribute to perinatal programming and new opportunities for preventive interventions may arise. For example, metabolites in milk may be specifically influenced by body weight reduction, dietary modification, or other lifestyle choices. Identification of factors related to the variance of metabolites and peptide hormones in HM is a promising tool for the elucidation of the physiologic processes of lactogenesis and determinants of HM composition. This could contribute to the implementation of measures to avoid adverse programming of long-term health during the perinatal period and might help to improve the long-term outcome of infants and mothers after complicated pregnancies.[67] Making use of the full potential will require a combination of determining small molecules, hormones, and macronutrients in HM.

REFERENCES

1. Prell C, Koletzko B. Breastfeeding and complementary feeding. Dtsch Arztebl Int 2016;113(25):435–44.
2. Koletzko B, Poindexter B, Uauy R. World review of nutrition and dietetics: nutritional care of preterm infants. Basel (Switzerland): Karger; 2014.
3. Agostoni C, Buonocore G, Carnielli VP, et al, ESPGHAN-Committee-on-Nutrition. Enteral nutrient supply for preterm infants: commentary from the European Society of Paediatric Gastroenterology, Hepatology and nutrition Committee on nutrition. J Pediatr Gastroenterol Nutr 2010;50(1):85–91.
4. Gidrewicz DA, Fenton TR. A systematic review and meta-analysis of the nutrient content of preterm and term breast milk. BMC Pediatr 2014;14:216.
5. Michaelsen KF, Skafte L, Badsberg JH, et al. Variation in macronutrients in human bank milk: influencing factors and implications for human milk banking. J Pediatr Gastroenterol Nutr 1990;11(2):229–39.
6. Rodriguez-Palmero M, Koletzko B, Kunz C, et al. Nutritional and biochemical properties of human milk, Part II: lipids, micronutrients, and bioactive factors. Clin Perinatol 1999;26(2):335–59.
7. Jensen RG. Handbook of milk composition. New York: Academic Press; 1995.
8. Prentice P, Ong KK, Schoemaker MH, et al. Breast milk nutrient content and infancy growth. Acta Paediatr 2016;105(6):641–7.
9. Andreas NJ, Hyde MJ, Gale C, et al. Effect of maternal body mass index on hormones in breast milk: a systematic review. PLoS One 2014;9(12):e115043.
10. Pico C, Oliver P, Sanchez J, et al. The intake of physiological doses of leptin during lactation in rats prevents obesity in later life. Int J Obes (Lond) 2007;31(8):1199–209.
11. Gorski JN, Dunn-Meynell AA, Hartman TG, et al. Postnatal environment overrides genetic and prenatal factors influencing offspring obesity and insulin resistance. Am J Physiol Regul Integr Comp Physiol 2006;291(3):R768–78.

12. Smilowitz JT, O'Sullivan A, Barile D, et al. The human milk metabolome reveals diverse oligosaccharide profiles. J Nutr 2013;143(11):1709–18.
13. Fields DA, Schneider CR, Pavela G. A narrative review of the associations between six bioactive components in breast milk and infant adiposity. Obesity (Silver Spring) 2016;24(6):1213–21.
14. Perng W, Gillman MW, Fleisch AF, et al. Metabolomic profiles and childhood obesity. Obesity (Silver Spring) 2014;22(12):2570–8.
15. Socha P, Grote V, Gruszfeld D, et al, European Childhood Obesity Trail Study Group. Milk protein intake, the metabolic-endocrine response, and growth in infancy: data from a randomized clinical trial. Am J Clin Nutr 2011;94(6): 1776S–84S.
16. Andreas NJ, Hyde MJ, Gomez-Romero M, et al. Multiplatform characterization of dynamic changes in breast milk during lactation. Electrophoresis 2015;36(18): 2269–85.
17. Villasenor A, Garcia-Perez I, Garcia A, et al. Breast milk metabolome characterization in a single-phase extraction, multiplatform analytical approach. Anal Chem 2014;86(16):8245–52.
18. Lonnerdal B, Hernell O. An opinion on "staging" of infant formula: a developmental perspective on infant feeding. J Pediatr Gastroenterol Nutr 2016;62(1):9–21.
19. Koletzko BV, Shamir R. Infant formula: does one size fit all? Curr Opin Clin Nutr Metab Care 2016;19(3):205–7.
20. Jensen RG. Lipids in human milk. Lipids 1999;34:1243–71.
21. Makela J, Linderborg K, Niinikoski H, et al. Breast milk fatty acid composition differs between overweight and normal weight women: the STEPS Study. Eur J Nutr 2013;52(2):727–35.
22. Nommsen LA, Lovelady CA, Heinig MJ, et al. Determinants of energy, protein, lipid, and lactose concentrations in human milk during the first 12 mo of lactation: the DARLING Study. Am J Clin Nutr 1991;53(2):457–65.
23. Quinn EA, Largado F, Power M, et al. Predictors of breast milk macronutrient composition in Filipino mothers. Am J Hum Biol 2012;24(4):533–40.
24. Koletzko B, Rodriguez-Palmero M, Demmelmair H, et al. Physiological aspects of human milk lipids. Early Hum Dev 2001;65:S3–18.
25. Koletzko B, Agostoni C, Bergmann R, et al. Physiological aspects of human milk lipids and implications for infant feeding: a workshop report. Acta Paediatr 2011; 100(11):1405–15.
26. Demmelmair H, Kuhn A, Dokoupil K, et al. Human lactation: oxidation and maternal transfer of dietary (13)C-labelled alpha-linolenic acid into human milk. Isotopes Environ Health Stud 2016;52(3):270–80.
27. Lattka E, Rzehak P, Szabo E, et al. Genetic variants in the FADS gene cluster are associated with arachidonic acid concentrations of human breast milk at 1.5 and 6 mo postpartum and influence the course of milk dodecanoic, tetracosenoic, and trans-9-octadecenoic acid concentrations over the duration of lactation. Am J Clin Nutr 2011;93(2):382–91.
28. Chang N, Jung JA, Kim H, et al. Macronutrient composition of human milk from Korean mothers of full term infants born at 37-42 gestational weeks. Nutr Res Pract 2015;9(4):433–8.
29. Koletzko B, von Kries R, Closa R, et al. Lower protein in infant formula is associated with lower weight up to age 2 y: a randomized clinical trial. Am J Clin Nutr 2009;89(6):1836–45.
30. Grunewald M, Hellmuth C, Demmelmair H, et al. Excessive weight gain during full breast-feeding. Ann Nutr Metab 2014;64(3–4):271–5.

31. Weber M, Grote V, Closa-Monasterolo R, et al. Lower protein content in infant formula reduces BMI and obesity risk at school age: follow-up of a randomized trial. Am J Clin Nutr 2014;99(5):1041–51.

32. Zhang Z, Adelman AS, Rai D, et al. Amino acid profiles in term and preterm human milk through lactation: a systematic review. Nutrients 2013;5(12):4800–21.

33. De Luca A, Hankard R, Alexandre-Gouabau MC, et al. Higher concentrations of branched-chain amino acids in breast milk of obese mothers. Nutrition 2016; 32(11–12):1295–8.

34. Rauschert S, Uhl O, Koletzko B, et al. Metabolomic biomarkers for obesity in humans: a short review. Ann Nutr Metab 2014;64(3–4):314–24.

35. Newgard CB, An J, Bain JR, et al. A branched-chain amino acid-related metabolic signature that differentiates obese and lean humans and contributes to insulin resistance. Cell Metab 2009;9(4):311–26.

36. Hellmuth C, Kirchberg FF, Lass N, et al. Tyrosine is associated with insulin resistance in longitudinal metabolomic profiling of obese children. J Diabetes Res 2016;2016:2108909.

37. San Gabriel A, Uneyama H. Amino acid sensing in the gastrointestinal tract. Amino Acids 2013;45(3):451–61.

38. Agostoni C, Terracciano L, Varin E, et al. The nutritional value of protein-hydrolyzed formulae. Crit Rev Food Sci Nutr 2016;56(1):65–9.

39. Li L, Xue J, Li HY, et al. Over-nutrient environment during both prenatal and postnatal development increases severity of islet injury, hyperglycemia, and metabolic disorders in the offspring. J Physiol Biochem 2015;71(3):391–403.

40. Desai M, Jellyman JK, Han G, et al. Maternal obesity and high-fat diet program offspring metabolic syndrome. Am J Obstet Gynecol 2014;211(3):237.e1-e13.

41. Martin Agnoux A, Antignac JP, Boquien CY, et al. Perinatal protein restriction affects milk free amino acid and fatty acid profile in lactating rats: potential role on pup growth and metabolic status. J Nutr Biochem 2015;26(7):784–95.

42. Agnoux AM, Antignac JP, Simard G, et al. Time window-dependent effect of perinatal maternal protein restriction on insulin sensitivity and energy substrate oxidation in adult male offspring. Am J Physiol Regul Integr Comp Physiol 2014;307(2): R184–97.

43. Savino F, Fissore MF, Liguori SA, et al. Can hormones contained in mothers' milk account for the beneficial effect of breast-feeding on obesity in children? Clin Endocrinol (Oxf) 2009;71(6):757–65.

44. Guilmeau S, Buyse M, Bado A. Gastric leptin: a new manager of gastrointestinal function. Curr Opin Pharmacol 2004;4(6):561–6.

45. Oliver P, Pico C, De Matteis R, et al. Perinatal expression of leptin in rat stomach. Dev Dyn 2002;223(1):148–54.

46. Schuster S, Hechler C, Gebauer C, et al. Leptin in maternal serum and breast milk: association with infants' body weight gain in a longitudinal study over 6 months of lactation. Pediatr Res 2011;70(6):633–7.

47. Miralles O, Sanchez J, Palou A, et al. A physiological role of breast milk leptin in body weight control in developing infants. Obesity (Silver Spring) 2006;14(8): 1371–7.

48. Dundar NO, Anal O, Dundar B, et al. Longitudinal investigation of the relationship between breast milk leptin levels and growth in breast-fed infants. J Pediatr Endocrinol Metab 2005;18(2):181–7.

49. Cammisotto PG, Gingras D, Renaud C, et al. Secretion of soluble leptin receptors by exocrine and endocrine cells of the gastric mucosa. Am J Physiol Gastrointest Liver Physiol 2006;290(2):G242–9.

50. Zepf FD, Rao P, Moore J, et al. Human breast milk and adipokines–A potential role for the soluble leptin receptor (sOb-R) in the regulation of infant energy intake and development. Med Hypotheses 2016;86:53–5.
51. Castillo-Laura H, Santos IS, Quadros LC, et al. Maternal obesity and offspring body composition by indirect methods: a systematic review and meta-analysis. Cad Saude Publica 2015;31(10):2073–92.
52. Weyermann M, Brenner H, Rothenbacher D. Adipokines in human milk and risk of overweight in early childhood: a prospective cohort study. Epidemiology 2007; 18(6):722–9.
53. Savino F, Fissore MF, Grassino EC, et al. Ghrelin, leptin and IGF-I levels in breast-fed and formula-fed infants in the first years of life. Acta Paediatr 2005;94(5): 531–7.
54. Lonnerdal B, Havel PJ. Serum leptin concentrations in infants: effects of diet, sex, and adiposity. Am J Clin Nutr 2000;72(2):484–9.
55. Carberry AE, Colditz PB, Lingwood BE. Body composition from birth to 4.5 months in infants born to non-obese women. Pediatr Res 2010;68(1):84–8.
56. Catli G, Olgac Dundar N, Dundar BN. Adipokines in breast milk: an update. J Clin Res Pediatr Endocrinol 2014;6(4):192–201.
57. Hovey RC, Aimo L. Diverse and active roles for adipocytes during mammary gland growth and function. J Mammary Gland Biol Neoplasia 2010;15(3):279–90.
58. Kamikawa A, Ichii O, Yamaji D, et al. Diet-induced obesity disrupts ductal development in the mammary glands of nonpregnant mice. Dev Dyn 2009;238(5): 1092–9.
59. Shehadeh N, Sukhotnik I, Shamir R. Gastrointestinal tract as a target organ for orally administered insulin. J Pediatr Gastroenterol Nutr 2006;43(3):276–81.
60. Lemas DJ, Young BE, Baker PR 2nd, et al. Alterations in human milk leptin and insulin are associated with early changes in the infant intestinal microbiome. Am J Clin Nutr 2016;103(5):1291–300.
61. Andreas NJ, Hyde MJ, Herbert BR, et al. Impact of maternal BMI and sampling strategy on the concentration of leptin, insulin, ghrelin and resistin in breast milk across a single feed: a longitudinal cohort study. BMJ Open 2016;6(7):e010778.
62. Mayfield J. Diagnosis and classification of diabetes mellitus: new criteria. Am Fam Physician 1998;58(6):1355–62, 1369–70.
63. Koldovsky O, Thornburg W. Hormones in milk. J Pediatr Gastroenterol Nutr 1987; 6(2):172–96.
64. Ley SH, Hanley AJ, Sermer M, et al. Associations of prenatal metabolic abnormalities with insulin and adiponectin concentrations in human milk. Am J Clin Nutr 2012;95(4):867–74.
65. Whitmore TJ, Trengove NJ, Graham DF, et al. Analysis of insulin in human breast milk in mothers with type 1 and type 2 diabetes mellitus. Int J Endocrinol 2012; 2012:296368.
66. Cesare Marincola F, Dessi A, Corbu S, et al. Clinical impact of human breast milk metabolomics. Clin Chim Acta 2015;451(Pt A):103–6.
67. De Magistris A, Marincola FC, Fanos V, et al. Nutrimetabolomics and adipocitokines in the "great obstetrical syndromes". Pediatr Endocrinol Rev 2015;13(2): 546–58.
68. Marincola FC, Noto A, Caboni P, et al. A metabolomic study of preterm human and formula milk by high resolution NMR and GC/MS analysis: preliminary results. J Matern Fetal Neonatal Med 2012;25(Suppl 5):62–7.
69. Pratico G, Capuani G, Tomassini A, et al. Exploring human breast milk composition by NMR-based metabolomics. Nat Prod Res 2014;28(2):95–101.

70. Longini M, Tataranno ML, Proietti F, et al. A metabolomic study of preterm and term human and formula milk by proton MRS analysis: preliminary results. J Matern Fetal Neonatal Med 2014;27(Suppl 2):27–33.
71. Spevacek AR, Smilowitz JT, Chin EL, et al. Infant maturity at birth reveals minor differences in the maternal milk metabolome in the first month of lactation. J Nutr 2015;145(8):1698–708.
72. Wu J, Domellof M, Zivkovic AM, et al. NMR-based metabolite profiling of human milk: a pilot study of methods for investigating compositional changes during lactation. Biochem Biophys Res Commun 2016;469(3):626–32.
73. Sundekilde UK, Downey E, O'Mahony JA, et al. The effect of gestational and lactational age on the human milk metabolome. Nutrients 2016;8(5).
74. Houseknecht KL, McGuire MK, Portocarrero CP, et al. Leptin is present in human milk and is related to maternal plasma leptin concentration and adiposity. Biochem Biophys Res Commun 1997;240(3):742–7.
75. Ucar B, Kirel B, Bor O, et al. Breast milk leptin concentrations in initial and terminal milk samples: relationships to maternal and infant plasma leptin concentrations, adiposity, serum glucose, insulin, lipid and lipoprotein levels. J Pediatr Endocrinol Metab 2000;13(2):149–56.
76. Uysal FK, Onal EE, Aral YZ, et al. Breast milk leptin: its relationship to maternal and infant adiposity. Clin Nutr 2002;21(2):157–60.
77. Bielicki J, Huch R, von Mandach U. Time-course of leptin levels in term and preterm human milk. Eur J Endocrinol 2004;151(2):271–6.
78. Bronsky J, Karpisek M, Bronska E, et al. Adiponectin, adipocyte fatty acid binding protein, and epidermal fatty acid binding protein: proteins newly identified in human breast milk. Clin Chem 2006;52(9):1763–70.
79. Bronsky J, Mitrova K, Karpisek M, et al. Adiponectin, AFABP, and leptin in human breast milk during 12 months of lactation. J Pediatr Gastroenterol Nutr 2011; 52(4):474–7.
80. Eilers E, Ziska T, Harder T, et al. Leptin determination in colostrum and early human milk from mothers of preterm and term infants. Early Hum Dev 2011;87(6): 415–9.
81. Fields DA, Demerath EW. Relationship of insulin, glucose, leptin, IL-6 and TNF-alpha in human breast milk with infant growth and body composition. Pediatr Obes 2012;7(4):304–12.
82. Savino F, Sorrenti M, Benetti S, et al. Resistin and leptin in breast milk and infants in early life. Early Hum Dev 2012;88(10):779–82.
83. Schueler J, Alexander B, Hart AM, et al. Presence and dynamics of leptin, GLP-1, and PYY in human breast milk at early postpartum. Obesity (Silver Spring) 2013; 21(7):1451–8.
84. Brunner S, Schmid D, Zang K, et al. Breast milk leptin and adiponectin in relation to infant body composition up to 2 years. Pediatr Obes 2015;10(1):67–73.
85. Quinn EA, Largado F, Borja JB, et al. Maternal characteristics associated with milk leptin content in a sample of Filipino women and associations with infant weight for age. J Hum Lact 2015;31(2):273–81.
86. Savino F, Sardo A, Rossi L, et al. Mother and infant body mass index, breast milk leptin and their serum leptin values. Nutrients 2016;8(6):383.

Preterm Human Milk Macronutrient and Energy Composition

A Systematic Review and Meta-Analysis

Francis B. Mimouni, MD[a,b,1], Ronit Lubetzky, MD[b,c,1],
Sivan Yochpaz, MD[c], Dror Mandel, MD[b,d],*

KEYWORDS

- Human milk • Breastfeeding • Macronutrients • Preterm

KEY POINTS

- The current systematic review allows the clinician to calculate in a more evidence-based manner the macronutrient and energy intakes of a preterm infant fed his own mother's milk.
- The numbers we provide here for all macronutrients and energy contents are reliable, since they are based on a very large sample of studies which all used the same methodology of pooled 24 hours human milk collection.
- Theoretical calculations on energy and macronutrient intake of preterm infant must be made according to a lactation time specific manner. This is particularly crucial for protein content which is essentially half's itself within 10–12 weeks.

INTRODUCTION

Human milk (HM) is a living and highly dynamic biological fluid that is nutrient specific to adapt to the needs of the growing human infant.[1] Its composition is notoriously variable and depends on several factors, only some of which are currently known.[2–9] For instance, there is striking mother-to-mother variability, which may be caused by differences in dietary habits but might also be related to other environmental or genetic variables.[2] These differences may explain the day-to-day[3] and day-to-night[4,5] variations in HM macronutrient content. Moreover, HM composition also varies as lactation progresses over time[6] or as maternal age increases[7,8] but seems to be unaffected by

[a] Department of Neonatology, Shaare Zedek Medical Center, 12 Shmuel Bait Street, Jerusalem 913102, Israel; [b] Sackler Faculty of Medicine, Tel Aviv University, Tel Aviv, Israel; [c] Department of Pediatrics, Dana Dwek Children's Hospital, Tel Aviv Sourasky Medical Center, 6 Weizman Street, Tel Aviv 64239, Israel; [d] Department of Neonatology, Dana Dwek Children's Hospital, Tel Aviv Sourasky Medical Center, 6 Weizman Street, Tel Aviv 64239, Israel
[1] These authors contributed equally to this article.
* Corresponding author.
E-mail address: dmandel@post.tau.ac.il

Clin Perinatol 44 (2017) 165–172
http://dx.doi.org/10.1016/j.clp.2016.11.010
perinatology.theclinics.com

breast size or breast asymmetry.[9] In 1978, it was reported for the first time that gestational age at delivery affects the composition of HM, and it was even argued that preterm HM, with its higher protein content, is more adapted to the nutritional needs of the preterm infant, as if there were physiologic mechanisms that may allow for this to happen.[10] In spite of the differences between term HM and preterm HM, it is now clear that even its own mother's milk alone cannot provide sufficient nutrition to the preterm infant, hence, the need for fortification. In recent years, there have been attempts to tailor the amount of fortification of HM based on bedside analysis of expressed HM, rather than by using calculations based on the known, theoretic content of the milk used. Unfortunately, this strategy requires expensive technology (near-infrared spectroscopy)[11] and is yet to show its superiority in terms of growth outcomes.

This systematic review of the macronutrient and energy composition of preterm HM will help enable the practicing neonatologist make informed and more precise nutritional decisions with regard to feeding the preterm infant.

MATERIALS AND METHODS

This systematic review was conducted in August 2016. Only studies reporting biochemical composition of human preterm milk (<37 weeks' gestational age) were included. One author searched MEDLINE, EMBASE, and Google Scholar using the key words: *preterm, prematurity, human milk, breast milk, macronutrients, fat, lipid, protein, carbohydrates, lactose, energy,* and *calories.* The references in studies identified as potentially relevant were also examined. Three authors screened titles and abstracts of all records identified by the search and coded records as "order" or "exclude." All records coded as order were assessed and the final decision was made about which records were ordered as full-text articles. The full texts were read to assess suitability for inclusion based on prespecified inclusion and exclusion criteria. Then the data were extracted independently using a data collection form to aid extraction of information on design, methods, and participants from each included study. Disagreements were discussed until a consensus was reached. If data from a given article were insufficient, the report was excluded from analysis. For the purpose of the meta-analysis, only articles that provided macronutrients and/or energy analysis from a pooled milk sample of a total 24 hours collection were retained, as suggested by Ballard and Morrow.[12] All studies reporting outcomes exclusively on term infants were excluded, but studies that reported preterm and term HM data (and excluded the term *data* from the same papers) were retained.

Analysis

Meta-analyses were conducted in all the studies that reported 1 or more of the following: total energy (kilocalories per deciliter), true protein (grams per deciliter), fat (grams per deciliter) and lactose (grams per deciliter). To help compare our analysis with the previous meta-analysis of Gidrewicz and Fenton[13] we also group the data into the following lactation days: 1 to 3 days (ie, colostrum), 4 to 7 days, week 2, week 3 to 4, week 5 to 6, week 7 to 9, and week 10 to 12. We noted for each study whether analyses were conducted using chemical methods (for protein, lactose, and fat) or near infrared spectroscopy (NIRS) and those calculating energy content using theoretic considerations versus those that used bomb calorimetry. The Minitab Statistical Package, version 16 (Minitab; State College, PA) was used for analyses. Meta-analyses were calculated and expressed as weighted averages with pooled standard deviations. Variation over time of macronutrients and energy was also studied using linear regression. Results are expressed as mean $\pm$ standard deviation, and a P-value of less than .05 was deemed significant.

RESULTS

Fig. 1 depicts a flow diagram of the literature search process. A total of 109 full-text articles was reviewed, of which 23 studies reported the outcomes that were of interest for the current study.[14–37] Three articles were excluded because they did not specify the exact timeframe of the sampling,[27–29] 6 others were excluded because they presented data in a way that did not allow for precise calculations of means and standard deviation,[30–35] and an additional study was excluded because it was the complete expression of only 1 breast.[36] A total of 13 articles was included in the final meta-analysis.[14–26]

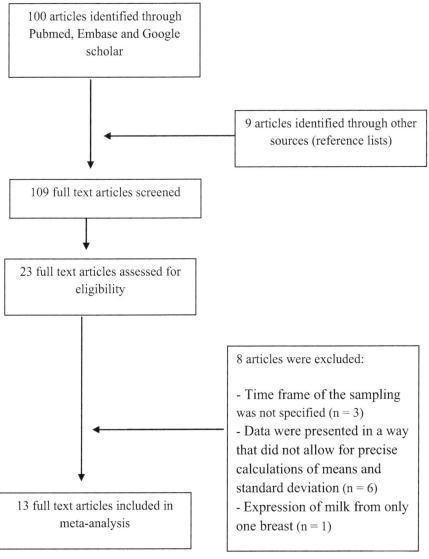

Fig. 1. Flow diagram of the analysis process.

Most studies used chemical methods. However, because NIRS provided results that were not significantly different from those obtained from chemical methods, NIRS and chemistry results were pooled in the analysis as were energy data because the percent difference between calculated and measured energy content was nearly null. **Table 1** depicts the means and standard deviations and sample size of macronutrients and energy content of HM at the various lactation periods described. Importantly, protein content decreases massively and significantly from day 1 to 3 to half this value at week 10 to 12 (**Fig. 2**; $R^2 = 0.93$, $P<.0001$). There was a significant linear increase in lactose, fat, and energy content during the same timeframe (**Figs. 3–5**; $R^2 = 0.80$, $P = .006$; $R^2 = 0.94$, $P = .02$; and $R^2 = 0.81$, $P = .006$, respectively).

DISCUSSION

The current systematic review should allow clinicians to calculate the macronutrient and energy intakes of a preterm infant fed his own mother's milk based on currently available evidence.

Many factors may influence the characteristics of HM. Woman-to-woman, day-to-night, and day-to-day differences and the various maternal dietary factors potentially may affect HM composition. The technology of bedside analysis of macronutrients and energy composition of HM exists, such as, NIRS, and its use is increasing, although methodologic concerns have been raised.[38] However, it would be extraordinarily time consuming and labor intensive to routinely perform these analyses on every single sample provided by the mother of a preterm infant. Thus, most institutions that do not have access to HM analysis technology use gross assumptions of the HM composition. These assumptions usually do not take into account the postnatal age of the child, which, as shown here, affects significantly the composition of HM. Over the first 12 weeks after delivery of a preterm infant, his or her mother's HM depicts a progressive decline of protein concentration together with a progressive increase

Table 1
Means and standard deviations and sample size of macronutrients and energy content of HM at a various lactation periods

	Protein (g/100 mL)	Lactose/Carbohydrates (g/100 mL)	Fat (g/100 mL)	Energy (kCal/100 mL)
Day 1–3	n = 163 2.57 ± 1.44	n = 143 6.2 ± 0.92	n = 173 2.52 ± 0.98	n = 143 58.8 ± 7.91
Day 4–7	n = 44 2.11 ± 0.44	n = 87 6.17 ± 0.49	n = 110 3.31 ± 1.27	n = 96 67.9 ± 14.1
Week 2	n = 383 1.98 ± 0.68	n = 389 6.72 ± 0.46	n = 426 3.19 ± 1.04	n = 417 69.1 ± 10.1
Week 3–4	n = 528 1.6 ± 0.5	n = 464 7.05 ± 0.51	n = 485 3.83 ± 1.01	n = 481 70.87 ± 9.34
Week 5–6	n = 330 1.43 ± 0.25	n = 354 7.14 ± 0.36	n = 371 4.04 ± 0.91	n = 354 73.97 ± 9.1
Week 7–9	n = 223 1.34 ± 0.2	n = 235 7.13 ± 0.38	n = 236 4.21 ± 0.92	n = 239 74.24 ± 8.77
Week 10–12	n = 120 1.26 ± 0.2	n = 120 7.12 ± 0.28	n = 120 4.25 ± 0.91	n = 120 74.53 ± 8.71

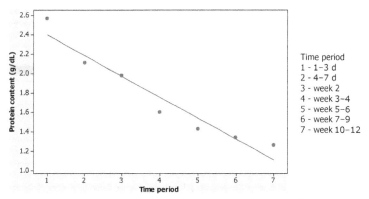

Fig. 2. Correlation between time of lactation and protein content ($R^2 = 0.93$, $P<.0001$).

in fat and energy concentrations. In contrast, carbohydrates first increase, then reach a steady state.

Our systematic review is not the first one on this topic. That of Gidrewicz and Fenton[13] published 2 years ago also provided the nutrient contents of preterm and term breast milk. In their systematic review, Gidrewicz and Fenton[13] were able to retrieve 41 studies that reported various constituents of HM. All retrieved studies were performed in developed countries mostly from the western world to decrease the bias of possible maternal malnutrition. Our systematic review allowed retrieval of all the above-mentioned articles plus 24 additional articles. Moreover, in their study, Gidrewicz and Fenton[13] retained for the meta-analysis all studies that used 24-hour breast milk collection only for energy and fat, because they felt that differences between foremilk and hindmilk and diurnally on protein are not important. Moreover, only 26 of the 41 retrieved studies in the report by Gidrewicz and Fenton[13] properly related to preterm infants, with a total impressive sample size of 843 infants. However, a careful examination of the tables finds that at various time points, the sample size for analysis was small. For instance, in the sample size for days 1 to 3 of lactation, they were not able to retrieve any sample for calculated energy content, and they had a sample size of 41 only at days 4 to 7. In comparison, in the current study, the authors were able to retrieve a sample size of 143 for energy content at days 1 to 3 and 96 at days 4 to 7. Thus, the authors feel confident that the numbers provided here for all macronutrients

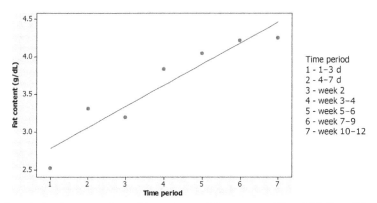

Fig. 3. Correlation between time of lactation and fat content ($R^2 = 0.94$, $P = .02$).

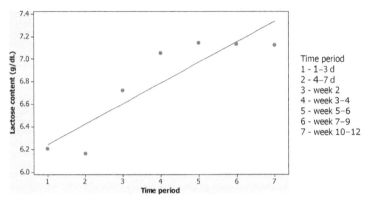

Fig. 4. Correlation between time of lactation and lactose content ($R^2 = 0.80$, $P = .006$).

and energy contents are more reliable, as they are based on a much larger sample size from studies that all used the same methodology of pooled 24-hour HM collection, thereby avoiding the biases of diurnal and hind-versus-foremilk variations. By the time this report was submitted for publication, another systematic review was published in September 2016.[37] The latter study included in its final analyses 24 articles because of laxer inclusion criteria. The results are expressed as week 1 results (thus does not differentiate between colostrum and transitional milk) and week 2 to 8, therefore, pooling all results after week 1, which does not provide the clinician an opportunity to detect the major but progressive compositional changes that occur during such an extended period.

The results provided here indicate specifically that theoretic calculation on energy and macronutrient intake of preterm infants must be made according to a lactation time-specific manner. This is particularly crucial for protein content, which essentially is cut in half within 10 to 12 weeks. The energy content and the fat content were strikingly related, a feature of HM that has been amply described in the past.[6] The increase in fat content over time that this meta-analysis describes is probably not limited to the first 12 weeks of lactation. The authors previously reported extraordinarily high concentrations of fat in prolonged (more than 1 year) lactation.[6] NIRS technology and chemical methods gave such similar results that for practical purposes the authors believe that if used at a bedside it is likely that the NIRS technology can be considered quite reliable.

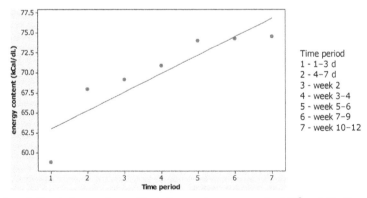

Fig. 5. Correlation between time of lactation and energy content ($R^2 = 0.81$, $P = .006$).

REFERENCES

1. American Academy of Pediatrics Section on Breastfeeding. Breastfeeding and the use of human milk". Pediatrics 2012;129:e827–41.
2. Harzer G, Haug M, Dieterich I, et al. Changing patterns of human milk lipids in the course of the lactation and during the day. Am J Clin Nutr 1983;37:612–21.
3. Mitoulas LR, Kent JC, Cox DB, et al. Variation in fat, lactose and protein in human milk over 24 h and throughout the first year of lactation. Br J Nutr 2002;88:29–37.
4. Lubetzky R, Littner Y, Mimouni FB, et al. Circadian variations in fat content of expressed breast milk from mothers of preterm infants. J Am Coll Nutr 2006;25: 151–4.
5. Lubetzky R, Mimouni FB, Dollberg S, et al. Consistent circadian variations in creamatocrit over the first 7 weeks of lactation: a longitudinal study. Breastfeed Med 2007;2:15–8.
6. Mandel D, Lubetzky R, Dollberg S, et al. Fat and energy contents of expressed human breast milk in prolonged lactation. Pediatrics 2005;116:e432–5.
7. Hausman Kedem M, Mandel D, Domani KA, et al. The effect of advanced maternal age upon human milk fat content. Breastfeed Med 2013;8:116–9.
8. Lubetzky R, Sever O, Mimouni FB, et al. Human milk macronutrients content: effect of advanced maternal age. Breastfeed Med 2015;10:433–6.
9. Pines N, Mandel D, Mimouni FB, et al. The effect of between-breast differences on human milk macronutrients content. J Perinatol 2016;36:549–51.
10. Atkinson SA, Bryan MH, Anderson GH. Human milk: difference in nitrogen concentration in milk from mothers of term and premature infants. J Pediatr 1978; 93(1):67–9.
11. Moran-Lev H, Mimouni FB, Ovental A, et al. Circadian macronutrients variations over the first 7 weeks of human milk feeding of preterm infants. Breastfeed Med 2015;10(7):366–70.
12. Ballard O, Morrow AL. Human milk composition: nutrients and bioactive factors. Pediatr Clin North Am 2013;60:49–74.
13. Gidrewicz DA, Fenton TR. A systematic review and meta-analysis of the nutrient content of preterm and term breast milk. BMC Pediatr 2014;14:216.
14. Atkinson SA, Bryan MH, Anderson GH. Human milk feeding in premature infants: protein, fat, and carbohydrate balances in the first two weeks of life. J Pediatr 1981;99(4):617–24.
15. Guerrini P, Bosi G, Chierici R, et al. Human milk: relationship of fat content with gestational age. Early Hum Dev 1981;5(2):187–94.
16. Hibberd CM, Brooke OG, Carter ND, et al. Variation in the composition of breast milk during the first 5 weeks of lactation: implications for the feeding of preterm infants. Arch Dis Child 1982;57(9):658–62.
17. Lemons JA, Moye L, Hall D, et al. Differences in the composition of preterm and term human milk during early lactation. Pediatr Res 1982;16(2):113–7.
18. Anderson DM, Williams FH, Merkatz RB, et al. Length of gestation and nutritional composition of human milk. Am J Clin Nutr 1983;37(5):810–4.
19. Ehrenkranz RA, Ackerman BA, Nelli CM. Total lipid content and fatty acid composition of preterm human milk. J Pediatr Gastroenterol Nutr 1984;3(5):755–8.
20. Lepage G, Collet S, Bouglé D, et al. The composition of preterm milk in relation to the degree of prematurity. Am J Clin Nutr 1984;40(5):1042–9.
21. Beijers RJ, Graaf FV, Schaafsma A, et al. Composition of premature breast-milk during lactation: constant digestible protein content (as in full term milk). Early Hum Dev 1992;29(1–3):351–6.

22. Maas YG, Gerritsen J, Hart AA, et al. Development of macronutrient composition of very preterm human milk. Br J Nutr 1998;80(1):35–40.
23. Faerk J, Skafte L, Petersen S, et al. Macronutrients in milk from mothers delivering preterm. Adv Exp Med Biol 2001;501:409–13.
24. Stoltz Sjöström E, Ohlund I, Tornevi A, et al. Intake and macronutrient content of human milk given to extremely preterm infants. J Hum Lact 2014;30(4):442–9.
25. Kreissl A, Zwiauer V, Repa A, et al. Human milk analyser shows that the lactation period affects protein levels in preterm breastmilk. Acta Paediatr 2016;105(6): 635–40.
26. Dritsakou K, Liosis G, Valsami G, et al. The impact of maternal- and neonatal-associated factors on human milk's macronutrients and energy. J Matern Fetal Neonatal Med 2016;1–7.
27. Steichen JJ, Krug-Wispé SK, Tsang RC. Breastfeeding the low birth weight preterm infant. Clin Perinatol 1987;14(1):131–71.
28. Groh-Wargo S, Valentic J, Khaira S, et al. Human milk analysis using mid-infrared spectroscopy. Nutr Clin Pract 2016;31(2):266–72.
29. Corvaglia L, Aceti A, Paoletti V, et al. Standard fortification of preterm human milk fails to meet recommended protein intake: bedside evaluation by near-infrared-reflectance-analysis. Early Hum Dev 2010;86(4):237–40.
30. Biochemical differences between preterm and term milk. Nutr Rev 1983;41(3): 79–80.
31. Cregan MD, De Mello TR, Kershaw D, et al. Initiation of lactation in women after preterm delivery. Acta Obstet Gynecol Scand 2002;81(9):870–7.
32. Atkinson SA, Anderson GH, Bryan MH. Human milk: comparison of the nitrogen composition in milk from mothers of premature and full-term infants. Am J Clin Nutr 1980;33(4):811–5.
33. Gross SJ, Geller J, Tomarelli RM. Composition of breast milk from mothers of preterm infants. Pediatrics 1981;68(4):490–3.
34. Morlacchi L, Mallardi D, Giannì ML, et al. Is targeted fortification of human breast milk an optimal nutrition strategy for preterm infants? An interventional study. J Transl Med 2016;14(1):195.
35. Polberger S, Räihä NC, Juvonen P, et al. Individualized protein fortification of human milk for preterm infants: comparison of ultrafiltrated human milk protein and a bovine whey fortifier. J Pediatr Gastroenterol Nutr 1999;29(3):332–8.
36. Bitman J, Wood DL, Miller RH, et al. Comparison of lipid composition of milk from half-Danish Jersey cows and United States Jersey cows. J Dairy Sci 1995;78(3): 655–8.
37. Boyce C, Watson M, Lazidis G, et al. Preterm human milk composition: a systematic literature review. Br J Nutr 2016;116(6):1033–45.
38. Fusch G, Rochow N, Choi A, et al. Rapid measurement of macronutrients in breast milk: how reliable are infrared milk analyzers? Clin Nutr 2015;34(3):465–76.

The Use of Multinutrient Human Milk Fortifiers in Preterm Infants

A Systematic Review of Unanswered Questions

Francis B. Mimouni, MD[a,b], Natalie Nathan, BSc[b,c],
Ekhard E. Ziegler, MD[d], Ronit Lubetzky, MD[b,c],
Dror Mandel, MD[b,e],*

KEYWORDS

- Human milk • Breastfeeding • Fortifier • Macronutrients

KEY POINTS

- There is little evidence that early introduction of human milk fortification compared with late fortification affects important outcomes such as early growth.
- There is no strong evidence that human milk–based fortifiers in otherwise exclusively human milk–fed preterm infants affect important outcomes.
- There is limited evidence that a bovine fortifier used with a combination of human milk and bovine-based formula places the infant at a higher risk of necrotizing enterocolitis.
- There is a definite need for additional studies, incorporating also long-term outcomes, to determine whether or not the use of human milk–based fortifiers improves outcomes.

INTRODUCTION

It has long been known that very low birth weight (VLBW) preterm infants fed exclusively breast milk cannot match intrauterine growth patterns and may end up with extrauterine growth restriction.[1,2] Efforts have been made to develop liquid or powder multinutrient products for the fortification of human breast milk.[3] These fortifiers

The authors have nothing to disclose.
[a] Department of Neonatology, Shaare Zedek Medical Center, 12 Shmuel Bait Street, Jerusalem 913102, Israel; [b] Sackler Faculty of Medicine, Tel Aviv Sourasky Medical Center, Tel Aviv University, Tel Aviv, Israel; [c] Department of Pediatrics, Dana Dwek Children's Hospital, Tel Aviv Sourasky Medical Center, 6 Weizman Street, Tel Aviv 6423906, Israel; [d] Department of Pediatrics, University of Iowa, Iowa City, IA, USA; [e] Department of Neonatology, Dana Dwek Children's Hospital, Tel Aviv Sourasky Medical Center, 6 Weizman Street, Tel Aviv 6423906, Israel
* Corresponding author. Department of Neonatology, Dana Dwek Children's Hospital, Tel Aviv Sourasky Medical Center, 6 Weizman Street, Tel Aviv 6423906, Israel.
E-mail address: dmandel@post.tau.ac.il

Clin Perinatol 44 (2017) 173–178
http://dx.doi.org/10.1016/j.clp.2016.11.011
0095-5108/17/© 2016 Elsevier Inc. All rights reserved.

increase nutrient intake and are expected to improve both growth and neurodevelopmental outcomes.[3] A recent systematic review within the Cochrane collaborative project aimed to determine whether multinutrient fortification of human breast milk improves important growth and developmental outcomes as compared with unfortified breast milk in preterm infants without increasing the risk of adverse effects, such as feeding intolerance or necrotizing enterocolitis (NEC).[4] This systematic review identified 14 randomized trials in which a total of 1071 infants participated. It concluded that individual trials were generally small and had weak methodology. Nevertheless, meta-analyses led to low-quality evidence that multinutrient fortification of breast milk increases in-hospital rates of growth by a mean daily weight gain of 1.81 g/kg (with a 95% confidence interval [CI] 1.23–2.40), by a mean weekly length gain of 0.12 cm (95% CI 0.07–0.17), and by a mean weekly head circumference gain of 0.08 cm/wk (95% CI 0.04–0.12). The meta-analyses did not show a positive effect of fortification on developmental outcomes. There was also low-quality evidence that fortification did not increase the risk of NEC in preterm infants with a typical relative risk (RR) 1.57 (95% CI 0.76–3.23). The investigators of this Cochrane review concluded that multinutrient fortified breast milk compared with unfortified breast milk does not significantly affect important outcomes, but that it leads to a slight increase of in-hospital growth rates. As often found in the conclusion of Neonatal Cochrane Systematic reviews,[5] the investigators of this important analysis concluded that the trials available "do not provide consistent evidence of effects on longer-term growth or development" and that "additional trials are needed to solve this issue."[4] This excellent review was published in 2016, and there was very little chance that we would be able to reach different conclusions because of additional, new data.

We thus elected to address other issues in our systematic review, issues that were purposely not addressed in the Cochrane review.[4] We specifically elected to determine whether studies (1) answered the question of early versus late introduction of fortifiers with regard to growth and/or other outcomes; and (2) had compared the efficacy/adverse effects of human milk–based fortifiers (HBF) with that of bovine fortifiers (BF) in otherwise exclusively human milk–fed infants.

MATERIALS AND METHODS

We conducted this systematic review in August 2016. We included only studies reporting the use of multinutrient human milk fortifiers. One author (NN) searched MEDLINE, EMBASE, and Google Scholar using the following key words: human milk, human milk fortifier, premature infant, preterm infant, human milk fortification. We also examined the references in studies identified as potentially relevant. Four authors (FB, NN, DM, and RL) screened titles and abstracts of all records identified by the search and coded records as "order" or "exclude." We then assessed all records coded as "order" and made the final decision about which records to order as full-text articles. We read the full texts to assess each article's suitability for inclusion on the basis of prespecified inclusion and exclusion criteria. Then the data were extracted independently by using a data collection form to aid extraction of information on design, methods, and participants from each included study. We assessed the quality of evidence at the outcome level using the Grading of Recommendations Assessment, Development, and Evaluation (GRADE) (http://www.gradeworkinggroup.org/) approach. Disagreements were discussed until a consensus was reached. If data from a given article were insufficient, the report was excluded from analysis. For the purpose of potential meta-analyses, we aimed to retain only articles that had studied the question of early versus late introduction of fortifiers and studies that compared the efficacy/adverse effects of HBF versus BF in otherwise exclusively human milk–fed preterm infants.

RESULTS

Our search allowed us to initially retrieve 2471 articles. The flow chart of **Fig. 1** depicts the retrieval and selection processes that were conducted to answer the 2 questions (see **Fig. 1**).

To answer the first question (early vs late introduction), only 5 trials were identified.[6–9] The first one, by Tillman and colleagues,[6] published in 2012, addressed the issue in a retrospective manner, as a pre-post comparison, and involved 53 early-fortification infants (from day 1 of feeding), as well as 42 delayed-fortification infants (when feedings reached 50–80 mL/kg per day). The inherent confounders associated with the retrospective study design did not allow this study to be included in a

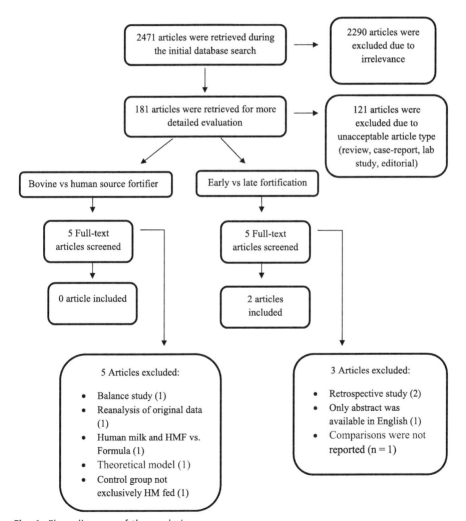

Fig. 1. Flow diagram of the analysis process.

meta-analysis. Nevertheless, the study did not find any differences in weight at 34 weeks postmenstrual age (PMA), but stated that the delayed-fortification group had a "higher incidence of elevated alkaline phosphatase." The study did not find significant differences in outcomes, such as feeding intolerance or NEC, but was underpowered to reach such conclusions in a definitive manner. The second study, by Maas and colleagues,[7] also addressed the issue in a retrospective manner, as a pre-post, comparison of nonconsecutive periods, and involved 206 preterm infants. Analyses did not focus on early versus late fortification, but rather on percentage of human milk in the total feeds. This study also was impossible to include in a meta-analysis, as no conclusion could be drawn from it with regard to the timing of fortification. The third article was retrieved from a non-Medline recorded article (*Iranian Journal of Pediatrics*) and its full text in the English language could not be obtained.[8] In its English abstract, the article stated that no anthropometric differences and no differences in adverse outcomes were found between the early-fortification and the late-fortification groups, but the abstract did not define what was meant by early or late. Its sample size was also relatively small (80 infants randomized) and the study is probably underpowered to detect small differences in effects or side effects. Another study, by Shah and colleagues,[9] consisted of a randomized controlled trial of early (beginning at an enteral intake of 20 mL/kg per day) versus late fortification (beginning at an enteral intake of 100 mL/kg per day). A population of 100 VLBW (<1500 g) infants was randomized to early (n = 50) and late (n = 50) groups. As expected, there were small but significant differences in protein intake between groups that persisted until week 4 of the study. In spite of that, no significant differences were found in anthropometric measurements (head circumference, length, weight, or weight velocity) or feeding intolerance, NEC, bronchopulmonary dysplasia (BPD), patent ductus arteriosus (PDA), or sepsis, although the study did not report post hoc type 2 errors, and was probably underpowered to detect small differences in effects as well as adverse effects. In a study by Sullivan and colleagues,[10] 2 subgroups of infants were randomized to early (40 mL/kg per day) versus late (100 mL/kg per day) introduction of an HBF, and the study also did not find differences in growth, feeding intolerance, or NEC.[10] It was stated only that the 2 groups did not differ between themselves, and quantitative comparisons were not reported. Nevertheless, and because of their heterogeneity, we felt that the study by Shah and colleagues[9] and the study by Sullivan and colleagues[10] could not be combined in a meta-analysis.

We therefore concluded from the first part of this systematic review that the limited available data do not provide strong evidence that early introduction of human milk fortification, compared late fortification, affects important outcomes, except that it leads to slightly increased initial protein intake.

To answer the second objective (HBF vs cow milk–based fortifier in otherwise exclusively human milk–fed preterm infants), we identified 5 articles.[10–14] Chronologically, the first report by Boehm and colleagues[11] compared a bovine-based commercial fortifier (at a concentration of 3 g per 100 mL fresh human milk) with powdered freeze-dried human milk plus minerals (at a concentration of 8 g per 100 mL fresh human milk). The study was conducted in a small number of infants (24 male VLBW infants) who were randomized to the BF group (n = 13) and the HBF group (n = 11). The study was very short in duration (14 days), and was not able (maybe in part because of its duration) to determine significant differences in weight or length gain. The HBF in that study seemed to have been custom-produced by the investigators and is not available commercially. This study was a balance study that did not find significant differences in nitrogen or fat intake, excretion, or retention and therefore was not retainable for a meta-analysis.

The second study, by Sullivan and colleagues,[10] recruited 207 infants fed their own mother's milk and randomized to 1 of 3 groups: one group received HBF when enteral intake was 40 mL/kg per day, the second one received HBF when enteral intake was 100 mL/kg per day, and the third one received BF when enteral intake was 100 mL/kg weight per day. The first 2 groups received donor human milk whenever their own mother's milk was not available, whereas the third group received a cow milk–based formula when mother's milk was not available. The 3 groups did not differ in weight, length, or head circumference patterns. When the outcomes of NEC and late-onset sepsis (LOS) were combined, there were very similar rates among the 3 groups. However, when only NEC was considered, both HBF groups had significantly lower rates, and all but 1 case of surgical NEC was found in the bovine preterm formula combined with human milk and bovine fortifier group. It must be noted that LOS in all 3 groups did not differ significantly ($P = .3$) but the lowest numbers were surprisingly in the bovine group, which had "masked" the effect on NEC when NEC and LOS were analyzed together. The power of the LOS analyses was not provided, and it is unclear whether a larger number of participants might have allowed for reaching statistical significance.

A reanalysis of the data of Sullivan and colleagues[10] (Ghandehari and colleagues[12]) was later published and also showed that total parenteral nutrition days were reduced in the HBF groups. Moreover, using the analysis of Sullivan and colleagues,[10] Ganapathy and colleagues[13] developed a theoretic model of costs of NEC and cost-effectiveness of exclusively human milk products in feeding extremely premature infants and concluded that a 100% human milk–based diet fortified with HBF may result in net savings on medical care resources by preventing NEC. Nevertheless, the study by Sullivan and colleagues,[10] as important as it is, does not allow to answer the question of superiority of an HBF over a BF in otherwise exclusively human milk–fed preterm infants. Because the group fed BF received a cow milk–based formula rather than donor human milk, the difference in feedings may have significantly affected the results. The last study, by Cristofalo and colleagues,[14] is a randomized trial of infants fed exclusively human milk and human milk–based products compared with infants fed formula and therefore could not be included in the analyses.

Thus, at this point, we conclude that there are limited data available and that the data do not provide strong evidence that HBF in otherwise exclusively human milk–fed preterm infants affects important outcomes. There is limited evidence that use of bovine fortifier with a combination of human milk *and bovine-based preterm formula* places the infant at a higher risk of NEC than use of HBF with exclusively human milk, which confirms previous observations on higher NEC risks in infants fed preterm formula as compared with human milk–fed preterm infants. However, the study design of this trial does not allow the conclusion that the use of human milk–based fortifier would reduce NEC risk as compared with bovine-based fortifier. There is a definite need for additional studies incorporating long-term outcomes to determine in a clean head-to-head comparison whether or not the use of human milk–based fortifiers might improve outcomes and reduce NEC and other adverse outcomes.

REFERENCES

1. Kashyap S, Schulze KF, Forsyth M, et al. Growth, nutrient retention, and metabolic response of low-birth-weight infants fed supplemented and unsupplemented preterm human milk. Am J Clin Nutr 1990;52:254–62.

2. Ehrenkranz RA, Younes N, Lemons JA, et al. Longitudinal growth of hospitalized very low birth weight infants. Pediatrics 1999;104:280–9.

3. Ziegler EE. Human milk and human milk fortifiers. In: Koletzko B, Poindexter B, Uauy R, editors. Nutritional care of preterm infants, vol. 110. Basel (Switzerland): Karger Publishers; 2014. p. 215–27.

4. Brown JV, Embleton ND, Harding JE, et al. Multi-nutrient fortification of human milk for preterm infants [review]. Cochrane Database Syst Rev 2016;(5):CD000343.

5. Mandel D, Littner Y, Mimouni FB, et al. Conclusiveness of the Cochrane neonatal reviews: a systematic analysis. Acta Paediatr 2006;95:1209–12.

6. Tillman S, Brandon DH, Silva SG. Evaluation of human milk fortification from the time of the first feeding: effects on infants of less than 31 weeks gestational age. J Perinatol 2012;32:525–31.

7. Maas C, Wiechers C, Bernhard W, et al. Early feeding of fortified breast milk and in-hospital-growth in very premature infants: a retrospective cohort analysis. BMC Pediatr 2013;13:178.

8. Sajjadian N, Alizadeh TP, Asgharyan FM, et al. A comparison between early and late breast milk fortification in preterm infants: a clinical trial study. Iran J Pediatr 2014;24:45.

9. Shah SD, Dereddy N, Jones TL, et al. Early versus delayed human milk fortification in very low birth weight infants—a randomized controlled trial. J Pediatr 2016; 174:126–31.

10. Sullivan S, Schanler RJ, Kim JH, et al. An exclusively human milk-based diet is associated with a lower rate of necrotizing enterocolitis than a diet of human milk and bovine milk-based products. J Pediatr 2010;156:562–7.

11. Boehm G, Müller DM, Senger H, et al. Nitrogen and fat balances in very low birth weight infants fed human milk fortified with human milk or bovine milk protein. Eur J Pediatr 1993;152:236–9.

12. Ghandehari H, Lee ML, Rechtman DJ, H2MF Study Group. An exclusive human milk-based diet in extremely premature infants reduces the probability of remaining on total parenteral nutrition: a reanalysis of the data. BMC Res Notes 2012;5:188.

13. Ganapathy V, Hay JW, Kim JH. Costs of necrotizing enterocolitis and cost-effectiveness of exclusively human milk-based products in feeding extremely premature infants. Breastfeed Med 2012;7:29–37.

14. Cristofalo EA, Schanler RJ, Blanco CL, et al. Randomized trial of exclusive human milk versus preterm formula diets in extremely premature infants. J Pediatr 2013; 163:1592–5.

Bioactive Proteins in Human Milk—Potential Benefits for Preterm Infants

Bo Lönnerdal, PhD

KEYWORDS

- Bioactive proteins • Protein digestibility • Human milk • Preterm infants

KEY POINTS

- Preterm milk contains high concentrations of several bioactive proteins.
- Significant amounts of these bioactive proteins survive digestion and are found intact in the stool.
- Bioactive proteins are likely to explain several of the advantageous outcomes described for preterm infants fed breast milk.

INTRODUCTION

Many components of breast milk are shown or suggested to provide bioactivities that are important for optimal health and development of the preterm infant. Among these are long-chain polyunsaturated fatty acids, complex oligosaccharides, bacteria with proposed beneficial effects provided with breast milk, nucleotides, and growth factors. The largest variety of bioactivities, however, is provided by proteins in breast milk (**Table 1**).[1,2] This article discusses these bioactivities and gives some examples of how milk proteins can improve infant outcomes. Clinical studies showing some of these benefits are presented and discussed.

PROTEIN DIGESTION IN TERM AND PRETERM INFANTS

To exert bioactivities in the gastrointestinal tract of infants, proteins need to retain an intact structure, or a significant portion thereof, that is, some resistance toward complete proteolysis for at least some time in the digestive process. Several human milk proteins have such resistance, among them secretory IgA (sIgA), lactoferrin, and lysozyme, which are present in significant quantities in the stool of breast-fed infants.

Disclosure: The author has participated as a clinical investigator, or advisory board member, or consultant or speaker for Mead Johnson Nutrition, Arla Foods, Semper, Hero, Albion, Valio, Humana, Biostime, Hipp, DSM, Triton, Nestec and Nestle Nutrition Institute.
Department of Nutrition, University of California, One Shields Avenue, Davis, CA 95616, USA
E-mail address: bllonnerdal@ucdavis.edu

Clin Perinatol 44 (2017) 179–191
http://dx.doi.org/10.1016/j.clp.2016.11.013
0095-5108/17/© 2016 Elsevier Inc. All rights reserved.

Table 1	
Bioactive human milk proteins	
Protein	**Bioactivity**
Lactoferrin	Bacteriostatic; bactericidal; immunomodulatory; cell proliferation and differentiation
α-lactalbumin	Prebiotic; antimicrobial; immunostimulatory; enhanced Fe and Zn absorption
sIgA	Transfer of maternal immunity; antibodies against bacteria and viruses
Lysozyme	Antibacterial activity; degradation of bacterial cell wall glycans
BSSL	Hydrolysis of triglycerides; fat absorption
Osteopontin	Immunomodulatory activity; brain function; intestinal development
Haptocorrin	Vitamin B12 absorption; antimicrobial activity
α_1-antitrypsin	Limit/slow down protein digestion
β-casein	Opioid activity; enhancing calcium absorption
κ-casein	Antibacterial activity by acting as structural analogues
MFGM proteins	Antibacterial and antiviral activities

Schanler and colleagues[3] found that very low-birth-weight infants fed pasteurized, lyophilized, mature human milk had markedly greater quantities of lactoferrin, lysozyme, and IgA in their stool than those fed cow's milk formula. Concentrations of total and sIgA were significantly correlated, and 95% of total IgA was sIgA. Fecal concentrations of specific sIgA antibodies to *Escherichia coli* O antigens correlated with the concentration of these antibodies in their milk. The investigators suggested that the larger quantities of these immune factors in the stool of infants fed breast milk is caused by increased ingestion but also raised the possibility of breast milk stimulating their endogenous synthesis. The same group also measured concentrations of these proteins in serum and found no difference between infants fed breast milk or cow's milk formula.[4] However, urinary excretion of these immune factors was significantly higher in infants fed breast milk than in those fed cow's milk formula, raising questions about the genesis of these proteins in the urine of infants fed breast milk. The authors of this report analyzed the presence of these immune factors in term, exclusively breast-fed infants and found significant quantities of lactoferrin and sIgA, which decreased with the age of the infant, but no detectable amounts of lysozyme.[5] Remarkably, during the first 2 weeks of age, nearly 70% of all soluble proteins in the feces consist of sIgA and lactoferrin, and this proportion decreases to about 20% to 30% at 4 to 5 months. In a carefully conducted nitrogen balance study on low-birth-weight infants,[6] the authors were able to calculate the survival rate for the major human milk bioactive proteins and found that these quantities were quite substantial and higher than what was observed in term infants.[7] As much as 25% and 9% of intake, respectively, of sIgA and lactoferrin were found in the fecal samples, whereas lysozyme and serum albumin (component of breast milk) were detected at lower amounts (~1% of intake). Immunoelectrophoresis and gel filtration chromatography confirmed that sIgA and lactoferrin were present in the stool in largely intact form, although there is a possibility of smaller peptides being formed, which are not immunoreactive. When comparing infants fed preterm milk only with those that received both preterm milk and cow's milk formula (50:50), the authors found that excretion of bioactive proteins was higher when formula was given and also that insoluble fecal nitrogen excretion was higher. This finding suggests that some cow milk proteins in formula which are difficult to digest form aggregates with breast milk proteins, enhancing their secretion but also most likely limiting their bioactivities in the gut. This finding, in turn, might explain why extremely premature infants fed an exclusively human milk–based diet are associated with significantly lower rates of necrotizing enterocolitis (NEC) and surgical NEC than those fed a preterm formula.[8]

The reasons for the lower digestibility of these proteins in preterm infants may be several: rapid transit time, comparatively high gastric pH (limiting pepsin activity), and low secretion of pancreatic enzymes. Another factor that may contribute is the presence of protease inhibitors in human milk, such as α_1-antitrypsin and α_1-antichymotrypsin,[9] which may limit the proteolysis of some bioactive proteins. The authors have shown that, in particular, α_1-antitrypsin is high in early milk and, therefore, most likely in breast milk from mothers delivering prematurely. The authors have shown in vitro, as a proof of concept, that human lactoferrin incubated with α_1-antitrypsin and exposed to digestion by pepsin and pancreatic enzymes is considerably more resistant against proteolysis than lactoferrin without α_1-antitrypsin.[9]

Also, the amounts of bioactive proteins found in the stool of breast-fed infants may be an underestimate of the amounts available at their point of action, which is likely in the small intestine. In a limited study on very young ileostomy- and colostomy-operated infants fed breast milk, the authors found an average of 32% of lactoferrin ingested in the excreted matter,[10] suggesting that a considerable proportion of lactoferrins escapes digestion in the upper gastrointestinal tract of infants.

ASSESSMENT OF BIOACTIVITIES OF MILK PROTEINS

Many studies exist on the bioactivities of human milk proteins. Most of these studies have, however, been performed in the laboratory using conventional assays or cell-based systems. Examples include the bacteriostatic/bactericidal activity of human lactoferrin, which can be demonstrated against a variety of pathogens, and the enzymatic activity of human bile salt–stimulated lipase (BSSL) showing its role in the digestion of various lipid substrates. Few studies have assessed the bioactivities of human milk proteins after heat treatment. With the increased use of banked human milk, in which pasteurization usually is required, this issue should be investigated in more detail. Although several studies have analyzed the concentrations of bioactive proteins like sIgA and lactoferrin in breast milk before and after pasteurization,[11] virtually no data exist on their *bioactivities* after such treatment. It is possible that the heat treatment will cause some aggregation of proteins, which will make them less detectable by immunologic methods (as they are based on exposed epitopes) and therefore indicates a loss of these proteins. However, low stomach pH, emulsifiers (bile salts), and digestive enzymes will cause dissociation of the same proteins—and thus restoration of their bioactivities—in the gastrointestinal tract. Freezer storage for extended time does not seem to affect concentrations of bioactive proteins like sIgA and lactoferrin.[12]

Assessment of bioactivities of human milk proteins in experimental animals requires larger quantities of the proteins, which are not commercially available in bulk quantity, and such models have, therefore, been used to a limited extent.

A novel and elegant way to explore the bioactivities of a specific milk protein is to use knockout mouse models. The expression of milk proteins vary considerably among species and the development of the offspring of rodents is quite different than that of the human infant, but if a particular protein is expressed at high levels in both the mouse and in humans, a knockout model is likely to give insight into the fundamental biological activities of that protein. As an example, the authors recently used an osteopontin knockout mouse model to assess osteopontin-related bioactivities. Both human and mouse milk have high concentrations of this protein, and their structures are similar. By using a design in which normal (wild-type) mouse pups were nursed by osteopontin knockout mothers with no detectable osteopontin in their milk or by normal (wild-type) mothers, we showed that osteopontin is important for brain development and cognitive function, immunity, and intestinal development.[13] Such results give important insight into the selection of appropriate biomarkers to use in clinical trials on added milk proteins.

BIOACTIVE PROTEINS IN HUMAN MILK

Concentrations of many bioactive proteins are higher in colostrum and early milk than later during lactation.[1,2] Interestingly, recent proteomics studies found that preterm human milk contains even higher concentrations of several of these proteins, for example, lactoferrin, BSSL, and lysozyme.[14] Thus, it is likely that bioactivities of many breast milk proteins will be high in the recipient preterm infant.

Lactoferrin

One of the first bioactivities ascribed to a human milk protein was the bacteriostatic effect of human lactoferrin on *E coli*.[15] Bullen and colleagues[15] found that the addition of iron to breast milk abolishes its bacteriostatic activity and subsequently showed that this was achieved by saturating the iron binding capacity of lactoferrin, which is present in breast milk in a largely unsaturated form (apo-lactoferrin). Lactoferrin is a major protein in breast milk and constitutes about 15% to 20% of the total protein content. But even if a major part of iron in human milk is bound to lactoferrin, it is only saturated to about 6% to 9%.[16] Because lactoferrin has an unusually high affinity constant for iron, it is capable of withholding iron from iron-requiring pathogens such as *E coli*. Apo-lactoferrin was subsequently found to also be bactericidal, killing several pathogens such as *Cholera vibrio* and *Streptococcus mutans*.[17] Lactoferrin was also found to have synergistic effects with lysozyme on the killing of gram-negative bacteria (see later discussion).

Lactoferrin has been found to bind to specific sites on small intestinal biopsies from human adults, and the potential existence of a lactoferrin receptor was suggested.[18] The authors subsequently isolated a receptor for human lactoferrin from human infant small intestine and characterized it biochemically[19] and subsequently cloned the gene for the human intestinal lactoferrin receptor.[20] This gene was found to be identical to that coding for intelectin, a lectin discovered in mouse small intestine. Both apo- and holo-lactoferrin bind to this receptor, become internalized, and activate different signaling pathways, and apo-lactoferrin eventually goes to the nucleus and is internalized.[21] It subsequently binds to specific segments of DNA, thus acting as a transcription factor.[22] This action most likely explains how lactoferrin affects cell proliferation and differentiation and also affects cytokine expression, thereby modulating the immune response. Buccigrossi and colleagues[23] found that lactoferrin at higher concentrations stimulates cell differentiation, whereas lower concentrations promote cell differentiation. Thus, higher concentrations in breast milk during early lactation, coupled with lower proteolytic degradation, may promote intestinal growth, whereas lower concentrations in later lactation and more efficient capacity to digest proteins may result in enhanced cell differentiation.

α-lactalbumin

Another major human milk protein is α-lactalbumin, which constitutes approximately 15% of the total protein content of breast milk. This protein forms a complex with galactosyltransferase in the mammary gland, forming lactose synthase that is responsible for lactose synthesis but is also secreted in the milk. Alpha-lactalbumin is comparatively easily digested, but during its digestion, peptides are formed that may provide bioactivities in the upper gastrointestinal tract (duodenum, jejunum).[24] These include a tripeptide that is immunomodulatory,[25] peptides that enhance iron and zinc absorption,[26] and antimicrobial peptides.[27] Eventually, however, α-lactalbumin will be almost completely digested in the small intestine and serve as a good source of essential amino acids, as no α-lactalbumin is found in the stool of breast-fed infants.

Secretory IgA

The human mammary gland synthesizes a special form of IgA, sIgA, which consists of 2 "regular" molecules of IgA bound together via 2 other proteins/peptides: the secretory component and the so-called J chain[28] which renders the sIgA molecule stability against proteolytic digestion, explaining why this molecule was found early in the stool of breast-fed infants. Elegant work finds that maternal immunity can be transferred into her milk and then to her breast-fed infant via the enteromammary pathway.[29] Thus, antibodies raised by the mother against pathogens in her environment can be transferred to her infant and bind to and prevent these bacteria and viruses from infecting it.

Lysozyme

For being an active enzyme, the concentration of lysozyme in breast milk is unusually high; it is 3000 times higher than in cow's milk.[30] Lysozyme can kill gram-positive bacteria by degrading the proteoglycan matrix of the bacterial cell wall. Because this protein is found in the stool of breast-fed infants, it is likely that it can exert this activity in infants. It is also possible that lysozyme can have a synergistic effect with lactoferrin in breast milk on gram-negative bacteria. Electron microscopy shows that lactoferrin first, by its high affinity toward lipopolysaccharide, binds this outer membrane constituent and creates holes/pores through which lysozyme can penetrate and degrade the inner proteoglycan matrix, thereby killing gram-negative bacteria.[31] As a proof-of-concept study, the authors treated Peruvian children hospitalized with acute diarrhea with recombinant human lactoferrin and lysozyme (see later discussion).

Bile Salt–Stimulated Lipase

Breast-fed infants are known to digest and use lipids efficiently. This is in part because of a high concentration of BSSL that can hydrolyze fatty acids from the sn-2 position in triglycerides.[32] The significance of this has been shown in a cross-over design on preterm infants that were fed either pasteurized or unpasteurized breast milk. Infants fed the pasteurized milk, in which the BSSL had been inactivated, had lower weight and length gain and also lower fat absorption than infants fed breast milk that had not been heat treated.[33]

Osteopontin

Originally discovered in bone, osteopontin is also present in significant amounts in breast milk.[34] This protein is heavily glycosylated and phosphorylated and binds to integrin receptors.[35] Osteopontin is a multifunctional protein involved in physiologic events, including cell-mediated immune responses[36] and anti-inflammatory responses.[37] Osteopontin is a key molecule inducing T-helper type 1 (Th1)-type immunity,[35,38] and increasing the Th1 response would enhance host defense against pathogens. It may, therefore, affect development of the newborn human infant.[13]

Human milk osteopontin is resistant to in vitro digestion by human neonatal gastric juice[39] and may, therefore, exert bioactivities in the upper gastrointestinal tract.

Haptocorrin

The major vitamin B12-binding protein in human milk is haptocorrin.[40] There is more haptocorrin in breast milk than there is vitamin B12, so it is largely in its unsaturated apo form.[41] Haptocorrin has strong antibacterial activity and may thus help prevent infections in breast-fed infants.[42] Haptocorrin also facilitates the uptake of vitamin B12 by human intestinal cells in culture and may, therefore, increase vitamin B12 absorption during early infancy when the synthesis of intrinsic factor is immature.[41] The concentration of haptocorrin in stool is likely too low to be detectable (its concentration in human milk is much lower than that of lactoferrin and lysozyme), but in vitro digestion studies using Western blot show that haptocorrin is resistant against digestion.[42]

α_1-antitrypsin

Although α_1-antitrypsin in the stool usually is a marker of disease, such as, protein-losing enteropathy, breast-fed infants excrete significant quantities of α_1-antitrypsin[43] because the concentration of α_1-antitrypsin is high in breast milk. The reason for this high concentration is not known, but it is hypothesized that α_1-antitrypsin limits the activity of trypsin to some extent and, therefore, allows a proportion of some difficult-to-digest bioactive milk proteins to exert their actions in the small intestine (see above).

β-casein

The major casein subunit in breast milk is β-casein, which is phosphorylated at one or more threonine or serine residues.[44] When these phosphorylated amino acid residues are structurally close to each other, they can chelate calcium thereby keeping calcium in a soluble form and possibly facilitating calcium absorption. Some studies in human adults using calcium isotopes find such an enhancement,[45] whereas others do not.[46] Such studies should also been done in infants in whom gastrointestinal conditions are quite different from those in adults.

κ-casein

The remaining part of casein in breast milk is mostly κ-casein,[47] with only a minor fraction consisting of α_{S1}-casein. In contrast to β-casein, κ-casein is heavily glycosylated with about 40% of its molecular mass being carbohydrate. These complex carbohydrates have structures similar to those on the surface of the small intestinal epithelial barrier, and they have therefore been suggested to act as "decoys," thereby preventing attachment and invasion of pathogens. For example, κ-casein can prevent the attachment of *Helicobacter pylori* to human gastric mucosa and thus possibly protect the breast-fed infant from *H pylori* infection.[48] It is known that breast-fed infants have a lower prevalence of *H pylori* infection than infants weaned early to solid foods.[49] Because lactoferrin[50] and sIgA both inhibit the growth of *H pylori*, it is possible that these 3 proteins work together to protect the infant.

Milk Fat Globule Membrane Proteins

The triglyceride core of the milk fat globule is surrounded by a membrane structure, actually formed by 3 membranes. The proteins in this milk fat globule membrane (MFGM) fraction constitute only 1% to 4% of the total protein content of human milk,[51] but proteomics analyses find that there are more than 160 different proteins, of which, many are unique for this membrane fraction.[52] Several of them like MUC1, lactadherin, butyrophilin, and xanthine oxidase have anti-infectious, anti-inflammatory and antioxidative activities.[53] For example, lactadherin inhibits the growth of rotavirus,[54] and a study in Mexico found that women with the highest concentrations of lactadherin in their milk had a lower prevalence of rotavirus infection in their infants.[55]

NOVEL SOURCES OF PROTEINS THAT MAY BE USED IN INFANT FORMULA
Recombinant Human Milk Proteins

Human milk proteins are, of course, not available in large quantities to be used for the manufacture of infant formula. Some of them, however, have been produced in recombinant form in a scale large enough to perform clinical trials. Among them are lactoferrin, which is produced in *Aspergillus*[56] and in rice[57]; lysozyme, which is also expressed in rice[58]; and BSSL, which is expressed in Chinese hamster ovary cells in culture.[59] Clinical trials of these proteins are described below. The *Aspergillus*-produced lactoferrin requires a high degree of purification for human consumption, as it is produced in a mold, whereas rice-produced lactoferrin requires a lower degree of purity, as the contaminants are rice starch and rice protein, common dietary ingredients in weaning foods for infants (and therefore less of a concern).

Bovine Milk Proteins or Milk Protein Fractions

Some proteins found in human milk are also found in cow's milk but usually at considerably lower concentrations. These proteins can be enriched or purified to various degrees and added to infant formula.[60] Examples of such proteins are lactoferrin, α-lactalbumin, osteopontin, and MFGM. There are usually differences in amino acid sequence, extent of glycosylation, the composition of the glycans, and extent and positions of phosphorylated amino acids between the human and bovine proteins. However, even if this is the case, these differences may not affect their biological activities (or only part of them when they have multiple functions). It is, therefore, important to characterize these proteins/protein fractions with regard to composition and bioactivities in vitro before conducting studies on larger experimental animals (eg, piglets, rhesus monkeys).

CLINICAL TRIALS ON BIOACTIVE MILK PROTEINS
Lactoferrin

Early studies on bovine lactoferrin added to infant formula and iron status and gut microbiota failed to find any effect of lactoferrin supplementation.[61,62] It was subsequently found that the bovine lactoferrin contained significant amounts of lipopolysaccharide (to which it has a strong binding affinity), which may have obscured the outcomes. More recent studies using more extensively purified bovine lactoferrin found positive effects on iron status and a reduction in upper respiratory infections in term infants.[63] Studies on preterm infants given bovine lactoferrin found a reduction in NEC and sepsis,[64] and further multicenter studies on this application are now being conducted. Recombinant human lactoferrin (produced in *Aspergillus*, called *talactoferrin*) has also been used in preterm infants,[65] and a randomized controlled trial showed no toxicity and a trend toward less infectious morbidity in the infants treated with talactoferrin.

Lactoferrin and Lysozyme

Because a synergistic antimicrobial effect of human lactoferrin and human lysozyme was found in vitro, the authors used recombinant forms of these proteins expressed in rice in an oral rehydration solution (ORS) to treat Peruvian children hospitalized with acute diarrhea. In this randomized, controlled trial, children were given either regular World Health Organization ORS or the rice-based World Health Organization ORS or that rice-based ORS with lactoferrin and lysozyme.[66] A significant reduction in duration of diarrhea, stool/diaper weight, and relapse of the diarrhea was found in the group given the ORS with lactoferrin and lysozyme. However, only the combination of the 2 proteins was tested, and it is not known if one of the proteins or the combination was responsible for the effect observed.

Bile Salt–Stimulated Lipase

Two randomized, double-blind clinical studies on preterm infants given recombinant BSSL (produced in mammalian cells) in pasteurized breast milk (no remaining BSSL activity) or preterm formula showed significantly improved growth and long-chain fatty acid absorption compared with placebo.[59] Disappointingly, however, a recent large phase 3 study failed to show any overall difference in growth velocity between preterm infants given recombinant BSSL and placebo, although there was a significant difference in a predefined subgroup of small-for-gestational-age infants.[67]

α-lactalbumin

Whey protein concentrates enriched in α-lactalbumin have been added to infant formulas for some time. The primary purpose for this was to add a good source of tryptophan, which is comparatively high in α-lactalbumin, when the protein content of infant formula was reduced.[24] Clinical studies on such formulas show that serum tryptophan is not lower than in breast-fed infants when α-lactalbumin–enriched whey protein is added to the formula.[68,69] Few of the bioactivities of α-lactalbumin have been evaluated in clinical trials, but studies on infant monkeys fed such formula show both increased iron and zinc status and shifts in the fecal microbiota.[26,70]

Milk Fat Globule Membrane Proteins

The MFGM fraction from cow's milk, which is commercially available from several dairy companies, not only contains proteins but also phospholipids, gangliosides, cholesterol, and sialic acid,[53] and it is, therefore, not possible to ascribe the clinical outcomes to any specific component. Several of the MFGM proteins have antimicrobial and anti-inflammatory activities, which may explain the effect on infections. The authors conducted a clinical trial on Swedish infants who were fed regular formula or formula supplemented with bovine MFGM from 6 weeks to 6 months of age.[71] A breast-fed reference group was also included. We found that infants fed the MFGM-supplemented formula had significantly better cognitive development at 12 months of age (as assessed by the Bailey III test) than those fed regular formula and that there was no difference between them and the breast-fed infants. We also found that infections were lower in the MFGM-supplemented group compared with those fed regular formula and again not different from the breast-fed infants.[72] This finding was especially pronounced for acute otitis media. Several other recent studies also found a positive effect of MFGM on cognitive development in infants and children.[73,74]

Osteopontin

The authors recently conducted a clinical trial on bovine osteopontin added to infant formula.[75] Bovine milk and human milk osteopontin have similar binding motifs and are both highly glycosylated and phosphorylated.[35] Cow's milk only contains about 18 mg/L of osteopontin, and the concentration infant formula is even lower (about 8 mg/L), whereas breast milk contains about 138 mg/L.[34] In our study,[75] infants were fed, from 1 month to 6 months of age, regular infant formula (low in osteopontin) or formula supplemented with either 65 mg/L of osteopontin (50% of human milk level) or 130 mg/L (100% of human milk level). Infants fed osteopontin-supplemented infant formula with the higher level had lower serum tumor necrosis factor-α levels than the other formula-fed groups and a cytokine profile more similar to that of breast-fed infants.[75] They also had significantly fewer days with fever, suggesting that the differences in serum cytokines affected the prevalence of infections.

SUMMARY

Human milk contains many bioactive proteins that are likely to be involved in the better outcomes of breast-fed infants compared with those fed infant formula. Bovine milk proteins or protein fractions may be able to provide some of these benefits and may, therefore, be used for preterm infants. Recombinant human milk proteins are likely to exert bioactivities similar to those of the native human milk proteins, but considerable research is needed before they can be used in routine care of preterm infants.

REFERENCES

1. Lönnerdal B. Nutritional and physiologic significance of human milk proteins. Am J Clin Nutr 2003;77:1537S–43S.
2. Lönnerdal B. Bioactive proteins in human milk: mechanisms of action. J Pediatr 2010;156(Suppl 2):S26–30.
3. Schanler RJ, Goldblum RM, Garza C, et al. Enhanced fecal excretion of selected immune factors in very low birth weight infants fed fortified human milk. Pediatr Res 1986;20:711–5.
4. Goldblum RM, Schanler RJ, Garza C, et al. Human milk feeding enhances the urinary excretion of immunologic factors in low birth weight infants. Pediatr Res 1989;25:184–8.
5. Davidson LA, Lönnerdal B. Persistence of human milk proteins in the breast-fed infant. Acta Paediatr Scand 1987;76:733–40.
6. Donovan SM, Atkinson SA, Whyte RK, et al. Partition of nitrogen intake and excretion in low birth-weight infants. Am J Dis Child 1989;143:1485–91.
7. Davidson LA, Donovan SM, Lönnerdal B, et al. Excretion of human milk proteins by term and premature infants. In: Atkinson SA, Lönnerdal B, editors. Protein and non-protein nitrogen in human milk. Boca Raton (FL): CRC Press, Inc.; 1989. p. 161–72.
8. Sullivan S, Schanler RJ, Kim JH, et al. An exclusively human milk-based diet is associated with a lower rate of necrotizing enterocolitis than a diet of human milk and bovine milk-based products. J Pediatr 2010;156:562–7.
9. Chowanadisai W, Lönnerdal B. Alpha-1-antitrypsin and antichymotrypsin in human milk: origin, concentrations, and stability. Am J Clin Nutr 2002;76:828–33.
10. Hambraeus L, Hjorth G, Kristiansson B, et al. Lactoferrin content in feces in ileostomy-operated children fed human milk. In: Barth CA, Schlimme E, editors. Milk proteins: nutritional, clinical, functional and technical aspects. Darmstadt (Germany): Steinkopff Verlag; 1989. p. 72–5.
11. Peila C, Moro GE, Bertino E, et al. The effect of holder pasteurization on nutrients and biologically-active components in donor human milk: a review. Nutrients 2016;8(477):1–19.
12. Ahrabi AF, Handa D, Codipilly CN, et al. Effects of extended freezer storage on the integrity of human milk. J Pediatr 2016;177:140–3.

13. Jiang R, Lönnerdal B. Biological roles of milk osteopontin. Curr Opin Clin Nutr Metab Care 2016;19:214–9.
14. Molinari CE, Casadio YS, Hartmann BT, et al. Proteome mapping of human skim milk proteins in term and preterm milk. J Proteome Res 2012;11:1696–714.
15. Bullen JJ, Rogers HJ, Leigh L. Iron-binding proteins in milk and resistance to Escherichia coli infection in infants. Br Med J 1972;1(5792):69–75.
16. Fransson GB, Lönnerdal B. Iron in human milk. J Pediatr 1980;96(3 Pt 1):380–4.
17. Arnold RR, Brewer M, Gauthier JJ. Bactericidal activity of human lactoferrin: sensitivity of a variety of microorganisms. Infect Immun 1980;28:893–8.
18. Cox TM, Mazurier J, Spik G, et al. Iron binding proteins and influx of iron across the duodenal brush border. Evidence for specific lactotransferrin receptors in the human intestine. Biochim Biophys Acta 1979;588:120–8.
19. Kawakami H, Lönnerdal B. Isolation and function of a receptor for human lactoferrin in human fetal intestinal brush-border membranes. Am J Physiol 1991; 261(5 Pt 1):G841–6.
20. Suzuki YA, Shin K, Lönnerdal B. Molecular cloning and functional expression of a human intestinal lactoferrin receptor. Biochemistry 2001;40:15771–9.
21. Lönnerdal B, Jiang R, Du X. Bovine lactoferrin can be taken up by the human intestinal lactoferrin receptor and exert bioactivities. J Pediatr Gastroenterol Nutr 2011;53:606–14.
22. Liao Y, Jiang R, Lönnerdal B. Biochemical and molecular impacts of lactoferrin on small intestinal growth and development during early life. Biochem Cell Biol 2012; 90:476–84.
23. Buccigrossi V, de Marco G, Bruzzese E, et al. Lactoferrin induces concentration-dependent functional modulation of intestinal proliferation and differentiation. Pediatr Res 2007;61:410–4.
24. Lönnerdal B, Lien EL. Nutritional and physiologic significance of alpha-lactalbumin in infants. Nutr Rev 2003;61:295–305.
25. Migliore-Samour D, Roch-Arveiller M, Tissot M, et al. Effects of tripeptides derived from milk proteins on polymorphonuclear oxidative and phosphoinositide metabolisms. Biochem Pharmacol 1992;44:673–80.
26. Kelleher SL, Chatterton D, Nielsen K, et al. Effects of glycomacropeptide and α-lactalbumin supplementation of infant formula on growth and nutritional status in infant rhesus monkeys. Am J Clin Nutr 2003;77:1261–8.
27. Pelligrini A, Thomas U, Bramaz N, et al. Isolation and identification of three bactericidal domains in the bovine α-lactalbumin molecule. Biochim Biophys Acta 1999;1426:439–48.
28. Lindh E. Increased resistance of immunoglobulin A dimers to proteolytic degradation after binding of secretory component. J Immunol 1975;114(1 Pt 2):284–6.
29. Goldman AS. Evolution of the mammary gland defense system and the ontogeny of the immune system. J Mammary Gland Biol Neoplasia 2002;7:277–89.
30. Chandan RC, Parry RM, Shahani KM. Lysozyme, lipase, and ribonuclease in milk of various species. J Dairy Sci 1968;51:606–7.
31. Ellison RT 3rd, Giehl TJ. Killing of gram-negative bacteria by lactoferrin and lysozyme. J Clin Invest 1991;88:1080–91.
32. Hernell O, Bläckberg L. Digestion of human milk lipids: physiologic significance of sn-2 monoacylglycerol hydrolysis by bile salt-stimulated lipase. Pediatr Res 1982;16:882–5.
33. Andersson Y, Sävman K, Bläckberg L, et al. Pasteurization of mother's own milk reduces fat absorption and growth in preterm infants. Acta Paediatr 2007;96: 1445–9.

34. Schack L, Lange A, Kelsen J, et al. Considerable variation in the concentration of osteopontin in human milk, bovine milk, and infant formulas. J Dairy Sci 2009;92: 5378–85.
35. Christensen B, Nielsen MS, Haselmann KF, et al. Post-translationally modified residues of native human osteopontin are located in clusters: identification of 36 phosphorylation and five O-glycosylation sites and their biological implications. Biochem J 2005;390:285–92.
36. Ashkar S, Weber GF, Panoutsakopoulou V, et al. Eta-1 (osteopontin): an early component of type-1 (cell-mediated) immunity. Science 2000;287(5454):860–4.
37. Hwang SM, Lopex CA, Heck DE, et al. Osteopontin inhibits induction of nitric oxide synthase gene expression by inflammatory mediators in mouse kidney epithelial cells. J Biol Chem 1994;69:11–5.
38. Nau GJ, Liaw L, Chupp GL, et al. Attenuated host resistance against Mycobacterium bovis BCG infection in mice lacking osteopontin. Infect Immun 1999;67: 4223–30.
39. Chatterton DEW, Rasmussen JT, Heegaard CW, et al. In vitro digestion of novel milk protein ingredients for use in infant formulas: research on biological functions. Trends Food Sci Technol 2004;15:373–83.
40. Sandberg DP, Begley JA, Hall CA. The content, binding, and forms of vitamin B_{12} in milk. Am J Clin Nutr 1981;34:1717–24.
41. Adkins Y, Lönnerdal B. Mechanisms of vitamin B12 absorption in breast-fed infants. J Pediatr Gastroenterol Nutr 2002;35:192–8.
42. Adkins Y, Lönnerdal B. Potential host-defense role of a human milk vitamin B_{12}-binding protein, haptocorrin, in the gastrointestinal tract of breast-fed infants, as assessed with porcine haptocorrin in vitro. Am J Clin Nutr 2003;77:1234–40.
43. Davidson LA, Lönnerdal B. Fecal alpha$_1$-antitrypsin in breast-fed infants is derived from human milk and is not indicative of enteric protein loss. Acta Paediatr Scand 1990;79:137–41.
44. Greenberg R, Groves ML. Human β-casein. Amino acid sequence and identification of phosphorylation sites. J Biol Chem 1984;259:5128–32.
45. Hansen M, Sandström B, Jensen M, et al. Casein phosphopeptides improve zinc and calcium absorption from rice-based but not from whole-grain infant cereal. J Pediatr Gastroenterol Nutr 1997;24:56–62.
46. Teucher B, Majsak-Newman G, Dainty JR, et al. Calcium absorption is not increased by caseinophosphopeptides. Am J Clin Nutr 2008;84:162–6.
47. Kunz C, Lönnerdal B. Human-milk proteins: analysis of casein and casein subunits by anion-exchange chromatography, gel electrophoresis, and specific staining methods. Am J Clin Nutr 1990;51:37–46.
48. Strömquist M, Falk P, Bergström S, et al. Human milk κ-casein and inhibition of Helicobacter pylori adhesion to human gastric mucosa. J Pediatr Gastroenterol Nutr 1995;21:288–96.
49. Roma E, Miele E. Helicobacter pylori infection in pediatrics. Helicobacter 2015; 20(Suppl 1):47–53.
50. Miehlke S, Reddy R, Osato MS, et al. Direct activity of recombinant human lactoferrin against Helicobacter pylori. J Clin Microbiol 1996;34:2593–4.
51. Lönnerdal B, Woodhouse LR, Glazier C. Compartmentalization and quantitation of protein in human milk. J Nutr 1987;117:1385–95.
52. Liao Y, Alvarado R, Phinney B, et al. Proteomic characterization of human milk fat globule membrane proteins during a 12 month lactation period. J Proteome Res 2011;10:3530–41.

53. Spitsberg VL. Invited review: bovine milk fat globule membrane as a potential nutraceutical. J Dairy Sci 2005;88:2289–94.
54. Kvistgaard AS, Pallesen LT, Arias CF, et al. Inhibitory effects of human and bovine milk constituents on rotavirus infections. J Dairy Sci 2004;87:4088–96.
55. Newburg DS, Peterson JA, Ruiz-Palacios GM, et al. Role of human milk lactadherin in protection against symptomatic rotavirus infection. Lancet 1998;18(351):1190–4.
56. Ward PP, Piddington CS, Cunningham GA, et al. A system for production of commercial quantities of human lactoferrin: a broad spectrum natural antibiotic. Biotechnology (N Y) 1995;13:498–503.
57. Suzuki YA, Kelleher SL, Yalda D, et al. Expression, characterization, and biologic activity of recombinant human lactoferrin in rice. J Pediatr Gastroenterol Nutr 2003;36:190–9.
58. Huang J, Wu L, Yalda D, et al. Expression of functional recombinant human lysozyme in transgenic rice cell culture. Transgenic Res 2002;11:229–39.
59. Casper C, Carnielli VP, Hascoet JM, et al. rhBSSL improves growth and LCPUFA absorption in preterm infants fed formula or pasteurized breast milk. J Pediatr Gastroenterol Nutr 2014;59:61–9.
60. Lönnerdal B. Infant formula and infant nutrition: bioactive proteins of human milk and implications for composition of infant formulas. Am J Clin Nutr 2014;99:712S–7S.
61. Fairweather-Tait SJ, Balmer SE, Scott PH, et al. Lactoferrin and iron absorption in newborn infants. Pediatr Res 1987;22:651–4.
62. Chierici R, Sawatzki G, Tamisari L, et al. Supplementation of an adapted formula with bovine lactoferrin. 2. Effects on serum iron, ferritin and zinc levels. Acta Paediatr 1992;81:475–9.
63. Manzoni P, Rinaldi M, Cattani S, et al. Bovine lactoferrin supplementation for prevention of late-onset sepsis in very low-birth-weight neonates. JAMA 2009;302:1421–8.
64. King JC Jr, Cummings GE, Guo N, et al. A double-blind, placebo-controlled, pilot study of bovine lactoferrin supplementation in bottle-fed infants. J Pediatr Gastroenterol Nutr 2007;44:245–51.
65. Sherman MP, Adamkin DH, Niklas V, et al. Randomized controlled trial of talactoferrin oral solution in preterm infants. J Pediatr 2016;175:68–73.
66. Zavaleta N, Figueroa D, Rivera J, et al. Efficacy of rice-based oral rehydration solution containing recombinant human lactoferrin and lysozyme in Peruvian children with acute diarrhea. J Pediatr Gastroenterol Nutr 2007;44:258–64.
67. Casper C, Hascoet JM, Ertl T, et al. Recombinant bile salt-stimulated lipase in preterm infant feeding: a randomized phase 3 study. PLoS One 2016;11(5):e0156071.
68. Davis AM, Harris BJ, Lien EL, et al. Alpha-lactalbumin-rich infant formula fed to healthy term infants in a multicenter study: plasma essential amino acids and gastrointestinal tolerance. Eur J Clin Nutr 2008;62:1294–301.
69. Sandström O, Lönnerdal B, Graverholt G, et al. Effects of alpha-lactalbumin-enriched formula containing different concentrations of glycomacropeptide on infant nutrition. Am J Clin Nutr 2008;87(4):921–8.
70. Bruck WM, Kelleher SL, Gibson GR, et al. rRNA probes used to quantify the effects of glycomacropeptide and alpha-lactalbumin supplementation on the predominant groups of intestinal bacteria of infant rhesus monkeys challenged with enteropathogenic Escherichia coli. J Pediatr Gastroenterol Nutr 2003;37:273–80.

71. Timby N, Domellöf E, Hernell O, et al. Neurodevelopment, nutrition, and growth until 12 mo of age in infants fed a low-energy, low-protein formula supplemented with bovine milk fat globule membranes: a randomized controlled trial. Am J Clin Nutr 2014;99:860–8.
72. Timby N, Hernell O, Vaarala O, et al. Infections in infants fed formula supplemented with bovine milk fat globule membranes. J Pediatr Gastroenterol Nutr 2015;60:384–9.
73. Gurnida DA, Rowan AM, Idjradinata P, et al. Association of complex lipids containing gangliosides with cognitive development of 6-month-old infants. Early Hum Dev 2012;88:595–601.
74. Veereman-Wauters G, Staelens S, Rombaut R, et al. Milk fat globule membrane (INPULSE) enriched formula milk decreases febrile episodes and may improve behavioral regulation in young children. Nutrition 2012;28:749–52.
75. Lönnerdal B, Kvistgaard AS, Peerson JM, et al. Growth, nutrition and cytokine response of breast-fed infants and infants fed formula with added bovine osteopontin. J Pediatr Gastroenterol Nutr 2016;62:650–7.

Human Milk Oligosaccharides and the Preterm Infant

A Journey in Sickness and in Health

Sara Moukarzel, PhD[a,b,1], Lars Bode, PhD[a,b,*]

KEYWORDS

- Human milk oligosaccharides • Glycans • Preterm infant • Nutrition • Microbiome
- Immune system

KEY POINTS

- Human milk oligosaccharides (HMOs) are the third most abundant component of human milk.
- Preterm infants consume several grams of approximately 200 structurally diverse HMOs daily from mother's own or donor milk. Formula-fed infants and infants on parenteral nutrition do not currently receive any HMOs.
- HMOs are proposed to support infant health, growth, and development by acting as prebiotics, antimicrobials, antiadhesives, and modulators of cell responses.
- Preclinical and cohort studies suggest HMOs are protective against necrotizing enterocolitis (NEC) in preterm infants.
- Larger mother-infant cohort and human intervention studies are limited, but recent technological advances in both HMO analysis and HMO synthesis help overcome hurdles and challenges.

INTRODUCTION

Preterm infants are a diverse group of babies with varying nutritional and medical needs, depending on the level of physiologic maturity at birth, birth weight, and neonatal morbidity, to name a few. Clinical care for all preterm infants, however, is focused on reducing short-term and long-term morbidity and mortality and promoting normal growth and development. Human milk not only is a source of nourishment but

Disclosure Statement: The authors have nothing to disclose.
[a] Department of Pediatrics, University of California, San Diego, 9500 Gilman Drive, La Jolla, CA 92093, USA; [b] Mother-Milk-Infant Center of Research Excellence, School of Medicine, University of California, San Diego, 9500 Gilman Drive, La Jolla, CA 92093, USA
[1] Present address: 9500 Gilman Drive, Mail Code 0715, San Diego, CA 92093-0715.
* Corresponding author. 9500 Gilman Drive, Mail Code 0715, San Diego, CA 92093-0715.
E-mail address: lbode@ucsd.edu

Clin Perinatol 44 (2017) 193–207
http://dx.doi.org/10.1016/j.clp.2016.11.014   perinatology.theclinics.com

also a life-saving and disease-preventing approach to preterm infant care.[1,2] Compared with formula-fed infants, human milk-fed preterm infants are less likely to develop nosocomial infection, NEC, late-onset sepsis, retinopathy of prematurity, and cognitive impairment.[3,4] Human milk feeding also may be protective against immune-mediated conditions, such as asthma, allergies, and inflammatory bowel disease,[5,6] and chronic noncommunicable diseases, such as cardiovascular disease and type 2 diabetes mellitus, later in life.[6,7] HMOs, the third most abundant component of human milk, may be one of the reasons why human milk supports and protects term and preterm infants.

This review outlines current and rapidly accumulating knowledge on the potential benefits of HMOs for human milk-fed infants and describes how individual HMOs are becoming available for human clinical studies and application.

FOOD FOR THOUGHT: A HUMAN BABY RECEIVES HUMAN MILK OLIGOSACCHARIDES

Milk is a remarkable biological fluid that has evolved over 150 million years to be a crucial source of nutrition and immunoprotection for infants, capable of sustaining life in an often pathogen-rich and nutrient-poor extrauterine environment. It is fascinating that some milk components evolved in a species-specific manner to meet species-dependent biological needs and levels of developmental maturity at term birth. An excellent example of this specificity is the presence of HMOs in milk. HMO structures and composition are far more complex than oligosaccharides in the milk of any other studied species, which includes cow milk on which most infant formula is based and also the milk of humans' closest relatives, nonhuman primates.[8,9] The reason why the human mammary gland invests energy to produce such a high amount and structural diversity of HMOs, with approximately 200 different structures identified so far, is an active area of research. The authors hypothesize that optimal health outcomes associated with HMOs are collectively achieved when infants consume a balanced combination of HMOs, as present in human milk. A particular biological benefit could be due to 1 or several HMOs interacting together. Knowledge of what HMO functions are and which particular HMOs contribute to these functions has increased substantially over the past decade. What a balanced HMO composition in milk is (which might be mother-infant specific), what affects it, and how it relates to infant outcomes, particularly in preterm infants, however, are far from being defined. Human milk components do not optimally meet the developmental needs of preterm infants, and how HMOs in preterm milk contribute to the preterm infant extrauterine metabolic adaptations is not known.

HUMAN MILK OLIGOSACCHARIDES: STRUCTURES, INFANT INTAKE, AND METABOLISM
Structures

HMOs are complex sugars present in free, unconjugated form in the milk aqueous phase. Approximately 200 HMOs with unique structures have been identified to date. HMOs consist of 5 monosaccharide building blocks: galactose (Gal), glucose (Glc), N-acetylglucosamine (GlcNAc), fucose (Fuc), and the sialic acid (Sia) derivative N-acetylneuraminic acid (Neu5Ac). All HMOs consist of lactose (Galβ1-4Glc) at the reducing end, which can be elongated by the addition of the following disaccharides: β1-3–linked or β1-6–linked lacto-N-biose (Galβ1-3GlcNAc-, type 1 chain) or N-acetyllactosamine (Galβ1-4GlcNAc-, type 2 chain). N-acetyllactosamine can be further extended by the addition of 1 or more of these 2 disaccharides. A β1-3 linkage between 2 disaccharides results in a linear chain elongation, whereas a β1-6 linkage results in chain branching. Lactose or the elongated/branched oligosaccharide chain can be fucosylated in α1-2, α1-3, or α1-4 linkages and/or sialylated in α2-3 or α2-6 linkages.[10]

One of the ways for categorizing HMOs is based on the presence or absence of Neu5Ac in the HMO molecule, resulting in a sialylated (acidic) or nonsialylated (neutral) HMO. Both acidic and neutral HMOs can be fucosylated. The ability to produce fucosylated HMOs is in part genetically determined, such that some but not all women express active fucosyltransferases. This depends on a woman's secretor and Lewis blood group status. The *Se* gene encodes an α1-2 fucosyltransferase (FUT2), responsible for catalyzing the addition of Fuc to Gal in an α1-2 linkage. Women who express this enzyme are referred to as *secretors* and produce milk with 2'-fucosylated HMOs, such as 2'-fucosyllactose (2'FL) and lacto-N-fucopentaose (LNFP) I. On the contrary, *nonsecretors* refers to women who are homozygous for mutated alleles of the *Se* gene, express inactive FUT2, and, therefore, produce milk without or with limited amounts of 2'-fucosylated HMOs. Approximately 20% of whites are homozygous for mutated FUT2-activating genes (20% are Nonsecretors).[11,12] The proportions of secretors and nonsecretors, however, seem to vary across populations potentially due to evolutionary selection pressures to produce milk with or without α1-2–fucosylated HMOs.[13,14] Fuc can also be added in an α1-3 or α1-4 linkage (dependent on the underlying type 1 or type 2 chain) by an α1-3/4–fucosyltransferase (FUT3), encoded by the *Le* gene. Women who express an active FUT3 enzyme produce HMOs, such as LNFPII with Fuc connected to GlcNAc by an α1-4 linkage. Although the expression of FUT3 is also partly genetically determined, the response to unexpressed FUT3 is not entirely all or none, such that α1-3–fucosylated HMOs and α1-4–fucosylated HMOs still are present but in significantly reduced amounts, which is likely due to the presence of an additional fucosyltransferase with somewhat redundant substrate specificity. Therefore, women can be grouped into 4 categories: secretors *Le* positive (both FUT2 and FUT3 are active), nonsecretors *Le* positive (FUT2 inactive, FUT3 active), secretors *Le* negative (FUT2 active, FUT3 inactive), and nonsecretors *Le* negative (both FUT2 and FUT3 are inactive). Driven in part by this genetic diversity, the composition of fucosylated HMOs varies significantly in milk samples from women across the 4 categories.[15–19]

In addition to Fuc, 1 or more Sias can be added to HMOs by several sialyltransferases, which connect Neu5Ac to the terminal Gal and/or to internal GlcNAc. Unlike FUT2 and FUT3 that can be completely inactive, complete loss of sialyltranferases activity and absence of particular sialylated HMOs in milk has not yet been reported. The more subtle variation in the composition of sialylated HMOs across milk samples may be due to differentially expressed genes relevant to sialylation (eg, sialyltransferases and transport proteins) across women. How environmental factors like maternal diet, lifestyle, or health conditions affect HMO composition is mostly unknown.

Intake

Although much attention is often given to the caloric, macronutrient, and micronutrient density of human milk, it is remarkable that human term infants consume approximately 10 g HMOs per day, assuming a daily milk volume intake of 800 mL. This often exceeds the amount of infant daily protein intake. HMO content is even higher in colostrum compared with mature milk, reaching or exceeding 20 g/L.[20,21] Over the course of lactation, HMO composition remains fairly constant in term milk but fluctuates in preterm milk.[21–23] Donor milk provides infants with HMOs that are not significantly altered after donor milk pasteurization.[24] HMO content and composition, however, differ across donor milk batches, secondary to normal variations in HMO production across donors.[23] On the contrary, formula-fed infants and infants on parenteral nutrition do not currently receive any HMOs. Most infant formula products are based on cow milk with no added HMOs. Synthetic and plant-based oligosaccharides, such as galacto-oligosaccharides (GOSs) and fructo-oligosaccharides (FOSs), are added in some preterm and term infant formula products to mimic the role of HMOs as prebiotics. Differences in oligosaccharide composition and abundance between human milk and formula, however, remain profound. For example, a breastfed term newborn infant consumes only approximately 15 mg/L of short chain GOSs (3', 4', and 6'-galactosyllactose).[25] Alternatively, GOS content varies among infant formula products but can reach approximately 7 g/L. FOSs are added to formula in much lower amounts than GOSs (approximately 1 g/L), but these oligosaccharides are not present in human milk.

Metabolism

HMO metabolism is likely complex, and describing 1 metabolic fate for all approximately 200 HMOs is an oversimplification of this complexity. Knowledge regarding the metabolism of individual HMOs remains limited, and key messages are summarized.

HMOs are only minimally degraded in the acidic stomach environment and are not digested in quantitative amounts by pancreatic and intestinal enzymes. A majority of HMOs reach the colon intact, although a small proportion of HMOs is absorbed into the systemic circulation. In the colon, HMOs are either metabolized by an infant's gut bacteria and/or excreted intact in the feces, depending on infant age, maturity at birth, blood group, and diet.[26–28]

During the first approximately 2 months of life, the colon becomes rapidly colonized with bacteria that undergo a process of diet-dependent adaptation, whereby bacterial communities capable of metabolizing available dietary compounds and their by-products, including oligosaccharides, thrive. Likely secondary to this adaptation process, HMOs from birth to 2 months are mainly excreted in the feces.[26,27] Fecal HMO composition is largely dependent on the HMOs in the infant diet. For example, feces of breastfed term and preterm infants at 2 months postpartum contain/lack various fucosylated HMOs, depending on their presence/absence in maternal milk. In turn, the composition of fucosylated HMOs in milk depends on the mother's secretor and Lewis status.[26–28]

In the months until complementary feeding begins (approximately 3–6 months), feces no longer contain HMOs with high resemblance to mother's milk composition. Instead, HMOs are predominantly degraded by gut bacteria, and feces mainly contain HMO degradation products and modified HMO structures.[26,27] With the introduction of complementary feeding at approximately 6 months of age, HMOs and their metabolic by-products decrease in an infant's feces. They are no longer detectable on cessation of human milk feeding.

In addition to HMO excretion in feces and metabolism by gut bacteria, an estimated minimum of 100 mg/d of HMOs is absorbed into the systemic circulation by a term breastfed infant (1% detectable in urine, estimated 10 g/d HMOs consumed). Indirect evidence for HMOs absorption in vivo stems from elegant stable isotope studies showing renal HMO excretion equivalent to 1% to 3% of term infant intake.[29,30] HMOs have been detected in plasma and urine of term breastfed infants[11,22,31] and in urine of those born preterm.[28,32] The composition of detected HMOs in urine suggests that several HMOs originate from mother's milk and are excreted intact, such as 2'FL and LNT.[33] Others, such as acetylated oligosaccharides, do not originate from mother's milk. They are likely due to a modification of HMOs by an infant's gut bacteria before absorption or by the infant after absorption, for example, liver or kidney metabolism.[26,28,34] Regardless of their origin, labeled HMOs can remain detectable in an infant's urine for at least 16 hours after labeled HMOs are no longer detectable in mother's milk.[33] The systemic effects of HMOs during this extended period merit investigation.

Earlier studies in tissue culture models by Gnoth and colleagues[35] suggest that neutral HMOs are absorbed via receptor-mediated transcytosis and paracytosis, whereas acidic HMOs are absorbed by paracytosis only. Whether or not the original observations from tissue culture models translate to human term and preterm infants remains unknown, and the specific molecular transport mechanisms remain to be elucidated.

Relative absorptions of synthetic 2'FL added to infant formula and 2'FL in human milk are estimated at 0.05% to 0.07% in term infants.[36] Differences between the composition of HMOs in feces and HMOs in urine of preterm infants suggest, however, that absorption efficiency may be different among individual HMOs.[28] With much to be learned about HMO metabolism, its apparent complexity suggests that HMOs and/or their metabolites may have functional roles within the gastrointestinal (GI) tract as well as systemically and in tissues and organs other than the gut. Research in cell culture and animal models suggest HMOs may protect and support term and preterm infants through their roles as prebiotics, antiadhesives, antimicrobials, and modulators of cell responses.

PROPOSED HUMAN MILK OLIGOSACCHARIDE FUNCTIONS BASED ON PRECLINICAL RESEARCH
Human Milk Oligosaccharides as Prebiotics

A majority of HMOs consumed by breastfed infants reach the colon intact where they act as metabolic substrates for specific bacteria with presumed health-promoting potential, such as *Bifidobacterium longum* subsp *infantis* (ATCC 15697) and select *B breve* (eg, SC95, SC154, SC568, and ATCC 15701).[37,38] Because these bacteria contain specific and comprehensive HMO utilization cassettes (enzymes, transporters, and so forth), they thrive at the expense of potentially pathogenic bacteria incapable of metabolizing HMOs at similar capacity. These potentially beneficial bacteria may reduce inflammation and GI infections in infants by modulating inflammation and immune epithelial cell responses. Evidence in support of this hypothesis stems from in vitro studies. For example, culturing *B infantis* with pooled HMOs (HMOs from pooled human milk), 6'-sialyllactose (6'SL), or a combination of 6'SL and 3-sialyllactose (3'SL) enhanced bacterial adhesion to intestinal epithelial cells.[39,40] In addition, human intestinal epithelial Caco-2 cells increased their expression of anti-inflammatory cytokine, interleukin 10, when exposed to *B infantis* (ATCC 15697) and *B bifidum* (ATCC 29521) that were previously cultured with HMOs compared with the same bacteria cultured on lactose.[40] Similarly, proinflammatory genes were down-regulated when Caco-2 cells are exposed to *B infantis* (ATCC 15697) and *B breve* (SC95) cultured on pooled HMOs.[39] This shift in anti-inflammatory and proinflammatory responses might be relevant to preterm infants.

Preterm infants have a less diverse gut bacterial composition, with higher levels of facultative anaerobes, such as *Enterobacteriaceae*, and lower levels of strict anaerobes, such as *Bifidobacterium* and *Bacteroides* compared with term infants during the first few weeks of life.[41,42] This dysbiosis is one of the crucial factors linked to preterm infant mortality and morbidity, including development of NEC and sepsis.[43,44] Underwood and colleagues[28] have recently reported statistically significant negative associations between fucosylated HMOs in milk fed to preterm infants and abundance of fecal *Enterobacteriales*, an order with several pathogens implicated in NEC and sepsis. HMOs from the same milk samples that were neither fucosylated nor sialylated were positively associated with potentially pathogenic bacteria in the feces. This suggests that keeping dysbiosis in check may be one means by which HMOs protect preterm infants. Perhaps a balanced HMO composition in milk is needed to shape the gut microbiome toward optimal trophic and protective effects.

In contrast, the authors' laboratory tested preclinical HMO efficacy in a rodent NEC model and identified 1 specific HMO called disialyllacto-N-tetraose (DSLNT) as the most protective oligosaccharide to improve survival and reduce pathology scores in neonatal rats.[45,46] The effects are highly structure-specific because the removal of the terminal Sia alone abolished the protective effects of DSLNT. Preclinical NEC models in rats, mice, or piglets, however, have significant limitations because they do not fully represent the pathology of the disorder in human preterm infants. Thus, interpretations solely based on results generated in these animal models have to be considered carefully before conducting human randomized clinical trials. To close this gap between preclinical and clinical studies, the authors conducted 2 independent mother-infant cohort analyses. The first study was a secondary data analysis in a South African cohort originally designed to dissect the role of prebiotics and probiotics on HIV infection and transmission via breastfeeding.[47] A subcohort of 184 mothers with very low-birth-weight preterm infants contained 8 NEC cases irrespective of HIV status. HMO composition analysis showed that infants who developed NEC received significantly less DSLNT with their mother's milk than infants who did not develop NEC. In contrast, none of the other 19 individual HMOs that had been quantifiable were significantly different between NEC cases and controls. The second study was conducted at 5 different neonatal ICUs in North America (United States and Canada) and specifically designed to test the hypothesis that DSLNT protects from NEC (Autran C, et al: Submitted for publication.). The study recruited a total of 200 mothers and their very low-birth-weight infants (<1500 g), followed the infants for the first 28 days of life, and collected milk samples that the infants received approximately every second day. Of the 200 infants, 8 infants developed NEC Bell stage 2 or 3. For each of these NEC cases, 5 control infants without NEC were matched based on study location, gestational age, birth weight, delivery mode, and race/ethnicity as well as sample availability over the course of the 28 days postpartum. HMO composition analysis in more than 650 milk samples revealed that infants who developed NEC received less DSLNT with their milk than those infants who did not develop NEC. Despite the small cohort and case size, data modeling allowed the authors to start predicting which infant develops NEC based on DSLNT threshold concentrations in the milk samples. If confirmed in larger cohorts, DSLNT threshold levels could become noninvasive screens to identify mother's own milk samples or donor milk batches that are deficient in DSLNT and potentially put infants at risk for developing NEC. Both cohorts independently identified high DSLNT levels associated with a lower risk for developing NEC, and in both cohorts none of the structurally related HMOs, such as lack of terminal Sia compared with DSLNT or lack of both Sias compared with DSLNT (LNT), correlated with NEC risk. Similarly, neither of these HMOs had a protective effect in the neonatal rat model. Because the effects of DSLNT seem highly structure-specific, the authors hypothesize that the underlying mechanism is not just a prebiotic effect with DSLNT serving as "food" for beneficial bacteria. Preliminary data from tissue culture models suggest that the effect is independent of bacteria altogether and that DSLNT acts on host cells via receptor-mediated pathways.

Human Milk Oligosaccharides as Antiadhesives

Breastfed infants have a lower incidence of infectious diseases caused by viruses, bacteria, fungi, and protozoan parasites compared with formula-fed infants[48,49] and this may be in part due to HMOs. Many pathogens require adhesion to the host mucosal surfaces as a prerequisite to initiate infection. Adhesion typically involves specific carbohydrate-dependent pathogen-host receptor interactions and can simplistically occur in the following 2 ways. Many pathogens express proteins, such as lectins and adhesins, which project from the pathogen's cell surface in threadlike structures called pili. Proteins at the tip of pili then adhere to oligosaccharide binding sites of host cell receptors, such as surface-bound mucin glycoproteins MUC1, MUC3, and MUC4 along the glycocalyx of the GI tract and secreted MUC2 in the GI tract mucus layer. This is how certain pathogenic strains of *Salmonella* and entero-pathogenic *Escherichia coli* (EPEC), for example, adhere to the mucosal surface of the human GI tract. Alternatively, the surface of pathogens can be directly covered with glycoproteins or other glycoconjugates, which themselves act as adhesion agents. Many HMOs resemble the structure of oligosaccharide moieties on host cell or pathogens surfaces. Accordingly, it is hypothesized that HMOs serve as soluble de-coys that bind to either host cell receptor and/or pathogen, blocking the adhesion process and thereby protecting infants from infection. Data in support of this mechanistic hypothesis so far stem from few in vitro studies with tissue culture binding assays and studies in mice. For instance, EPEC attachment to cultured epithelial cells was significantly reduced in the presence of pooled HMOs. Additionally, EPEC colonization was lower in neonatal mice supplemented with pooled HMOs compared with unsupplemented mice.[50] Similarly, colonization of lactating mice with *Campylobacter jejuni* was inhibited with pooled HMO feeding. In vitro experiments and experiments with transgenic mice suggest 2'-fucosylated HMOs may be among the specific antiadhesives against *C jejuni*.[51] HMOs also prevented attachment of *Entamoeba histolytica*, the amebiasis-causing protozoan parasites, to human intestinal cells and inhibited their cytotoxicity.[52] In tissue culture assays, invasion of *Candida albicans* on premature intestinal epithelial cells was reduced when treated with physiologic concentrations of pooled HMOs,[53] raising the question of whether 1 or several HMOs can help treat and/or prevent life-threatening candidiasis, particularly among extremely low-birth-weight preterm infants.

Human Milk Oligosaccharides as Modulators of Cell Responses

HMOs are not only food for bugs and antiadhesives but they also act as signaling molecules directly interacting with the host. In tissue culture models, HMOs modulate intestinal cell proliferation, differentiation, and apoptosis via receptor binding and MAPK (mitogen-activated protein kinases)-signalling.[54] Physiologic concentrations of individual or combinations of sialylated HMOs (2'FL, 3'SL, and 6'SL) enhance differentiation and inhibit proliferation of epithelial cell models of the crypt-villus axis in a similar fashion to pooled HMOs.[55] Broadly, the authors hypothesize that the consistent exposure of an infant's intestinal epithelial cells to large amounts of HMOs (infants fed every 3–4 hours) promotes normal gut development via HMO-dependent signaling pathways. Further studies are needed to determine whether the lack of HMO exposure among formula-fed and parenterally fed preterm infants disrupts normal gut development.

In addition to epithelial cells, HMOs have been shown to interact directly with immune cells, altering their responses to a stimulus. For example, 2'FL directly inhibits lipopolysaccharide-mediated inflammation during *E coli* invasion of mature and immature intestinal epithelial cells.[56] Beyond the intestine and keeping in mind that several hundred micrograms of HMOs reach the systemic circulation, allergen-specific T cells from individuals with peanut allergy produce fewer type 2 helper T-cell cytokines when cultured with sialylated HMOs. This suggests the latter may mediate a more balanced immune response to allergen exposure among allergy-prone infants.[57] The authors have shown that sialylated HMOs also block the invasion of uropathogenic *E coli* strain (UPEC) to bladder epithelial cells by suppressing intracellular signaling of apoptotic pathways in epithelial cells. As a consequence, bladder epithelial cells become resistant to UPEC invasion and survive. In summary, HMOs are highly abundant complex carbohydrates in milk proposed to support infant health, growth, and development by acting as prebiotics, antiadhesives, and modulators of cell responses.

RECENT ADVANCES IN HUMAN MILK OLIGOSACCHARIDE ANALYSIS AND HUMAN MILK OLIGOSACCHARIDE SYNTHESIS

The past 5 years have witnessed an immense increased interest in HMO-focused cohort and intervention studies, which is driven by at least 3 major developments. First, accumulating evidence from in vitro and animal studies (discussed previously) provide more and more convincing evidence to suggest that HMOs provide infants with substantial health benefits. Second, technical advances in rapid HMO composition analysis now enable correlation and association studies in large mother-infant cohorts. For example, 5 years ago it took approximately a week to analyze HMO composition in fewer than a dozen samples. Today, several different analytical platforms allow analyzing HMO composition in more than 150 samples per week, and the analysis is more sensitive, robust, and reliable. Third, advances in the synthesis of individual HMOs chemically, chemoenzymatically, or in bioengineered microbes make HMOs accessible in quantities required for preclinical studies in larger animals (eg, piglets) and with longer exposure periods to probe long-term outcomes. In addition, chemical and chemoenzymatic synthesis generates HMO libraries that cover a more comprehensive chemical space of different structurally distinct HMOs to enable structure-activity relationship studies, similar to conventional drug discovery approaches. Most importantly, these recent advances in HMO synthesis provide individual HMOs for randomized controlled trials to study the short-term and long-term benefits of select HMOs in human term and preterm infants.

Human Milk Oligosaccharide Composition Analysis in Mother-Infant Cohort Studies

Six cohort studies so far implicate HMOs in term infant survival and immunoprotection. First, incidence of diarrhea caused by *C jejuni* during the first 2 years of life was more common in infants fed human milk low in 2'FL.[58] Second, LNFPII concentrations in human milk at 2 weeks postpartum were negatively associated with infants' incidence of respiratory and GI problems by 6 weeks and 12 weeks of age (n = 49 mother-infant dyads; $P<.05$).[59] Third, Sprenger and colleagues[60] reported significant negative associations between 2'FL concentrations in human milk collected at approximately 2 days postpartum and incidence of any allergic disease, eczema, and IgE-associated disease at 2 years of age, if the child was born by cesarean section and had a high hereditary risk for developing allergies. Fourth, in a case-control study designed to assess the relationship between immunologic factors in human milk and development of cow milk allergy (CMA) within the first 18 months of life, samples of milk fed to infants with CMA (n = 39) were significantly lower in 6'SL, DSLNT, LNFPI, and LNFPIII compared with infants without CMA (n = 41).[61] The likelihood for having CMA was almost 7-fold higher among infants fed milk low in LNFPIII (<60 nM; multiple comparisons—adjusted odds ratio 6.7; 95% CI, 2.0–22). Similarly, milk fed to infants with atopic dermatitis (AD) was lower in 6'SL and DSLNT levels compared with infants without AD. Fifth, survival rate during the first 2 years of life was significantly higher in infants fed human milk high in several fucosylated HMOs, including 2'FL, in a cohort of more than n = 150 Zambian HIV-uninfected infants breastfed by HIV-infected mothers.[62] Sixth, HIV transmission through breastfeeding during the first 4 months of life was less likely to occur in infants fed human milk containing total HMOs above the group median (1.87 g/L).[63] In this case-control study, HIV-infected women (n = 93) who transmitted HIV (cases) and HIV-infected women (n = 86) who did not transmit HIV (controls) were included. Milk samples were analyzed at 1 month postnatal prior to HIV transmission, and statistical adjustments for maternal CD4 count and breast milk HIV RNA concentrations were made.

Not only is HMO intake associated with immune-related outcomes during infancy in several cohort studies, but also HMOs may potentially influence noncommunicable disease risk later in life. For example, the authors tested the hypothesis that interindividual variation in HMO composition in the mother's milk influences the infant's metabolic phenotype either directly or indirectly through changes in the microbiome. In a cohort of 25 mother-infant pairs, HMO diversity, evenness, and LNFPI concentration in milk were negatively associated with infant body weight at 1 month. At 6 months, LNFPI concentration was negatively associated with infant body weight, lean mass, and fat mass. Conversely, other HMOs, such as DSLNT and LNFPII, were positively associated with fat mass at 6 months.[64] Studies that include the infant gut microbiome and metabolome are currently under way. On the other side of the metabolic spectrum, human milk samples from mothers of stunted Malawian infants (n = 204) were significantly lower in several sialylated and fucosylated HMOs compared with samples from mothers of healthy infants (n = 99).[65] If HMO composition in milk affects human infant growth and body composition, the extent to which HMO intake has an impact on risk for developing obesity later in life merits investigation. In line with the developmental origins of health and disease theory,[66] several studies have reported breastfeeding as modestly protective against childhood and adolescent obesity. The authors speculate specific HMOs cause a less-obesogenic infant phenotype by shaping the gut bacterial composition/function and/or acting as signaling molecules. Charbonneau and colleagues[65] supplemented gnotobiotic mice and piglets with bovine sialylated oligosaccharides (approximately 88% 3'SL and 6'SL) after colonizing the animals with bacterial strains from a stunted Malawian infant and feeding a prototypic Malawian diet. This resulted in a bacteria-dependent increase in body weight and lean body mass and alterations in metabolic pathways associated with liver and muscle energy and nutrient metabolism.

Although cohort studies do not determine causality, they bring researchers 1 step closer toward accurately identifying specific HMOs with a beneficial or potentially detrimental clinical impact in humans. For example, although total HMO content in milk seems protective against HIV transmission through breastfeeding, the proportion of milk 3'SL, in particular, is associated with an increase in transmission risk.[63] This raises the question of whether increased infant consumption of 3'SL per se or an interaction between several consumed HMOs modulates HIV transmission through breastfeeding. Another issue regarding HMO balance in milk can be addressed in future cohort studies: mice fed milk deficient in 3'SL during infancy are less susceptible to dextran sulfate sodium–induced colitis during adulthood compared with 3'SL-fed mice.[67] Because 3'SL is a natural oligosaccharide in mouse milk (and in milk of other mammalian species, including humans), the proinflammatory properties of 3'SL found in mice may seem counterintuitive. Nonetheless, their balanced presence in milk with other HMOs may be important to mediate a healthy infection-resolving inflammatory response. An exacerbated proinflammatory response may potentially result from feeding milk enriched in 3'SL at the expense of lower anti-inflammatory HMOs, such as 2'FL.

Feeding Human Milk Oligosaccharides to Human Neonates

Larger cohort and intervention studies are made possible largely due to the recent large-scale availability of several individual HMOs for commercial and research use and due to advancements in analytical methods allowing high-throughput HMO analysis. The first HMO to become commercially available in the near future is 2'FL, recently registered as a safe ingredient for infant and toddler formula in Europe (novel food application) and the United States (generally recognized as safe). Several other individual HMO products are currently under review. Consumption of 2'FL added to infant formula (2 experimental concentrations of 0.2 g/L 2'FL and 1 g/L 2'FL; n = 81 infants and n = 83 infants, respectively; both formulas were isocaloric, approximately 643 kcal/L) was recently reported as safe and tolerable in term infants approximately 5 days to 4 months old.[36] Two comparative groups, a formula-fed group nonsupplemented with 2'FL (n = 84) and a breastfed group (n = 90), were also included in the study. The proportion of infants in both supplemented groups who had adverse events (eg, infections and illnesses during the 4 months) were not significantly different from the formula-fed nonsupplemented group. Average stool consistency, number of stools per day, and percent of feedings associated with spitting up or vomit did not differ significantly between the 3 formula-fed groups, particularly after 28 days postnatal. Overall, no significant differences in gender-stratified average weight, length, and head circumference were found among the 4 groups during the 4-months period. Average plasma 2'FL concentrations were highest in the breastfed group, with the highest consumption of 2'FL from maternal milk, consecutively followed by the 2'FL (1 g/L) supplemented group, 2'FL (0.2 g/L) supplemented group, and nonsupplemented group. Relative absorption (concentration of 2'FL in plasma relative to 2'FL consumed), however, was similar across the groups at approximately 0.05%.

SUMMARY

Preclinical and cohort studies suggest HMOs support infant health, growth, and development by acting as prebiotics, antiadhesives, and cell response modulators. NEC is just one of the detrimental medical conditions among preterm infants for which risk of occurrence may be significantly reduced by feeding specific HMOs. Candidiasis, sepsis, and several other conditions highly relevant to preterm infants might also benefit from either specific individual HMOs or complex HMO mixtures.

Although individual HMOs become available for clinical application, for example, 2'FL as a general and more natural prebiotic or DSLNT to prevent NEC, it is important to emphasize that HMOs are naturally consumed in complex mixtures and not as single structure entities. Feeding infants just 1 or 2 of the many different HMOs might carry a risk of driving the development of microbial communities or/and the immune system out of balance, with potentially adverse long-term effects. Thus, in most cases, human milk feeding is the superior choice because it contains a mixture of many different HMOs with a wide range of potentially beneficial effects for term infants as well as preterm infants.

The ultimate goal is to understand which and how HMOs support infants during their journey through sickness and health. Clinically translating this knowledge may then help reduce term and preterm infant morbidity and mortality and allow infants to achieve their full potential for growth and development.

Best Practices

What is the current practice?

Care objectives
1. Reduce preterm infant mortality and morbidity
2. Promote adequate growth and development

General feeding guidelines
- The American Academy of Pediatrics recommends all preterm infants receive human milk or pasteurized donor milk if mother's own milk is unavailable or contraindicated.
- Fortification of human milk with protein, minerals, and vitamins is recommended for infants to ensure optimal nutrient intake for infants less than 1500 g at birth.
- A dietary requirement for HMOs is not established. Preterm infant HMO intake (content and composition) is not currently included in clinical algorithms, including protocols for milk fortification.

What changes in current practice are likely to improve outcomes?

- There is currently insufficient evidence to recommend changes in practice with respect to HMOs.

Summary statement

- Recent advances in HMO composition analysis and HMO synthesis are key drivers for mother-infant cohort studies and infant intervention studies designed to generate additional evidence in support of screening human milk and human milk products and using individual HMOs or mixtures of different HMOs to improve preterm infant care.

REFERENCES

1. Moro GE, Arslanoglu S, Bertino E, et al. XII. Human milk in feeding premature infants: consensus statement. J Pediatr Gastroenterol Nutr 2015;61(Suppl 1): S16–9.
2. Cleminson JS, Zalewski SP, Embleton ND. Nutrition in the preterm infant: what's new? Curr Opin Clin Nutr Metab Care 2016;19(3):220–5.
3. Bhatia J. Human milk and the premature infant. Ann Nutr Metab 2013;62(Suppl 3):8–14.
4. Schanler RJ. Evaluation of the evidence to support current recommendations to meet the needs of premature infants: the role of human milk. Am J Clin Nutr 2007; 85(2):625s–8s.
5. Klement E, Cohen RV, Boxman J, et al. Breastfeeding and risk of inflammatory bowel disease: a systematic review with meta-analysis. Am J Clin Nutr 2004; 80(5):1342–52.
6. Walker WA, Iyengar RS. Breast milk, microbiota, and intestinal immune homeostasis. Pediatr Res 2015;77(1–2):220–8.
7. Horta BL, Loret de Mola C, Victora CG. Long-term consequences of breastfeeding on cholesterol, obesity, systolic blood pressure and type 2 diabetes: a systematic review and meta-analysis. Acta Paediatr 2015;104(467):30–7.
8. Goto K, Fukuda K, Senda A, et al. Chemical characterization of oligosaccharides in the milk of six species of New and Old World monkeys. Glycoconj J 2010; 27(7–9):703–15.
9. Urashima T, Odaka G, Asakuma S, et al. Chemical characterization of oligosaccharides in chimpanzee, bonobo, gorilla, orangutan, and siamang milk or colostrum. Glycobiology 2009;19(5):499–508.
10. Bode L. Human milk oligosaccharides: every baby needs a sugar mama. Glycobiology 2012;22(9):1147–62.

11. Goehring KC, Kennedy AD, Prieto PA, et al. Direct evidence for the presence of human milk oligosaccharides in the circulation of breastfed infants. PLoS One 2014;9(7):e101692.

12. Kelly RJ, Rouquier S, Giorgi D, et al. Sequence and expression of a candidate for the human Secretor blood group alpha(1,2)fucosyltransferase gene (FUT2). Homozygosity for an enzyme-inactivating nonsense mutation commonly correlates with the non-secretor phenotype. J Biol Chem 1995;270(9):4640–9.

13. Castanys-Munoz E, Martin MJ, Prieto PA. 2'-fucosyllactose: an abundant, genetically determined soluble glycan present in human milk. Nutr Rev 2013;71(12):773–89.

14. Ferrer-Admetlla A, Sikora M, Laayouni H, et al. A natural history of FUT2 polymorphism in humans. Mol Biol Evol 2009;26(9):1993–2003.

15. Blank D, Dotz V, Geyer R, et al. Human milk oligosaccharides and Lewis blood group: individual high-throughput sample profiling to enhance conclusions from functional studies. Adv Nutr 2012;3(3):440S–9S.

16. Stahl B, Thurl S, Henker J, et al. Detection of four human milk groups with respect to Lewis-blood-group-dependent oligosaccharides by serologic and chromatographic analysis. Adv Exp Med Biol 2001;501:299–306.

17. Smilowitz JT, O'Sullivan A, Barile D, et al. The human milk metabolome reveals diverse oligosaccharide profiles. J Nutr 2013;143(11):1709–18.

18. Thurl S, Munzert M, Henker J, et al. Variation of human milk oligosaccharides in relation to milk groups and lactational periods. Br J Nutr 2010;104(9):1261–71.

19. Chaturvedi P, Warren CD, Altaye M, et al. Fucosylated human milk oligosaccharides vary between individuals and over the course of lactation. Glycobiology 2001;11(5):365–72.

20. Coppa GV, Pierani P, Zampini L, et al. Oligosaccharides in human milk during different phases of lactation. Acta Paediatr Suppl 1999;88:89–94.

21. Gabrielli O, Zampini L, Galeazzi T, et al. Preterm milk oligosaccharides during the first month of lactation. Pediatrics 2011;128(6):e1520–31.

22. De Leoz ML, Wu S, Strum JS, et al. A quantitative and comprehensive method to analyze human milk oligosaccharide structures in the urine and feces of infants. Anal Bioanal Chem 2013;405(12):4089–105.

23. Marx C, Bridge R, Wolf AK, et al. Human milk oligosaccharide composition differs between donor milk and mother's own milk in the NICU. J Hum Lact 2014;30(1):54–61.

24. Bertino E, Coppa GV, Giuliani F, et al. Effects of holder pasteurization on human milk oligosaccharides. Int J Immunopathol Pharmacol 2008;21(2):381–5.

25. Sumiyoshi W, Urashima T, Nakamura T, et al. Galactosyllactoses in the milk of Japanese women: changes in concentration during the course of lactation. J Appl Glycosci 2004;51(4):341–4.

26. Albrecht S, Schols HA, van Zoeren D, et al. Oligosaccharides in feces of breast- and formula-fed babies. Carbohydr Res 2011;346(14):2173–81.

27. Albrecht S, Schols HA, van den Heuvel EG, et al. Occurrence of oligosaccharides in feces of breast-fed babies in their first six months of life and the corresponding breast milk. Carbohydr Res 2011;346(16):2540–50.

28. Underwood MA, Gaerlan S, De Leoz ML, et al. Human milk oligosaccharides in premature infants: absorption, excretion, and influence on the intestinal microbiota. Pediatr Res 2015;78(6):670–7.

29. Rudloff S, Obermeier S, Borsch C, et al. Incorporation of orally applied (13)C-galactose into milk lactose and oligosaccharides. Glycobiology 2006;16(6):477–87.

30. Rudloff S, Kunz C. Milk oligosaccharides and metabolism in infants. Adv Nutr 2012;3(3):398S–405S.
31. Ruhaak LR, Stroble C, Underwood MA, et al. Detection of milk oligosaccharides in plasma of infants. Anal Bioanal Chem 2014;406(24):5775–84.
32. Rudloff S, Pohlentz G, Diekmann L, et al. Urinary excretion of lactose and oligosaccharides in preterm infants fed human milk or infant formula. Acta Paediatr 1996;85(5):598–603.
33. Dotz V, Rudloff S, Blank D, et al. 13C-labeled oligosaccharides in breastfed infants' urine: individual-, structure- and time-dependent differences in the excretion. Glycobiology 2014;24(2):185–94.
34. Dotz V, Rudloff S, Meyer C, et al. Metabolic fate of neutral human milk oligosaccharides in exclusively breast-fed infants. Mol Nutr Food Res 2015;59(2):355–64.
35. Gnoth MJ, Rudloff S, Kunz C, et al. Investigations of the in vitro transport of human milk oligosaccharides by a Caco-2 monolayer using a novel high performance liquid chromatography-mass spectrometry technique. J Biol Chem 2001;276(37):34363–70.
36. Marriage BJ, Buck RH, Goehring KC, et al. Infants fed a lower calorie formula with 2′FL show growth and 2′FL uptake like breast-fed infants. J Pediatr Gastroenterol Nutr 2015;61(6):649–58.
37. LoCascio RG, Ninonuevo MR, Freeman SL, et al. Glycoprofiling of bifidobacterial consumption of human milk oligosaccharides demonstrates strain specific, preferential consumption of small chain glycans secreted in early human lactation. J Agric Food Chem 2007;55(22):8914–9.
38. Ruiz-Moyano S, Totten SM, Garrido DA, et al. Variation in consumption of human milk oligosaccharides by infant gut-associated strains of Bifidobacterium breve. Appl Environ Microbiol 2013;79(19):6040–9.
39. Kavanaugh DW, O'Callaghan J, Butto LF, et al. Exposure of Bifidobacterium longum subsp. Infantis to milk oligosaccharides increases adhesion to epithelial cells and induces a substantial transcriptional response. PLoS One 2013;8(6):e67224.
40. Chichlowski M, De Lartigue G, German JB, et al. Bifidobacteria isolated from infants and cultured on human milk oligosaccharides affect intestinal epithelial function. J Pediatr Gastroenterol Nutr 2012;55(3):321–7.
41. Arboleya S, Binetti A, Salazar N, et al. Establishment and development of intestinal microbiota in preterm neonates. FEMS Microbiol Ecol 2012;79(3):763–72.
42. Cong X, Xu W, Janton S, et al. Gut microbiome developmental patterns in early life of preterm infants: impacts of feeding and gender. PLoS One 2016;11(4):e0152751.
43. Torrazza RM, Neu J. The altered gut microbiome and necrotizing enterocolitis. Clin Perinatol 2013;40(1):93–108.
44. Groer MW, Luciano AA, Dishaw LJ, et al. Development of the preterm infant gut microbiome: a research priority. Microbiome 2014;2:38.
45. Yu H, Lau K, Thon V, et al. Synthetic disialyl hexasaccharides protect neonatal rats from necrotizing enterocolitis. Angew Chem Int Ed Engl 2014;53(26):6687–91.
46. Jantscher-Krenn E, Zherebtsov M, Nissan C, et al. The human milk oligosaccharide disialyllacto-N-tetraose prevents necrotising enterocolitis in neonatal rats. Gut 2012;61(10):1417–25.
47. Van Niekerk E, Autran CA, Nel DG, et al. Human milk oligosaccharides differ between HIV-infected and HIV-uninfected mothers and are related to necrotizing

enterocolitis incidence in their preterm very-low-birth-weight infants. J Nutr 2014; 144(8):1227–33.

48. Duijts L, Ramadhani MK, Moll HA. Breastfeeding protects against infectious diseases during infancy in industrialized countries. A systematic review. Matern Child Nutr 2009;5(3):199–210.

49. Lawrence RM, Pane CA. Human breast milk: current concepts of immunology and infectious diseases. Curr Probl Pediatr Adolesc Health Care 2007;37(1): 7–36.

50. Manthey CF, Autran CA, Eckmann L, et al. Human milk oligosaccharides protect against enteropathogenic Escherichia coli attachment in vitro and EPEC colonization in suckling mice. J Pediatr Gastroenterol Nutr 2014;58(2):165–8.

51. Ruiz-Palacios GM, Cervantes LE, Ramos P, et al. Campylobacter jejuni binds intestinal H(O) antigen (Fuc alpha 1, 2Gal beta 1, 4GlcNAc), and fucosyloligosaccharides of human milk inhibit its binding and infection. J Biol Chem 2003; 278(16):14112–20.

52. Jantscher-Krenn E, Lauwaet T, Bliss LA, et al. Human milk oligosaccharides reduce Entamoeba histolytica attachment and cytotoxicity in vitro. Br J Nutr 2012;108(10):1839–46.

53. Gonia S, Tuepker M, Heisel T, et al. Human milk oligosaccharides inhibit Candida albicans invasion of human premature intestinal epithelial cells. J Nutr 2015; 145(9):1992–8.

54. Kuntz S, Rudloff S, Kunz C. Oligosaccharides from human milk influence growth-related characteristics of intestinally transformed and non-transformed intestinal cells. Br J Nutr 2008;99(3):462–71.

55. Holscher HD, Bode L, Tappenden KA. Human milk oligosaccharides influence intestinal epithelial cell maturation in vitro. J Pediatr Gastroenterol Nutr 2016. [Epub ahead of print].

56. He Y, Liu S, Kling DE, et al. The human milk oligosaccharide 2'-fucosyllactose modulates CD14 expression in human enterocytes, thereby attenuating LPS-induced inflammation. Gut 2016;65(1):33–46.

57. Eiwegger T, Stahl B, Haidl P, et al. Prebiotic oligosaccharides: in vitro evidence for gastrointestinal epithelial transfer and immunomodulatory properties. Pediatr Allergy Immunol Pulmonol 2010;21(8):1179–88.

58. Morrow AL, Ruiz-Palacios GM, Altaye M, et al. Human milk oligosaccharides are associated with protection against diarrhea in breast-fed infants. J Pediatr 2004; 145(3):297–303.

59. Stepans MB, Wilhelm SL, Hertzog M, et al. Early consumption of human milk oligosaccharides is inversely related to subsequent risk of respiratory and enteric disease in infants. Breastfeed Med 2006;1(4):207–15.

60. Sprenger N, Odenwald H, Kukkonen AK, et al. FUT2-dependent breast milk oligosaccharides and allergy at 2 and 5 years of age in infants with high hereditary allergy risk. Eur J Clin Nutr 2016. [Epub ahead of print].

61. Seppo A, Autran C, Bode L, et al. Human milk oligosaccharides and development of cow's milk allergy in infants. J Allergy Clin Immunol 2016. [Epub ahead of print].

62. Kuhn L, Kim HY, Hsiao L, et al. Oligosaccharide composition of breast milk influences survival of uninfected children born to HIV-infected mothers in Lusaka, Zambia. J Nutr 2015;145(1):66–72.

63. Bode L, Kuhn L, Kim HY, et al. Human milk oligosaccharide concentration and risk of postnatal transmission of HIV through breastfeeding. Am J Clin Nutr 2012;96(4):831–9.

64. Alderete TL, Autran C, Brekke BE, et al. Associations between human milk oligosaccharides and infant body composition in the first 6 mo of life. Am J Clin Nutr 2015;102(6):1381–8.
65. Charbonneau MR, O'Donnell D, Blanton LV, et al. Sialylated milk oligosaccharides promote microbiota-dependent growth in models of infant undernutrition. Cell 2016;164(5):859–71.
66. Silveira PP, Portella AK, Goldani MZ, et al. Developmental origins of health and disease (DOHaD). J Pediatr (Rio J) 2007;83(6):494–504.
67. Fuhrer A, Sprenger N, Kurakevich E, et al. Milk sialyllactose influences colitis in mice through selective intestinal bacterial colonization. J Exp Med 2010; 207(13):2843–54.

"Bed Side" Human Milk Analysis in the Neonatal Intensive Care Unit

A Systematic Review

Gerhard Fusch, PhD[a], Celia Kwan, BHSc[a], Gynter Kotrri, BHSc[a],
Christoph Fusch, MD, PhD, FRCPC[a,b],*

KEYWORDS

- Infrared spectroscopy • Fortification • Preterm • Method validation • Growth
- Nutrition • Macronutrient

KEY POINTS

- Currently, there is an increase in human milk analyzers usage to measure the macronutrient content in breast milk before supplementation with fortifiers.
- These devices allow for a rapid analysis of milk, serving as a means to overcome the variability of nutritional content in breast milk and improve growth outcomes.
- It is crucial to introduce good laboratory and clinical practice when using these devices; otherwise their use can affect the growth outcomes of preterm infants.

INTRODUCTION

Optimal protein, fat, and lactose content in breast milk is crucial to the healthy growth of neonates, especially those with a very low birth weight.[1] Specifically for very low birth weight infants, macronutrient content in native breast milk is insufficient and needs to be fortified to meet their caloric and nutritional needs.[2] However, human milk shows a large variation in its macronutrient content.[3] The content varies between mothers, within the same mother, through the lactation period, during the same day, and even during feeds.[3] The current practice to fortify breast milk with standard amounts of fat, protein and carbohydrates may, therefore, not be adequate to overcome this variability in macronutrient content and meet the nutritional needs of preterm infants.[4]

Disclosure Statement: The authors have nothing to disclose.
[a] Division of Neonatology, Department of Pediatrics, McMaster University, 1280 Main Street West, Hamilton, Ontario L8S 4L8, Canada; [b] Department of Pediatrics, Paracelsus Medical School, General Hospital of Nuremberg, Breslauer Straße 201, Nuremberg 90471, Germany
* Corresponding author. Division of Neonatology, Department of Pediatrics, 1280 Main Street West, Room HSC-4F5, Hamilton, Ontario L8S 4K1, Canada.
E-mail address: fusch@mcmaster.ca

Currently, there is a trend in using infrared (IR) human milk analyzers to measure the macronutrient content in breast milk to tailor fortification.[4,5] These devices allow for a rapid analysis of milk, thus serving as a means to individually fortify breast milk to overcome the variability of nutritional content in breast milk and improve the quality of growth in infants.[4,5] Currently, there are 2 types of IR milk analyzers on the market: the mid-IR and the near-IR human milk analyzers. Owing to the complexity of milk composition, IR analyzers need to make certain assumptions about the composition of the substrate measured, the so-called matrix. For reliable analysis, it is assumed that the composition of this matrix is constant within certain limits. However, these IR devices were developed originally for the use in dairy industry.[5] They must, therefore, be validated using a sufficient number of human milk samples and principles of good laboratory practice should be applied.[5]

However, there is currently no agreement on standard procedures to validate or calibrate these devices.[5] There are also no human milk sample standards available for those interested in calibrating their devices.[6] Different devices also have different features and sample preparation requirements. Hence, this article reviews the current evidence about the use of human milk analyzers to improve neonatal nutrition.

METHODS

A literature search was conducted in PubMed, Embase (1974 to August 2, 2016), Ovid Health Star (1966 to August 2, 2016), Ovid MEDLINE(R) In-Process and Other Non-Indexed Citations, Ovid MEDLINE(R) Daily, and Ovid MEDLINE(R) (1946 to August 2, 2016). The following keywords were searched: "Miris" OR "human milk analyzer" OR "((Unity) OR Spectra Star) AND human milk" OR "Calais analyzer" OR "breast milk spectroscopy macronutrients" OR "Miris analyzer" OR "breast milk macronutrient" OR "energy content breast milk" OR "breast milk formula AND fortif* AND low birth weight infants" OR "near-infrared-reflectance-analysis" OR "human milk anal* macronutrient" OR "breast milk anal* macronutrient" OR "milkoscan" OR "Lactoscope." Titles and abstracts were screened to identify if studies were relevant for full-text screening, after which full texts were included if they met the prespecified inclusion criteria.

Selection Criteria

Article titles and abstracts were screened for full-text review. Only original studies in English, German, French, and Chinese were included. Duplicates of articles found in each database, as well as abstracts for conference proceedings were excluded. Studies were considered eligible during title and abstract screening if (1) human milk analyzers were mentioned in the title or the abstract, (2) measurement of macronutrient content was mentioned, or (3) the study investigated variability of macronutrient content in human milk.

Information Collection

Two authors (G.K. and C.K.) screened titles and abstracts independently. Disagreements for full-text article review were resolved through discussion between the 2 authors. When necessary, a third party (G.F.) was consulted to reach a consensus. Articles considered eligible at the title and abstract screening stage were evaluated at the full-text review stage independently by the 2 authors, using identical inclusion and exclusion criteria.

Information Extraction

Following selection of eligible articles, the following information was extracted from each study: (1) model of milk analyzer used (company and date of manufacture), (2) setting of the manufacturer used for measurement (wavelength of IR spectra of device, calibration of the device), (3) previous validation of the device for measurement of human milk, (4) handling and storage condition of milk samples during collection and before measurement, (5) sample preparation for measurement, (6) sample size, (7) characteristic of breast milk samples used in study (gestational age, lactation period), (8) purpose of the study, and (9) study results and clinical conclusions asserted by the authors.

RESULTS

Sixty-two studies fulfilled our inclusion criteria. **Table 1** provides an overview of the results.

Milk Analyzer Models

Eight different milk analyzers were identified in the included articles: the Human Milk Analyzer by MIRIS[7] (Uppsala, Sweden) (n = 33),[5,6,8–38] the Milkoscan[39] (Foss, Hillerod, Denmark) (n = 10),[40–49] the Unity Scientific Spectrastar[50] (Brookfield, CT) (n = 9),[4,5,51–57] the Calais Human Milk Analyzer[58] (Cleveland, OH) (n = 3),[3,59,60] the near-IR reflectance analysis (NIRA) (NIRA, Fenir 8820; Esetek Instruments, Marino, Roma, Italy) (n = 3),[61–63] the Delta Lactoscope[64] (n = 1)[65] (Drachten, the Netherlands), the AcuDairy Mid-Range Infrared instrument from Analytical Technologies[66] (n = 1)[67] (Westfield, NY), and the York Dairy Analyzer from Metron Instruments[68] (n = 1)[69] (Bedford Heights, OH). Two studies did not specify the milk analyzer they have used.[70,71]

Purposes of Included Studies

A summary of the studies can be found in **Tables 2–4**; these tables group the studies according to their aims. The first group (n = 14) includes studies[5,6,8–11,40,41,51,52,59–61,65] whose main aim is to evaluate IR milk analyzers (ie, investigating the accuracy and precision of the device) (see **Table 2**). The second group (n = 40) includes studies[3,8,12–34,42–48,52–54,62,67,69–71] whose main aim is to investigate the effect of different conditions on the macronutrient content of breast milk, using milk analyzers as the method of measurement (see **Table 3**). The third group (n = 11) includes trials[4,35–38,42,49,55–57,63] that used milk analyzers in a clinical setting (see **Table 4**).

In the second group, the 29 following conditions were studied to understand their impact on the macronutrient content of breast milk: feeding methods (n = 4),[45,46,53,69] various containers (n = 1),[19] left or right breast (n = 2),[18,27] breast size (n = 1),[27] maternal handedness (n = 1),[27] lactation period/stage (n = 8),[16,25,26,29,32,33,47,70] pooling of milk (n = 2),[23,54] delivery type (n = 2),[17,34] bariatric surgery (n = 1),[15] premature infants (n = 6),[12,16,21,23,33,48] fortification (n = 5),[3,13,42,62,71] pasteurization (n = 3),[22,45,52] milk bank (n = 2),[44,67] freezing and thawing (n = 6),[14,19,20,22,43,45] homogenization (n = 2),[14,24] dilution of samples (n = 1),[8] maternal age (n = 1),[28] diurnal variations (n = 1),[29] milk expression method (manual expression vs electric pump) (n = 1),[30] lactational mastitis (n = 1),[31] gestational age (n = 1),[33] birth weight (n = 1),[33] postpregnancy body mass index (n = 1),[33] gestational diabetes (n = 1),[33] birth height (n = 1),[34] infant sex (n = 1),[34] postpartum age (n = 1),[34] and administration by gavage and continuous infusion (n = 1).[43] Multiple mentions are possible within each study. Among the second and third groups, there are 12 studies[4,32,37,42–44,48,49,54,57,62,70] that have used previously validated IR milk analyzers, and 35 studies[3,12–17,19–31,33–36,38,45–47,53,55,56,63,67,69,71] that have not previously validated their milk analyzers.

Table 1
Overview of results

		Number of Studies
Brand of Analyzer used[a,b]	MIRIS	33
	Unity Scientific Spectrastar	9
	Milkoscan	10
	Calais	3
	NIRA	3
	Delta Lactoscope	1
	Acudairy	1
	York Dairy Analyzer	1
	Not specified	2
Purpose of Study[a]	Evaluate IR milk analyzers	14
	Investigate the effect of different conditions on the macronutrient content of breast milk	40
	Clinical trials that use milk analyzers in a clinical study	11
Evaluation of the device – method to measure fat	Modified Folch method	1
	Spectroscopic esterified fatty acid method	1
	Gerber method	2
	Roese-Gottlieb method	2
	Bligh and Dyer method	1
	Mojonnier method	4
	Modified Mojonnier method	2
	Not specified	1
Evaluation of the device – method to measure protein[a]	Kjeldahl method	9
	Bradford Method	2
	Modified Bradford method using a commercial protein reagent	1
	Elemental analysis	2
	Not specified	1
Evaluation of the device – method to measure lactose[c]	High-performance liquid chromatography	5
	Enzymatic spectroscopic method	1
	Chloramine-T method	1
	Automated orcinol method	1
	Enzymatic Assay	1
	High-pH anion exchange chromatography with pulsed amperometric detector	1
	UPLC-MS/MS	2
	Not specified	1
Evaluation of the device – results on accuracy[a,c]	Fat IR measurements are accurate	10
	Fat IR measurements are inaccurate	5
	Protein IR measurements are accurate	10
	Protein IR measurements are inaccurate	4
	Lactose IR measurements are accurate	2
	Carbohydrate IR measurements are accurate	1
	Lactose IR measurements only accurate between 6-7g/dL	1
	Lactose IR measurements correlate moderately to those obtained from reference methods	1
	Lactose/Carbohydrate IR measurements are inaccurate representations of true lactose values	5
Evaluation of the device – results on precision	Fat IR measurements are precise	9
	Protein IR measurements are precise	9
	Lactose IR measurements are precise	5
	Lactose IR measurements are not precise	1

(continued on next page)

Table 1 (continued)		Number of Studies
Sample Storage Temperature[a]	4°C	9
	-5°C	1
	-20 to -30°C	25
	-80°C	9
	Not stored – measured fresh	6
	Not reported	20
Sample storage period prior to analyses[a]	24h	7
	48h	1
	72h	1
	1 wk	1
	3 mo	2
	8-83 d	1
	30-180 d	1
	6 months	1
	No limit	1
	Not stored – measured fresh	6
	Not reported	45
Sample thawing temperature[a]	4°C	2
	25°C	1
	37°C	7
	38°C	1
	40°C	24
	45°C	1
	50°C	1
	Variable temperatures[d]	2
	Thawed in microwave	2
	Not reported	22
Homogenization technique[a]	Calais internal homogenizer	1
	Sonicator	24
	Vortex	2
	Shaking samples by hand	3
	Unspecified stirring method	1
	Manual homogenization	1
	Unspecified homogenization technique	7
	Unhomogenized	1
	Homogenization not reported	25
Homogenization time/rate[a]	Shaken 10 times	1
	10s	1
	15s	2
	20s	1
	30s	1
	3 × 10 s	2
	1.5s/mL	13
	Volume dependant[e]	1
	Not reported	42

Abbreviations: IR, infrared; UPLC-MS/MS, ultraperformance liquid chromatography tandem massspectrometry.

[a] Multiple mentions were possible.
[b] One study used two devices (MIRIS and Unity Scientific).
[c] Not all evaluation studies investigated the accuracy of protein or lactose measurements.
[d] Ranges 25 to 33°C, and 20 to 40°C reported.
[e] Homogenization time depends on the sample volume in this study: 30s/mL for 2.5mL and 5s/mL for 4-74 mL.

Table 2
Studies that aim to validate their milk analyzers

Author, Year	Purpose of Study (What Was Measured and for What Purpose)?	Results of Study/ Conclusion	Used Milk Analyzer Model and Setting	Calibration of Device	Sample Size and Characteristics (eg. Term, Preterm)	Sample Preparation/ Handling and Storage (eg. Homogenized, Vortexed, Frozen, Thawed, How Much Volume in Analyzer?)
Menjo et al,[8] 2009	Examine if the macronutrient values measured by human milk analyzer are comparable with those measured by conventional methods Discover whether we could dilute the milk sample used for the human milk analyzer measurement if the amount of milk available for testing was insufficient	When comparing the human milk analyzer and conventional methods, all 3 nutrients exhibited a significantly positive correlation ($P<.001$); lactose content was reliable on the condition that it is 6–7 g/dL When comparing diluted and nondiluted samples, fat and protein had expected values after dilution whereas lactose did not (it was overestimated) HMA yields reliable measurements	Human Milk Analyzer (MIRIS)		32 samples from 16 mothers (1 from each breast) for comparison between HMA and conventional methods 23 samples for effect of dilution purpose, measured in triplicate	2 mL of breast milk used for analysis, but if the amount of OMM is not meeting the infant's need, then a smaller measurement would be better Samples stored at −20°C as soon as possible, and remained until analysis For the HMA, samples were thawed and warmed at 37°C, then stirred before measured Repeated measurements 3 times Mixed samples with water to dilute and investigate effect
Casadio et al,[9] 2010	Compare the macronutrient levels determined by the HMA with those derived from traditional laboratory methods, over a wide range of composition (diluted samples, high-fat samples)	There was a small but statistically significant difference in the levels of fat, protein, lactose, total solids, and energy for all samples For higher macronutrient levels, a trend to greater differences between the HMA and the laboratory method was seen	Human milk analyzer (MIRIS)	Factory calibration, optimized to measure human milk with normal biological variation	Thirty 100-mL human milk samples, 4 dilutions each Samples obtained from 13 term and 7 preterm mothers at various stages of lactation	Sample were frozen before analysis and were thawed/ warmed to 40°C Samples were then homogenized (1.5 s/mL) by an ultrasonic vibrator and measured in duplicate (3 mL/measurement)

Study	Objective	Findings/Comments	Device	Mode	Samples	Processing
Silvestre et al,[10] 2014	To evaluate the suitability of a rapid method for the analysis of macronutrients in human milk as compared with the analytical methods applied by cow's milk industry	The use of an IR HMA for the analysis of lipids, proteins and lactose in human milk proved satisfactory as regards the rapidity, simplicity and the required sample volume. The instrument afforded good linearity and precision in application to all three nutrients. However, accuracy was not acceptable when compared with the reference methods, with overestimation of the lipid content and underestimation of the amount of proteins and lactose contents. The use of mid-IR HMA might become the standard for rapid analysis of human milk once standardization and rigorous and systematic calibration is provided	Human Milk Analyzer (MIRIS)	Operated in "processed milk" mode, indicated for frozen samples (different calibration for fresh and frozen milk in device)	Mature milk from 39 donors, delivered at term	Kept frozen at −20°C until processed. Thawed at room temperature, then warmed up to 40°C and homogenized (1.5 s/mL) before analysis. 2 mL used for analysis
Sauer & Kim,[51] 2011	To demonstrate that the real-time nutritional analysis of human milk carbohydrate, fat and protein with NIR	This study demonstrates the feasibility of the use of NIR for nutrient analysis of human milk. NIR offers the potential for analysis and adjustable	SpectraStar 2400 (Unity Scientific)	Calibrated and validated during this study	42 samples used to create calibration, 10 samples used to validate the machine	Frozen or room temperature milk samples were prewarmed to 40°C in a digital water bath and gently shaken by hand to prevent milk fat from

(continued on next page)

Table 2
(continued)

Author, Year	Purpose of Study (What Was Measured and for What Purpose)?	Results of Study/Conclusion	Used Milk Analyzer Model and Setting	Calibration of Device	Sample Size and Characteristics (eg, Term, Preterm)	Sample Preparation/Handling and Storage (eg, Homogenized, Vortexed, Frozen, Thawed, How Much Volume in Analyzer?)
	spectrophotometric methods is accurate	fortification of human milk to optimize nutrient intake for the high-risk neonate				separating out Use 1 mL for analysis Samples then stored at −20°C then sent out for reference chemical analysis
Michaelsen et al,[40] 1988	To evaluate the precision and accuracy of an IR analyzer for measuring protein, fat, carbohydrate, and energy content of human milk	Precision of IR results are high for all 4 components Close linear covariation between IR results and reference results, except covariation between IR carbohydrate results and results of lactose assay was poor	MilkoScan 104 (Foss Electric)	N/A	N = 30 (including preterm milk, term milk, colostrum, milk from women donating to milk bank, and pooled milk from the bank)	6 mL of milk for analysis Only pooled milk was frozen before it was apportioned Each specimen heated to 37°C, then divided under constant agitation into 9 subsamples, which were frozen separately at −20°C for later analysis Analyses done in duplicate, analyzing 2 subsamples frozen separately Specimens heated to 40°C and agitated before measurement
Smilowitz et al,[65] 2014	Evaluate accuracy and precision of a FT mid-IR spectroscope	The agreement between the FT mid-IR spectroscope analysis and reference methods was high for protein and fat and moderate for lactose and energy	Delta Lactoscope FTIR Advanced Mid-IR Dairy Analyzer (Advanced Instruments)	First calibrated for human milk total protein, fat, and lactose using undiluted and diluted raw milk Component Calibration Standards (Eurofins DQCI, USA)	116 breast milk samples across lactation stages from women who delivered at term (n = 69) and preterm (n = 5) Term means >37 wk,	Samples cold-thawed overnight at 4°C On each test day, 10 milk samples were fully thawed at room temperature for 2 h and placed in a heated water bath until the sample reached 38°C

	Purpose	Device/Method	Study design	Samples	Sample preparation
(continued study)				preterm is between 26–36 wk	The composition of these bovine calibrants was determined by the Kjeldahl method (total nitrogen multiplied by 6.25; protein for human milk), the gravimetric Mojonnier method (fat), and HPLC (lactose) and by oven drying to constant weight (total solids). To determine how the use of human milk calibration influences human milk component measurements, a subset of human milk samples from the study (n = 14) that spanned the range of protein, fat, and lactose of interest was used to recalibrate the instrument	Each milk sample was vortexed at the maximum speed for 20 s to ensure the sample was evenly mixed. Each sample split into 2 aliquots: one sent to Eurofins for analysis using chemical reference methods, and one diluted and heated to 38°C, then revortexed at maximum speed for 20 s and analyzed by FT mid-IR spectroscopy
Billard et al,[6] 2015	To compare HMA results with results from biochemical Reference Methods for a large range of protein, fat, and carbohydrate contents and to establish a	New calibration curves were developed for the MIRIS HMA, allowing accurate measurements in large ranges of macronutrient content. This is necessary for reliable use of this device in individualizing nutrition for preterm	Human Milk Analyzer (MIRIS)	Purpose is to develop new calibration curves. Hence, measurements from HMA here are obtained through the HMA's calibration mode for processed milk according to the manufacturer's instructions	Raw human milk samples were obtained from the local human milk bank	Samples kept in aliquots of 30–50 mL at −20°C. Samples were pools of milk from 3 to 5 donors from the biobank. They were heated for 10 min at 50°C in a hot water bath, pooled, and homogenized (5 s/mL) before being aliquoted in 2.5 mL and

(continued on next page)

Table 2
(continued)

Author, Year	Purpose of Study (What Was Measured and for What Purpose)?	Results of Study/Conclusion	Used Milk Analyzer Model and Setting	Calibration of Device	Sample Size and Characteristics (eg, Term, Preterm)	Sample Preparation/Handling and Storage (eg, Homogenized, Vortexed, Frozen, Thawed, How Much Volume in Analyzer?)
	calibration adjustment	newborns A homogenization step with a disruptor coupled to a sonication step was necessary to obtain better accuracy of the measurements				stored at −20°C Before being processed with the HMA, the 2.5-mL milk sample was sonicated (30 s/mL, 2 times for 30 s on followed by 15 s off and again 15 s on, 40% amplitude)
Rigourd,[41] 2010	To validate a rapid method of measurement of human milk macronutrient composition (protein, fat, lactose) To answer the question: is there a variability in composition of different human milk batches	Human milk has a significant variability in protein and fat The Milkoscan minor calibration adapts well to HMA after a simple adjustment for protein and fat, and can be used to rapidly analyze human milk composition	MilkoScan Minor (FOSS)	Calibration was done according to the recommendations of the FOSS society using 15 samples that have been measured using reference methods	98 samples	N/A
Corvaglia et al,[61] 2008	To validate NIR reflectance analysis (NIRA) as a fast, reliable and suitable method for routine evaluation of	A strong agreement was found between the results of traditional methods and NIRA for both fat and nitrogen content	NIRA (Fenir 8820; Esetek Instruments)	Calibrated using 97 samples Validated using 60 samples	124 samples of expressed human milk (55 from preterm mothers and 69 from term mothers)	Samples stored in refrigerator

						Preterm = 26–32 wk; term = 37–41 wk
	human milk's nitrogen and fat content	NIRA can be used as a quick and reliable tool for routine monitoring of macronutrient content of human milk and for devising individualized human milk fortification regimens in the feeding of very premature infants				
Fusch et al,[5] 2015	Validate 2 milk analyzers for breast milk analysis with reference methods and to determine an effective sample pretreatment	For fat analysis, (A) measured precisely but not accurately (B) measured precisely and accurately For protein analysis, (A) was precise but not accurate whereas (B) was both precise and accurate For lactose analysis, both devices (A) and (B) showed 2 distinct concentration levels and measured, therefore, neither accurately nor precisely Macronutrient levels were unchanged in 2 independent samples of stored breast milk (20°C measured with IR; 80°C measured with wet chemistry) over a period of 14 mo	SpectraStar, (Unity Scientific), and Human Milk Analyzer (MIRIS)	Unity InfoStar version 3.9.0 for SpectraStar and XMA-SW version 2.0.1 for HMA Before analysis, a daily calibration check was performed using the calibration solution (MIRIS check)	Validating using 1188 breast milk samples collected from 63 mothers of preterm and term infants Samples were collected on 2 different occasions to cover different time points of lactation and various gestational ages at the time of sample collection	Initially, all samples were homogenized for 3 × 10 s Samples stored at −80°C for analysis Stored samples were warmed to 37°C in a water bath and homogenized for 3 × 10 s before analysis

(continued on next page)

Table 2
(continued)

Author, Year	Purpose of Study (What Was Measured and for What Purpose)?	Results of Study/ Conclusion	Used Milk Analyzer Model and Setting	Calibration of Device	Sample Size and Characteristics (eg, Term, Preterm)	Sample Preparation/ Handling and Storage (eg, Homogenized, Vortexed, Frozen, Thawed, How Much Volume in Analyzer?)
Zhu et al,[11] 2016	To compare the accuracy and precision of HMA method with fresh milk samples in the field studies with chemical methods with frozen samples in the laboratory	The protein, fat, and total solid levels were significantly correlated between the 2 methods The mean protein content was significantly lower and the mean fat level was significantly greater when measured using HMA method Thus, linear recalibration could be used to improve mean estimation for both protein and fat Overall, HMA might be used to analyze macronutrients in fresh human milk with acceptable accuracy and precision after recalibrating fat and protein levels of field samples	Human Milk Analyzer (MIRIS)	The unprocessed calibration procedure was used for fresh sample analysis according to the manufacturer's recommendation (MIRIS) A daily calibration check and cleaning steps every 10 analyses were performed using the calibration solution and cleaning solution, respectively Both solutions were supplied by the manufacturer	151 subjects recruited There were 99, 100, and 89 samples analyzed for protein, lactose, and fat to cover greater intersubject variation, respectively	Fresh milk samples were warmed to 40°C in a water bath before analysis One fresh milk sample (~2 mL) was injected into the analysis cell and measured for each subject For chemical methods: The remaining milk samples were aliquoted into 15 mL centrifuge tubes and were stored at −20°C in the field for further analysis in the laboratory The frozen samples were shipped to the China CDC laboratory in frozen conditions and were stored at −80°C until analysis with the reference methods in the laboratory All samples were thawed and homogenized using MIRIS ultrasonic oscillatory mixing machine for 30 s Then protein, lactose, fat, and moisture were determined using the

Source	Objective	Device	Findings	Measurement/Analysis	Samples	Sample Preparation
Kotrri et al,[52] 2016	To test a correction algorithm for a NIR milk analyzer for fat and protein measurements, and examine the effect of pasteurization on the IR matrix and the stability of fat, protein, and lactose	SpectraStar (Unity Scientific)	The correction algorithm generated for our device was found to be valid for unpasteurized and pasteurized breast milk. Pasteurization had no effect on the macronutrient levels and the IR matrix of breast milk. These results show that fat and protein content can be accurately measured and monitored for unpasteurized and pasteurized breast milk. Of additional importance is the implication that donated human milk, generally low in protein content, has the potential to be target fortified	Measurement values generated through NIR analysis were compared against those obtained through chemical reference methods to test the correction algorithm for the NIR milk analyzer. A correction algorithm was previously generated by plotting NIR measurement values against those generated through chemical reference methods. The inverse linear function of each of the resulting regression equations was used as the correction algorithm for readout generated by the NIR milk analyzer	50 samples (V = 60 mL)	Pasteurized and unpasteurized samples were then aliquoted (V = 1.5 mL each) and subsequently stored at −20°C temperature. For analysis, aliquoted samples were thawed at 37°C for 5 min and homogenized using an ultrasonic vibrator (VCX 130; Chemical Instruments AB; Sollentuna, Sweden) for 15 s
Groh-Wargo et al,[59] 2016	To compare mid-IR spectroscopy to reference laboratory milk analysis	Calais Milk Analyzer	No significant differences were detected between the macronutrient content of human milk obtained by MIR vs	The MIR analyzer was calibrated by the manufacturer to human milk values. To ensure a wide range of	Mothers with low-birth-weight infants (<2 kg at birth)	Pooled and frozen at −20°C. Only 1 freeze–thaw cycle for the milk analyzed. Milk was thawed overnight in a refrigerator

reference methods, respectively. All samples were run in duplicate

(continued on next page)

Table 2
(continued)

Author, Year	Purpose of Study (What Was Measured and for What Purpose)?	Results of Study/ Conclusion	Used Milk Analyzer Model and Setting	Calibration of Device	Sample Size and Characteristics (eg, Term, Preterm)	Sample Preparation/ Handling and Storage (eg, Homogenized, Vortexed, Frozen, Thawed, How Much Volume in Analyzer?)
		reference laboratory analysis Conclusions: MIR analysis seems to provide an accurate assessment of macronutrient content in expressed human milk from mothers of preterm infants		nutrient content, the calibration set included 6 samples of donor milk and 6 samples from mothers of preterm infants recruited for the current study Calibration samples were not used in the analysis comparing MIR spectroscopy to laboratory values		To solubilize and distribute the fat in the milk, the sample was first inverted several times to mix well and then was warmed to 40°C (104°F) in a water bath to ensure that a representative sample was presented to the analyzer pipette The Calais has an internal "ball and seat" high-pressure (3500 psi) mechanism that homogenizes the sample before analysis is performed 15-mL aliquot used for Calais milk analyzer analysis

| O'Neill et al,[60] 2013 | Test the hypothesis that a human milk analyzer (HMA) would provide more accurate data for fat and energy content than analysis by the creamatocrit | Mean fat content and mean energy by the creamatocrit were significantly higher than by HMA Comparison of biochemical analysis with HMA of the subset of milk samples showed no statistical difference for fat and energy | HMA (Calais) | Specifically calibrated to human milk with a series of 6 pooled human milk samples with varying concentrations of each compound; nutrient content of the calibrators was assayed by a certified reference laboratory (Mojonnier for fat, Kjeldahl for protein, and HPLC for carbohydrates) | 51 well-mixed samples of previously frozen expressed human milk were obtained after thawing | All milk samples were prewarmed at 40°C for 10 min before analysis, and were analyzed within minutes |

Abbreviations: (A), SpectraStar; (B), MIRIS; FT, Fourier transform; HMA, human milk analysis; HPLC, high-pressure liquid chromatography; IR, infrared; N/A, not applicable; NIR, near-infrared.

Table 3
Studies that aim to use milk analyzers to measure clinical samples under various clinical conditions

Author, Year	Purpose of Study (What Was Measured and for What Purpose?)	Results of Study/Conclusion	Model of Milk Analyzer Used and Setting	Calibration of Device	Sample Size and Characteristics (eg, Term, Preterm)	Sample Preparation/Handling and Storage (eg, Homogenized, Vortexed, Frozen, Thawed, How Much Volume in Analyzer?)
de Halleux et al,[42] 2013	To show the variability in human milk composition from an infant's OMM or pooled human milk from the milk bank. To evaluate the advantages of individual fortification on nutritional intakes over standard fortification	The variability in contents of fat, protein, and energy was high for all types of human milk samples. Compared with standard fortification, Individual fortification significantly reduced the variability in nutritional intakes	Milkoscan Minor (Foss)	In a previous paper, this group talked about the importance of calibration and validation	428 OMM, 138 human milk pools from single donors, 224 pools from multiple donors, and 14 pools from colostral milk	10 mL of human milk used for analysis. Human milk transported under aseptic HACCP conditions. OMM kept at 4°C and used within 72 h. DHM frozen and pasteurized by Holder method, and warmed by thawing to 37°C before analysis
Abranches et al,[43] 2014	To analyze the changes in human milk macronutrients: fat, protein, and lactose in natural human milk (raw), frozen and thawed, after administration simulation by gavage and continuous infusion	The fat content was significantly reduced after administration by continuous infusion ($P<.001$) during administration of both raw and thawed samples. No changes in protein and lactose content was observed between the 2 forms of infusion. However, the thawing	Milkoscan Minor (Foss)	Previously validated for human milk	34 human milk samples	The milk was extracted by manual expression or electric pump and stored in glass vials. Of the total collected volume, 50 mL were used, which were divided into 3 aliquots of 10 mL and 1 aliquot of 20 mL. The latter was frozen at −20°C for 24 h and thawed in a microwave for 45 s. The analysis of natural human milk was

Source	Aim	Results	Method	Validation	Samples	Notes
		process significantly increased the levels of lactose and milk protein				performed immediately after the extraction
Corvaglia et al,[62] 2010	To evaluate in a NICU setting if human milk protein content after standard fortification meets the recommended intake	After FF, protein content was >3 g/dL in none of the samples, and <2.33 g/dL in 16 of 34 samples. After LF, protein content was >3 g/dL in none of the samples and <2.33 g/dL in 32 of 34 Human milk protein content after standard fortification fails to meet the recommended intake for preterm infants in approximately one-half of the cases	NIR Reflectance-Analysis — NIRA	Previously calibrated and validated to human milk; specifically, nitrogen and fat content were evaluated in 124 human milk samples, collected from 55 mothers of preterm newborns and from 69 mothers of term newborns, by both NIRA and reference methods (Gerber for fat and Kjeldhal for nitrogen)	34 preterm human milk samples collected from 34 mothers who were feeding their preterm infants (gestational age between 24-33 wk)	N/A
Michaelsen et al,[70] 1994	The aim of the present analysis is to describe the nutritional role of breastfeeding We wanted to give a detailed description of human milk intake and protein, fat, carbohydrate, and energy contents in human milk, together with an analysis of influencing factors	The results of this study give a detailed description of milk intake, macronutrient concentration, and intake in a cohort of Copenhagen infants The cohort can be regarded as being reasonably representative of healthy, full-term Copenhagen infants	IR method used, but no milk analyzer explicitly mentioned	We previously evaluated IR analysis for determination of protein, fat, carbohydrate, and energy and found the method accurate	91 healthy term infants Milk samples were collected 4 d after delivery, 14 d after delivery, then every 2 wk up to 3 mo after delivery, and thereafter monthly as long as the mother was breastfeeding	Samples kept frozen at −20°C in the home until analyzed

(continued on next page)

Table 3
(continued)

Author, Year	Purpose of Study (What Was Measured and for What Purpose)?	Results of Study/ Conclusion	Model of Milk Analyzer Used and Setting	Calibration of Device	Sample Size and Characteristics (eg, Term, Preterm)	Sample Preparation/ Handling and Storage (eg, Homogenized, Vortexed, Frozen, Thawed, How Much Volume in Analyzer?)
Michaelsen et al,[44] 1990	Protein, fat, and carbohydrate concentration in expressed human bank milk was determined by IR analysis of 2554 samples from 224 mothers to monitor the content of macronutrients in the milk from the milk bank	The protein and fat contents increased slightly with increasing body mass index of the mother, the protein content decreased with increasing amounts of milk delivered to the milk bank, and the fat content was higher in mothers delivering large amounts of milk Thus, by continuous monitoring of macronutrient content in human bank milk it is possible to develop a "high-protein" milk with sufficient protein and energy content to cover the needs of preterm infants with very low birth weights (<1500 g)	Milkoscan 104 IR milk analyzer (Foss Electric)	Previously evaluated this method and found very close linear covariation between IR results and reference methods for protein, fat, and energy The validation (in the previous paper) uses 30 samples of human milk This includes preterm and term milk, colostrum, and donor milk	2554 samples from 224 mothers	Milk was pooled together, stirred, then stored at −25°C until analysis At the time of analysis, samples were heated to 40°C, stirred mechanically, and measured by IR analysis
He et al,[12] 2014	To study the dynamic changes in macronutrients and	The levels of macronutrients and energy in milk from	Human Milk Analyzer (MIRIS)		339 human milk samples from 170 women who	Samples (5 mL) stored at 4°C and homogenized before analyzed with milk

	energy in human milk from mothers of premature infants	mothers of premature infants vary significantly between colostrum, transitional milk, and mature milk Protein levels are significantly higher in colostrum from premature infants' mothers than in colostrum from term infants' mothers		delivered preterm or full-term infants	analyzer 2–3 mL of milk injected in analyzer for analysis
Cooper et al,[13] 2013	Compare macronutrient content between formula milk and donated human expressed breast milk ± fortification to investigate whether DEBM meets current recommended macronutrient requirements To demonstrate potential variability in nutritional intake of DEBM	Results confirm the nutritional variability of donated human expressed breast milk and demonstrate the potential of nutritional analysis to target the use of donor milk according to energy content No significant difference in composition of milk between term and preterm mothers No significant differences in milk composition expressed at different postnatal ages At volumes of 180 mL/kg/day 119 samples (66%) would have provided minimum preterm energy	Human Milk Analyzer (MIRIS) N/A	179 samples from 42 unique donors	Single donor milk samples were pooled Sequential donated milk samples were analyzed over a 3-mo period Aliquots from a single donor were pooled, pasteurized, frozen and stored as per the NICE guidelines Before analysis, samples were warmed to 37°C and homogenized using an ultrasound probe (20,000 Hz, 1.5 s/mL)

(continued on next page)

Table 3
(continued)

Author, Year	Purpose of Study (What Was Measured and for What Purpose?)	Results of Study/Conclusion	Model of Milk Analyzer Used and Setting	Calibration of Device	Sample Size and Characteristics (eg, Term, Preterm)	Sample Preparation/Handling and Storage (eg, Homogenized, Vortexed, Frozen, Thawed, How Much Volume in Analyzer?)
		requirements without fortification however protein levels were low and even with fortification 39% of samples would fail to meet the recommended preterm requirements				
Garcia-Lara et al,[14] 2012	Determine the effect of freezing time up to 3 mo on the content of fat, total nitrogen, lactose, and energy + assess whether ultrasonic homogenization of samples enables a more suitable reading of breast milk macronutrients with a human milk analyzer	Observed a decline in the concentration of fat and energy content by 3 mo of freezing at −20°C Total nitrogen and lactose contents revealed a variable, low-magnitude, and not constant reduction with freezing time The absolute concentration of all macronutrients and calories was greater with ultrasonic homogenization Correct homogenization is fundamental for correct nutritional analysis	Human Milk Analyzer (MIRIS)	Calibrated by manufacturer, using a set of reference breast milk samples with different fat, protein, and lactose contents that were analyzed with benchmark biochemical methods: the Roese–Gottlieb method (fat), the Kjeldahl method (total nitrogen), and high-performance liquid chromatography (lactose) Habitual use of MIRIS CHECK solution provided by manufacturer for normal use of the instrument avoids the need for recalibration	61 breast milk samples from 59 mothers 46% of mothers gave birth before week 32 of gestation, 21% between weeks 32 and 36, and 33% at week 37 or later Stage of lactation: The 25th, 50th, and 75th percentile values were 13, 18, and 41 d, respectively Minimum = 5 d, maximum = 389 d	Samples collected with a volume of ≥35 mL, then immediately stored in a refrigerator at <5°C for a maximum period of 24 h before their analyses Stored in glass flask with sterile plastic cap For homogenization, samples were heated at 40°C and temperature was verified with a thermometer with certified calibration Sample was stirred by means of rocking the sample in an arclike fashion 10 times 12 aliquots of 2.5 mL were prepared and placed in polypropylene test tubes Frozen at −20°C Each aliquot was heated at 40°C and stirred by

					rocking in an arclike fashion twice. Ultrasound processor was applied to one-half of the samples at 75% amplitude and 1.5 s/mL. Used Coulter counter to measure size of breast milk fat globules. Put 2 mL of breast milk into homogenizer
Jans et al,[15] 2015	Investigate macronutrient and energy content of breast milk from women with bariatric surgery	Human Milk Analyzer (MIRIS)	A higher fat, energy, and a slightly higher carbohydrate milk content was found in the surgical group compared with the nonsurgical group. The nutritional value of breast milk after bariatric surgery seems to be at least as high as in nonsurgical controls. Significantly lower carbohydrate in total study population compared with reference values from UK Food composition	Sample from 16 lactating women and 36 nonsurgical controls. Lactating women who delivered at term (≥ 37 gestational weeks) were invited. Samples gathered 4 d after delivery. Gathered 5 mL after infant was fed for 3 min	Samples immediately frozen at -80°C. Samples analyzed 24 h before sampling with a food record
Hsu et al,[16] 2014	Investigate the changes in composition of breast milk from mothers with preterm infants (gestation age < 35 wk) during	Human Milk Analyzer (MIRIS)	There were increases in lactose, lipid, calorie, phosphate concentration, and decrease in protein and secretory IgA. No significant difference in most	80 fresh milk samples from 17 mothers who had delivered preterm infants was collected longitudinally for 4–6 wk. 30 fresh milk samples	After expression, samples were immediately stored in the refrigerator and analyzed within 24 h. 5 mL used in HMA. Before analysis, milk heated to 40°C in a water bath

(continued on next page)

Table 3
(continued)

Author, Year	Purpose of Study (What Was Measured and for What Purpose)?	Results of Study/Conclusion	Model of Milk Analyzer Used and Setting	Calibration of Device	Sample Size and Characteristics (eg, Term, Preterm)	Sample Preparation/Handling and Storage (eg, Homogenized, Vortexed, Frozen, Thawed, How Much Volume in Analyzer?)
	the first 4–6 wk of lactation Fat, protein, lactose, energy, minerals (calcium and phosphate), and immune components (secretory IgA, leptin, lysozyme, and lactoferrin) content were measured	components of breast milk between preterm and full-term mothers			from 15 mothers of full-term infants was also collected at the 1st week and 4th week Each participant gave 20 mL breast milk each time on days 5–7, days 12–14, days 19–21, days 26–28, days 33–35, and days 39–42 after delivery	and homogenized Each sample analyzed twice
Radmacher et al,[3] 2013	To use real-time human milk macronutrient analysis to calculate final composition following fortification Measured for fat, protein and lactose	Lactose was similar in PHM and DHM Protein in PHM showed the expected decline as lactation progressed DHM protein was significantly lower vs PHM Fat was highly variable and lowest in DHM Using standard fortification protocols, not all fortified milks met targets for protein	Mid-IR spectrometry (Calais Human Milk Analyzer)		Mother's own preterm milk or purchased pooled DHM were obtained after thawing 83 discrete milk samples for very low birth weight infants and 6 DHM samples from a regional milk bank were analyzed	Analysis performed the same day the milk was thawed

Study	Purpose	Device	Validation	Sample collection	Sample processing	Results
Dizdar et al,[17] 2014	To determine the effect of delivery type on macronutrient content of colostral milk. Milk protein, fat, carbohydrate, and energy levels were measured	Human Milk Analyzer (MIRIS)	Correlation coefficient was 0.92 for human milk analyzer and high-pressure liquid chromatography method in one study (referenced study from Menjo 2009)	Colostral milk samples from 204 term lactating mothers who gave birth by vaginal (n = 111) or cesarean delivery (n = 93) were obtained on the 2nd postpartum day. 4 mL were obtained from mothers	Eppendorf tubes were used for collection and unfrozen fresh milk samples were analyzed within 2 h after sample collection. Samples aliquoted into 2, then 2 mL into analyzer. Each sample measured twice	and energy. Individualized fortification resulted in milks closer to target recommendations. Vaginal delivery is associated with higher colostrum protein content. Colostral fat, carbohydrate, and energy levels were similar between groups
Khan et al,[18] 2013	To investigate short-term changes in breast milk composition between left and right breasts, over a 3-wk period within the first 6 mo of lactation	Human Milk Analyzer (MIRIS)	Using HMA calibration mode of processed (homogenized) milk	The left and right breasts of the mothers of healthy, term infants (n = 23) were simultaneously expressed with an electric breast pump for 15 min, on 3 occasions within 3 wk. Milk samples (5 mL) were collected from the total expression volume of each breast at each session. Milk samples were collected at each session from each	Samples stored at −20°C until further analysis. 2 mL used for analysis. Before analysis, all samples were thawed, warmed to 40°C in a digital water bath, and homogenized (1.5 s per 1 mL of sample) using an ultrasonic processor VCX130. All samples analyzed in duplicate	Over the 3 weekly sessions, no significant changes were found in macronutrient contents. The macronutrient concentration was similar for the left and right breasts; however, milk composition varied markedly between mothers. Mean 24-h fat content was consistently lower than the mean fat content from a single expression

(continued on next page)

Table 3
(continued)

Author, Year	Purpose of Study (What Was Measured and for What Purpose)?	Results of Study/ Conclusion	Model of Milk Analyzer Used and Setting	Calibration of Device	Sample Size and Characteristics (eg, Term, Preterm)	Sample Preparation/ Handling and Storage (eg, Homogenized, Vortexed, Frozen, Thawed, How Much Volume in Analyzer?)
					breast at the beginning (pre, 1–2 mL), middle (mid, 5 mL), and end (post, 1–2 mL) of the expression session	session by approximately 13 g/L
Chang et al,[19] 2012	To evaluate the impact of various containers on the nutrient concentrations in human milk	There was a significant decrease in the fat content after the storage, freezing, and thawing processes There were statistically significant increases in protein and carbohydrate concentrations in all containers ($P = .021$ and 0.001, respectively); however, there were no significant differences between the containers in terms of fat, protein, carbohydrate, or energy contents	Human Milk Analyzer (MIRIS)	N/A	42 breast milk samples collected from 18 healthy lactating mothers All infants are full term, aging from 1–23 mo	Samples obtained were immediately stored in glass containers in a refrigerator for no more than 3 d before analysis Samples were homogenized using a homogenizer for 1.5 s/mL Baseline determined, then samples divided and stored in 9 different commercial milk containers Each container stored at −20°C for 48 h, then put into refrigerator at 4°C for 12 h to thaw After removal from refrigerator, samples subjected to same homogenization and analysis 3 mL of milk used, and measured in triplicate

Study	Objective	Analyzer	Calibration	Samples	Processing	Conclusions
Brooks et al,[69] 2013	To compare the differences in lipid loss from 24 samples of banked DHM among 3 feeding methods: DHM given by syringe pump over 1 h, 2 h, and by bolus/gravity gavage	York Dairy analyzer	The analyzer is calibrated against chemical assays in cooperation with the US Dairy Association in Carrolton, TX, biannually and tested daily against a control for stability. The instrument is calibrated with bias and slope as well as automatic linear regression	24 samples of banked DHM	Samples warmed to 37°C using a warmer, then poured into a glass flask and hard swirled to mix. After testing the daily control sample, samples were uniformly warmed to 40°C, homogenized and analyzed	Unlike gravity feedings, the timed feedings resulted in a statistically significant loss of fat as compared with their controls
Lev et al,[20] 2014	To test the null hypothesis that human milk freezing and storage for a range of 1–10 wk at −80°C does not affect human milk fat, protein, lactose, and energy contents	Human Milk Analyzer (MIRIS)	N/A	60 samples from 20 mothers of preterm infants	After extraction, samples were stored in polyethylene tubes in a refrigerator at <5°C for a maximum period of 24 h. Stored at −80°C for 8–83 d. Samples are thawed by heating at 40°C in a thermostatic bath and homogenized before analysis	Freezing at −80°C significantly decreases the energy content of human milk, both from fat and carbohydrates. Because quantitatively the decrease in macronutrients was much higher than that published for human milk storage at −20°C, our results do not support freezing human milk at −80°C as the gold standard for long-term storage
Vieira et al,[45] 2011	To determine the effect of various process (Holder pasteurization, freezing and thawing and feeding method) on the	MilkoScan Minor (Foss Analytical)	Previously calibrated for human milk measurements using Kjeldahl method for protein, Chloramine-T for lactose and Gerber for fat	57 samples analyzed in first step (pasteurization) 228 in offer step	Samples frozen at −20°C, then slow thawed (water bath at 40°C for 10 min) or quick thaw (microwave oven for 45 s)	The repeated processes that DHM is submitted before delivery to newborn infants cause a reduction in the fat and protein concentration

(continued on next page)

Table 3
(continued)

Author, Year	Purpose of Study (What Was Measured and for What Purpose)?	Results of Study/ Conclusion	Model of Milk Analyzer Used and Setting	Calibration of Device	Sample Size and Characteristics (eg. Term, Preterm)	Sample Preparation/ Handling and Storage (eg. Homogenized, Vortexed, Frozen, Thawed, How Much Volume in Analyzer?)
	macronutrient concentration of human milk	The magnitude of this decrease is higher on the fat concentration				
Zachariassen et al,[21] 2013	Determine the content of macronutrients in human milk (human milk) from mothers who gave birth very prematurely, and to investigate possible associations between macronutrients and certain maternal and infant characteristics	Protein content in human milk varies considerably between mothers, and decreases within weeks after very preterm birth Previous breastfeeding experience and low gestational age were associated with a lower protein and a higher fat and energy content in human milk, respectively Interindividual differences in human milk content possibly influences nutrition and this raises the question of the need for an individualized approach when fortifying human milk for preterm infants	Human Milk Analyzer (MIRIS)	Initially recalibrated with reference milk analyzed with the methodologies of Rose-Gottlieb (fat), Kjeldahl (protein), dry oven (solids/lactose) at a certified laboratory for official controls of foods under the Danish Ministry of Food, Agriculture, and Fisheries in Aarhus, Denmark	736 human milk samples from 214 mothers of preterm infants with gestational age of <32 wk These mothers expressed milk for analysis 2 wk after birth, every second week until discharge, at term, at 2, and at 4 mo of corrected age	Samples were frozen as soon as possible after 24 h of collection For analysis, samples were defrosted in a refrigerator, heated in warm water until reaching a temperature of 40°C and homogenized before analysis Every human milk sample contained human milk for 2–5 analyses A mean value was calculated for each human milk sample
Garcia-Lara et al,[22] 2013	Explore the effect of Holder pasteurization and frozen storage	Holder pasteurization decreased fat and energy content of human milk	Human Milk Analyzer (MIRIS)	The instrument was calibrated by the manufacturer for optimum measurement of breast milk within its	34 samples of frozen breast milk donated by 28 women	No limit on freezing time before pasteurization Samples stored at −20°C until processing, then

	at −20°C after pasteurization on fat, total nitrogen, lactose, and energy content of breast milk Both procedures are practiced routinely in human milk banks	Frozen storage at −20°C of pasteurized milk significantly reduced fat, lactose, and energy content of human milk	normal biological variation For internal calibration, machine uses a Check solution provided by the manufacturer This solution corrects any instrument transmission-level problems Regarding external calibration, the device was initially calibrated and tested at the factory (Roese-Gottlieb for fat; Kjeldahl for total nitrogen; high performance liquid chromatography for lactose) To recalibrate it, every year at least 2 human milk samples of different concentrations are analyzed with HMA and are sent to a Spanish ENAC Certified Laboratory, which follows the instructions contained in the norm UNE-EN ISO/IEC 17025: 2005 for physical and chemical analysis in human milk The laboratory analyses are Roese-Gottlieb for fat, Kjeldahl for total nitrogen, and gravimetry for total solids Lactose value is obtained by subtracting fat and total nitrogen values from the total solid value			thawed and heated to 40°C using a thermostatic bath; the temperature of the samples was measured continuously by a thermometer with certified calibration Samples were then homogenized for 1.5 s/mL
Anderssen et al,[23] 2015	Evaluate the reproducibility of macronutrient	The domestic pooling of 24-h expressed human milk for	Human Milk Analyzer (MIRIS)	Calibrated with human milk standards for macronutrients	120 samples from 28 new mothers expressed their	Sample was stored in the refrigerator, and the rest were stored in the freezer

(continued on next page)

Table 3
(continued)

Author, Year	Purpose of Study (What Was Measured and for What Purpose)?	Results of Study/ Conclusion	Model of Milk Analyzer Used and Setting	Calibration of Device	Sample Size and Characteristics (eg, Term, Preterm)	Sample Preparation/ Handling and Storage (eg, Homogenized, Vortexed, Frozen, Thawed, How Much Volume in Analyzer?)
	measurements of domestic pooled human milk from mothers with preterm infants and to see how the results affected human milks	macronutrient analysis was a simple and reliable way of obtaining representative data Standard fortification implies there is a risk of undernutrition and overnutrition, and individual fortification may improve the nutrition of preterm infants			breast milk for 24 h on 2 consecutive days and repeated the process at weakly intervals	Samples are heated to 40°C and homogenized before analysis
Garcia-Lara et al,[24] 2014	Compared the loss of fat based on the use of 3 different methods for homogenizing thawed human milk during continuous feeding	When thawed human milk is continuously infused, a smaller fat loss is observed when syringes are agitated hourly vs when ultrasound or a baseline homogenization is used	Human Milk Analyzer (MIRIS)	Machine calibrated for fat against Roese-Gottlieb reference method Calibration was done in an independent laboratory for 5 milk samples	N = 16	Stored in a freezer at −20°C until they were ready for processing Thawed in a thermostatic bath at 40°C Homogenized, stored for 48 h After that: Samples were shaken in an arclike fashion to mimic clinical routine
Yang et al,[25] 2014	To measure breast milk energy and macronutrient concentrations of healthy urban	Stage of lactation was a strong factor affecting milk composition Minimal evidence was	Human Milk Analyzer (MIRIS)	N/A	A stratified sample including 150 mothers from each of the 3 cities (30 each of whom were	Milk samples were collected from one breast between 9:00 and 11:00 AM Milk was then gently swirled and 40 mL was taken for

	Objective	Findings	Instrument	Recalibration/Notes	Samples analyzed	Population / Sample handling
	Chinese mothers at different lactation stages, to expand the database of milk composition of Chinese population, and to examine whether dietary or other maternal factors can affect the levels of macronutrients in breast milk	found for associations between maternal current dietary intake and milk macronutrient concentration, consistently with prior research. Maternal body mass index was associated positively with milk fat content, to a greater extent than did dietary intake. All other maternal characteristics were not significant for milk composition. These findings suggest that milk composition is generally weakly associated with maternal factors except for stage of lactation, and is likely to be more susceptible to long-term maternal nutritional status than short-term dietary fluctuation			at 5–11 d, 12–30 d, 31–60 d, 61–120 d, and 121–240 d postpartum, respectively). Included breastfeeding mothers aged 18–45, were primigravida and healthy, and had delivered a single healthy baby; excluded those who did not deliver their babies at term. Total of 436 mothers with 86, 85, 88, 90, and 87 from each postpartum time point, respectively, were examined	analyses of individual samples. The samples were placed on freezer packs, and delivered within 2 h to the analytical laboratories where they were aliquoted and stored at −80°C. 2 mL from each sample was thawed and warmed to 40°C before analysis. The quantities of the components were measured in a single run
Wojcik et al,[67] 2009	Banked donor milk may be a reasonable substitute for mother's milk for human infants	Banked donor milk differs from freshly expressed, mature milk in nutrient content and energy	AcuDairy IR 5150 (Analytical Technologies)	"Because it was originally intended for use with dairy milk, the instrument was specifically recalibrated, with the assistance of the	These analyses are of single-donor donations pooled from that donor's individual	Samples were held at Prolacta for up to 3 mo at −30°C before testing. Although there is no way to trace how long samples

(continued on next page)

Table 3
(continued)

Author, Year	Purpose of Study (What Was Measured and for What Purpose)?	Results of Study/ Conclusion	Model of Milk Analyzer Used and Setting	Calibration of Device	Sample Size and Characteristics (eg, Term, Preterm)	Sample Preparation/ Handling and Storage (eg, Homogenized, Vortexed, Frozen, Thawed, How Much Volume in Analyzer?)
	No data on the macronutrient composition of banked donor milk have been reported This study determined the composition of donated milk from a large number of banked donor milk samples and compared it with the reported values for macronutrients in mature breast milk	value This difference may be owing to MOM being produced and consumed on a 24-h basis, whereas banked milk represents just a portion of what is expressed over that same period The most notable difference manifests itself in the total energy value Unformulated banked donor milk alone, similar to mother's milk alone, does not have sufficient macronutrient content or energy density to sustain a very low birth weight preterm infant		manufacturer, to meet the requirements for assessing nutrient content of human milk"	collection bottles The containers of each donor's frozen milk were received, thawed, pooled, and a sample was then drawn for analysis of protein and lipids, as well as calculation of carbohydrates and energy There were 415 samples from 273 unique donors	were held in each donor's freezer, this fact is applicable to all milk banking situations The instrument uses about 7 mL per sample Quality control was performed through the use of negative control, which involves zeroing the instrument per the manufacturer's instructions
Krcho et al,[71] 2015	Compared changes in the concentrations of the main constituents of	Dry matter and energy content increased the most after fortification	"This device is approved by European standard 98/79/EC, and uses	No mention	30 samples obtained from mothers of preterm infants (gestational age	Samples were stored at room temperature and then heated to 40°C just before analysis

Reference	Purpose	Findings/Conclusion	Device	Results	Sample	Population
Stoltz Sjöström et al,[46] 2014	This study aimed to describe the types and amounts of human breast milk before and after fortification	Although protein also increased, the magnitude of this increase was small relative to the increases in the other components. Lipid concentrations did not significantly change with fortification. Protein is needed for adequate growth in premature infants; however, fortification of breast milk from the mothers of preterm infants resulted in only a small increase in this essential nutrient. Based on these results, we conclude that fortification of human milk must be individually adjusted based on continuous analysis of breast milk composition. Customized fortification would provide more optimal nutrition to preterm infants to support better growth and development	MilkoScan 4000 (FOSS) and infrared spectroscopy to measure the absorption of infrared radiation". Both of these mid-IR techniques were calibrated for human milk	Protein content in MOM decreased significantly from 2.2 to 1.2 g/	Nutritional content in 821 MOM samples was analyzed. From a 24-h collection of expressed MOM, a 10-mL sample was transferred to	28-36 wk; birthweight 900-2470 g)

(continued on next page)

Table 3
(continued)

Author, Year	Purpose of Study (What Was Measured and for What Purpose)?	Results of Study/ Conclusion	Model of Milk Analyzer Used and Setting	Calibration of Device	Sample Size and Characteristics (eg, Term, Preterm)	Sample Preparation/ Handling and Storage (eg, Homogenized, Vortexed, Frozen, Thawed, How Much Volume in Analyzer?)
	enteral feeds given to Swedish extremely preterm infants during hospitalization and to investigate the energy and macronutrient contents in human milk given to these infants	100 mL during the first 112 postpartum days, whereas fat and energy content were highly variable within and between MOM samples In addition, 354 samples of donor milk were analyzed Content of protein, fat, and energy in pooled donor milk (n = 129) was lower compared with single donor milk Swedish extremely preterm infants receive MOM to a large extent during hospitalization Protein, carbohydrates, and energy in MOM changed significantly with time Weekly analyses of MOM during the first month of lactation would allow more individualized nutritional support for these vulnerable infants	MilkoScan 133 (FOSS)			a plastic tube, which was prepared with 20 µL of Bronopol BASF SE (Protectol BN, Ludwigshafen, Germany), which is used as an antimicrobial Samples were then sent by overnight mail and analyzed at the central laboratory

	Objective	Results	Human Milk Analyzer		Sample	Methods
Kreissl et al,[26] 2016	To determine the relationship between protein content and lactation period	The wide variations in macronutrient content were not influenced by the gestational age of the infant and the lactation day results from 70 of the mothers correlated inversely with the protein content. Variations in macronutrients were high in the breast milk of women who delivered preterm babies and the protein content decreased with lactation	Human Milk Analyzer (MIRIS)	The MIRIS Human Milk Analyzer is calibrated against standard methods	83 samples of 24-h pooled human milk from 76 mothers who delivered preterm infants weighing under 1500 g at <32 wk of gestational age	A pretest phase was performed to establish a standardized procedure for sampling, handling, heating and measuring the expressed human milk. To start with, the sample was warmed to 20°C–40°C and vortexed to homogenize all the components properly. Then, 3 mL of human milk was analyzed using the MIRIS unit
Mokha & Davidovics,[53] 2016	To assess macronutrient losses using human milk as continuous tube feeds as done in the inpatient and home setting using a feeding bag and pump	Significant fat losses were observed at all rates at hours 1–4, averaging to 73% at 5 mL/h. Caloric losses correlated strongly with fat losses. Significant gains in the fat content (+116% at hour 4 at 5 mL/h) were seen in the preinfusion aliquots (feeding bags). Horizontal positioning and continuous agitation of the feeding bag only partially limited fat losses	SpectraStar (Unity Scientific)	N/A	249 samples from volunteers who had term deliveries	The expressed milk was collected, dated, and frozen in bisphenol A–free, polypropylene containers until transfer to the study bank, where they were stored for up to 3 mo at −20°C until analysis. The amount of human milk required for analysis was thawed overnight at 4°C, pooled, warmed to a temperature of 25°C in an incubator on the day of the experiments, and then divided into aliquots

(continued on next page)

Table 3
(continued)

Author, Year	Purpose of Study (What Was Measured and for What Purpose)?	Results of Study/ Conclusion	Model of Milk Analyzer Used and Setting	Calibration of Device	Sample Size and Characteristics (eg, Term, Preterm)	Sample Preparation/ Handling and Storage (eg, Homogenized, Vortexed, Frozen, Thawed, How Much Volume in Analyzer?)
		Fat delivery at 5 mL/h was significantly enhanced to 87% when the feeding bag was placed in an inverted position and improved further up to 98% with higher infusion rates No carbohydrates and proteins losses were seen Conclusions: Enabling the delivery of the human milk from the top of the feeding bag optimizes fat delivery and limits losses				At the time of sampling, the containers were shaken by hand; 3-mL samples were drawn using a glass pipette at hours 0–4 and homogenized, and 1 mL was used for analysis
Pines et al,[27] 2016	To compare macronutrients content of human milk from both breasts, taking into account the self-reported preferential feeding ('dominant') breast, breast size, and handedness (right vs left)	Macronutrients content of mid expression of human milk is unaffected by maternal handedness, breast size, or breast side dominance	Human Milk Analyzer (MIRIS)	N/A	57 mothers We excluded mothers who suffered from acute mastitis, febrile illness, chronic disease such as diabetes, asthma, inflammatory bowel diseases, and those who underwent previous plastic surgery of the	Immediately after expression, samples were stored in a home freezer for a maximum period of 24 h before being stored at −20°C until thawed and analyzed Just before analysis, each frozen sample was initially heated at 40°C in a thermostatic bath Samples of 1–3 mL were then homogenized by the MIRIS milk refresher

| Chang et al,[47] 2015 | To measure the concentrations of macronutrients and to evaluate their changes according to lactation period in breast milk from lactating Korean women | MilkoScan FT-2 (Foss Analytical) | N/A | "The mean macronutrient composition per 100 mL of mature breast milk was 7.1 g for lactose, 1.4 g for protein and 3.0 g for fat, and energy content was 61.1 kcal" "The protein concentration was significantly lower in milk samples at 1–2 wk (2.0 g/dL) to 2–3 mo (1.4 g/dL) than those at 0–1 wk (2.2 g/dL), but it was similar among samples from 3–4 mo to 7–8 mo (1.3 g/dL)" "Mean lipid levels varied among different lactational period groups (2.7–3.2 g/dL), but presented no significant difference" "Lactose concentration in the milk samples did not differ with lactation period" "Maternal body mass | 2632 healthy lactating women (mean age, 32.0 ± 3.3 y), where the lactating period was up to a period of 8 mo breast or any surgery in the chest or the upper limbs | The breast milk samples were stored at −20°C until analysis The frozen samples were thawed in a refrigerator and heated in water bath until 37°C then homogenized before analysis (Uppsala, Sweden) using an ultrasonic technique |

(continued on next page)

Table 3
(continued)

Author, Year	Purpose of Study (What Was Measured and for What Purpose?)	Results of Study/Conclusion	Model of Milk Analyzer Used and Setting	Calibration of Device	Sample Size and Characteristics (eg, Term, Preterm)	Sample Preparation/Handling and Storage (eg. Homogenized, Vortexed, Frozen, Thawed, How Much Volume in Analyzer?)
		index was positively related to protein and lipid breast milk contents, but was negatively related to lactose content" "General linear models examining the associations between maternal variables and milk macronutrient content revealed that lactation period had a major impact on protein and lipid, but not on lactose content in breast milk"				
Kotrri et al,[52] 2016	To test a correction algorithm for a NIR milk analyzer for fat and protein measurements, and examine the effect of pasteurization on the IR matrix and the stability of fat, protein, and lactose	The correction algorithm generated for our device was found to be valid for unpasteurized and pasteurized breast milk Pasteurization had no effect on the macronutrient levels	SpectraStar (Unity Scientific)	Measurement values generated through NIR analysis were compared against those obtained through chemical reference methods to test the correction algorithm for the NIR milk analyzer A correction algorithm was previously generated by	50 samples (V = 60 mL)	Pasteurized and unpasteurized samples were then aliquoted (V = 1.5 mL each) and subsequently stored at −20°C temperature For analysis, aliquoted samples were thawed at 37°C for 5 min and homogenized using an

	Objective	Analyzer/Method	Results	Samples	Details
			and the IR matrix of breast milk. These results show that fat and protein content can be accurately measured and monitored for unpasteurized and pasteurized breast milk. Of additional importance is the implication that donated human milk, generally low in protein content, has the potential to be target fortified	plotting NIR measurement values against those generated through chemical reference methods. The inverse linear function of each of the resulting regression equations was used as the correction algorithm for readout generated by the NIR milk analyzer	ultrasonic vibrator (VCX 130; Chemical Instruments AB; Sollentuna, Sweden) for 15 s
Menjo et al,[8] 2009	Examine if the macronutrient values measured by human milk analyzer are comparable with those measured by conventional methods. Discover whether we could dilute the milk sample used for the human milk analyzer measurement if the amount of milk available for testing was insufficient	Human Milk Analyzer (MIRIS) Used mode for nonhomogenized measurement	When comparing the human milk analyzer and conventional methods, all 3 nutrients exhibited a significantly positive correlation ($P<.001$); lactose content was reliable on the condition that it is 6–7 g/dL When comparing diluted and nondiluted samples, fat and protein had expected values after dilution whereas	32 samples from 16 mothers (1 from each breast) for comparison between HMA and conventional methods 23 samples for effect of dilution purpose, measured in triplicate	2 mL of breast milk used for analysis, but if the amount of OMM is not meeting the infant's need, then a smaller measurement would be better Samples stored at −20°C as soon as possible, and remained until analysis For the HMA, samples were thawed and warmed at 37°C, then stirred before measured Repeated measurements 3 times Mixed samples with water to

(continued on next page)

Table 3
(continued)

Author, Year	Purpose of Study (What Was Measured and for What Purpose)?	Results of Study/ Conclusion	Model of Milk Analyzer Used and Setting	Calibration of Device	Sample Size and Characteristics (eg, Term, Preterm)	Sample Preparation/ Handling and Storage (eg, Homogenized, Vortexed, Frozen, Thawed, How Much Volume in Analyzer?)
						dilute and investigate effect
						lactose did not (it was overestimated) HMA yields reliable measurements
Faerk et al,[48] 2001	To present data on the protein, carbohydrate, fat, and energy content of preterm human milk from a large study of preterm infants with gestational age of <32 wk	Protein concentration decreased significantly with time (P<.00001) Carbohydrate, fat and energy concentration was significantly lower in the first 2 wk after delivery, after which they increased to a constant level Macronutrient level in milk is not associated with gestational age (P = .3)	Milkoscan 104 IR (Foss Electric)	Analyzer used is calibrated for human milk and validated for protein, carbohydrate and fat	476 milk samples from 101 mothers delivering before the 32nd gestational week, and 88 milk samples from 88 mothers delivering at term	N/A
Lubetzky et al,[28] 2015	To study macronutrient content in human milk collected in older (≥35 y) compared younger (<35 y) mothers	Fat content in colostrum and carbohydrate content in mature milk are significantly higher in the older mothers group	Human Milk Analyzer (MIRIS)	N/A	72 lactating mothers (38 older and 34 younger) were recruited within the first 3 of delivery Their newborns' gestational age at birth ranged from 37 to 42 wk Each mother	Immediately after extraction, samples were stored at <5°C for a maximum period of 24 h, then stored at −80°C until analysis Before analyses, samples were heated at 40°C and then homogenized using an ultrasonic technique

Moran-Lev et al,[29] 2015	To evaluate diurnal variations of macronutrients and energy content of preterm human milk over the first 7 wk of lactation and test the hypothesis that values obtained during a morning sample are predictive of those obtained from an evening sample	Mean fat and energy contents of all samples obtained during the whole period were significantly higher in evening samples (P<.0001) There were no significant differences between morning and evening carbohydrates and protein contents Concentrations of protein, carbohydrates, and fat from morning samples were predictive of evening concentrations to different extents (R2 = 0.720, R2 = 0.663, and R2 = 0.20, respectively; P<.02) In repeated-measures analysis of variance performed on 11 patients who completed the whole	Human Milk Analyzer (MIRIS)	N/A	32 mothers of preterm infants (26–33 wk in gestational age) who routinely expressed all their milk every 3 h from the beginning of the second to the seventh week after delivery One aliquot was obtained from the first morning expression and the second from the evening expression	Immediately after extraction, samples were stored in a refrigerator at <5°C for a maximum period of 24 h before being stored at −20°C until thawed and analyzed Just before analysis, each frozen sample was initially heated at 40°C in a thermostatic bath Samples were then homogenized by the MIRIS (Uppsala, Sweden) milk refresher using an ultrasonic technique
					contributed 3 samples in total, at the following time points: 72h after labor, 7 d, 14 d postpartum	

(continued on next page)

Table 3
(continued)

Author, Year	Purpose of Study (What Was Measured and for What Purpose)?	Results of Study/ Conclusion	Model of Milk Analyzer Used and Setting	Calibration of Device	Sample Size and Characteristics (eg, Term, Preterm)	Sample Preparation/ Handling and Storage (eg, Homogenized, Vortexed, Frozen, Thawed, How Much Volume in Analyzer?)
		7-wk period, over time, there was a significant decrease in fat, energy, and protein contents, whereas carbohydrates content remained unchanged Day-night differences remained significant only for fat content				
Stellwagen et al,[54] 2013	To test the hypothesis that pooling MOM for 24 h compared with individual pump session collection of milk would provide a more consistent nutrient content and ease mother's work load without leading to an increase in bacterial content in milk	24-h pooling of human milk reduces nutrient and caloric variability without increasing bacterial counts	SpectraStar (Unity Scientific)	Previously validated	19 mothers who were expressing milk for their infants	Milk collected was refrigerated for a maximum of 24 h before analysis 3 mL of sample were warmed to 40°C and 1 mL was used for analysis using an IR milk analyzer
Mangel et al,[30] 2015	To evaluate the effect of milk expression method (manual	The fat and energy contents of milk obtained through	Human Milk Analyzer (MIRIS)	N/A	Data on 21 mothers of 21 newborns 48–72 h after	At least 2 mL of breast milk was collected per method of expression

Study	Aim	Results	Device		Sample	Notes
	expression vs electric pump) on the composition of breast milk	manual expression were higher than those obtained by pump. There were no significant differences in protein or carbohydrate content of milk obtained by either method of expression. The difference in fat content between milk obtained by the 2 methods was not correlated with mother's age, delivery method, gestational age at delivery, parity, or the interval between delivery and the time the sampled milk was obtained			delivery were collected and analyzed. The women were randomly assigned to express breast milk manually followed by pump, or in reverse order	Samples were stored at −20°C for 48 h and then preserved at −80°C until analysis. The sample were assayed in duplicate, and the average of the 2 results was used for analysis
Say et al,[31] 2016	To examine the effect of mastitis during lactation on the macronutrient content of breast milk	Fat, carbohydrate, and energy levels were statistically lower in the milk samples of mothers with mastitis compared with the mothers without mastitis	Human Milk Analyzer (MIRIS)	N/A	The study recruited 30 term lactating mothers: 15 mothers diagnosed with mastitis and 15 healthy mothers	4 mL of fresh breast milk was collected in Eppendorf tubes and divided equally into 2 aliquots. Each sample was analyzed twice, and average values were used for further analysis
Thakkar et al,[32] 2016	To share data from an observatory, single-center, longitudinal trial assessing the constituents of human milk	The protein content decreased with evolving stages of lactation from an average of 1.45–1.38 g/100 mL	Human Milk Analyzer (MIRIS)	HMA	50 mothers	Stored at −80°C

(continued on next page)

Table 3
(continued)

Author, Year	Purpose of Study (What Was Measured and for What Purpose)?	Results of Study/ Conclusion	Model of Milk Analyzer Used and Setting	Calibration of Device	Sample Size and Characteristics (eg. Term, Preterm)	Sample Preparation/ Handling and Storage (eg. Homogenized, Vortexed, Frozen, Thawed, How Much Volume in Analyzer?)
Dritsakou et al,[33] 2016	To test the impact of specific maternal- and neonatal-associated factors on human milk's macronutrients and energy	A significant inverse correlation of fat, protein, and energy content with gestational age and birth weight was established. Fat and energy were lower in colostrum, increased in transitional milk and decreased on the 30th day's mature milk compared with transitional. The rate of protein decline from colostrum to mature milk was lower in premature deliveries compared with that of full-terms, resulting in greater contents of protein in preterm mature milk. The upmost amounts of carbohydrates were found in mature milk of preterm deliveries	Human Milk Analyzer (MIRIS)	N/A	630 samples of raw milk and 95 samples of donor pasteurized milk were delivered from a total of 305 mothers	Raw milk was kept in the refrigerator without being frozen at 0°C to 4°C. We conducted manual homogenization of the 24-h quantity of milk

Reference	Aim	Results	Device		Sample	Storage
		A positive correlation was found between maternal age and fat contents In women with higher post-pregnancy body mass index levels greater analogies of fat and energy were presented In women suffering diet-controlled gestational diabetes (GD), lower protein and higher fat and energy levels were found			478 human milk samples	Stored in plastic containers at −20°C The samples were thawed at 45°C for homogenization using MIRIS sonicator
Hahn et al,[34] 2016	To analyze the macronutrient of human milk (human milk) and to find out the various maternal-infantile factors that can affect human milk composition	Various maternal–infant factors were found to be associated with human milk composition changes; higher fat: Cesarean section and birth height; higher protein: postpartum age; higher carbohydrate: vaginal delivery and female infant; higher calorie: postpartum age, female infant, and birth height	Human Milk Analyzer (MIRIS)	N/A		

Abbreviations: DEBM, donor expressed breast milk; DHM, donor human milk; HACCP, hazard analysis and critical control point; IgA, immunoglobulin A; IR, infrared; MOM, mother's own milk; N/A, not applicable; NICE, National Institute for Health and Care Excellence; NICU, neonatal intensive care unit; NIR, near infrared; OMM, own mother's milk; PHM, pasteurized human milk.

Table 4
Clinical studies that use milk analyzers

Author, Year	Purpose of Study (What Was Measured and for What Purpose)?	Results of Study/Conclusion	Model of Milk Analyzer Used and Setting	Calibration of Device	Sample Size and Characteristics (eg, Term, Preterm)	Sample Preparation/ Handling and Storage (eg, Homogenized, Vortexed, Frozen, Thawed, How Much Volume in Analyzer?)
de Halleux et al,[49] 2007	Assess IR laser technology as a method to analyze human milk composition rapidly, before fortification Evaluate the benefit of adjustable fortification compared with standard fortification	Individualized fortification of human milk improves growth rate in preterm infants (21 g/kg/d) to a level close to formula fed infants After adjustable human milk fortification based on human milk analysis using Milkoscan, we observe a more stable protein content and a lower amount of added fortifier decreasing the risk of hyperosmolarity Furthermore, the energy content is higher following of the fat human milk adjusted content	MilkoScan (Foss)	Article talks about the importance of calibrating and validating the device before using it for measurement purposes	N/A	N/A
de Halleux & Rigo,[42] 2013	To show the variability in human milk composition from an infant's OMM or pooled human milk from the milk bank To evaluate the advantages of individual fortification on nutritional intakes over standard fortification	The variability in contents of fat, protein, and energy was high for all types of human milk samples Compared with standard fortification, individual fortification significantly reduced the variability in nutritional intakes	MilkoScan Minor (Foss)	In previous paper, this group talked about the importance of calibration and validation	428 OMM, 138 human milk pools from single donors, 224 pools from multiple donors, and 14 pools from colostral milk	10 mL of human milk used for analysis Human milk transported under aseptic HACCP conditions OMM kept at 4°C and used within 72 h Donor human milk frozen and pasteurized by Holder method, and warmed by thawing to 37°C before analysis

Hair et al,[55] 2014	To evaluate whether premature infants who received an exclusive human milk-based diet and a human milk-derived cream supplement (cream) would have weight gain (g/kg/d) at least as good as infants receiving a standard feeding regimen (control)	Premature infants who received human milk-derived cream to fortified human milk had improved weight and length velocity compared with the control group Human milk-derived cream should be considered an adjunctive supplement to an exclusive human milk-based diet to improve growth rates in premature infants	SpectraStar 2400RTW (Unity Scientific)			78 infants
Tabata et al,[56] 2015	This study evaluated fat loss in enteral nutrition using current strategies for providing high-risk infants fortified human milk	The addition of H2MF and cream to human milk provides both the benefits of bioactive elements from mother's milk and increased fat delivery, making the addition of H2MF and cream an appropriate method to improve infant weight gain	SpectraStar (Unity Scientific)	Followed procedure from SpectraStar for analysis	Human milk collected from 5 mothers, pooled into a 4-L container	Stored in freezer at -20°C, then thawed with warm water and agitated using a laboratory vortexer at 500 rpm to ensure homogeneity before analysis Before analysis, samples warmed to 25°C–33°C and homogenized using a probe sonicator for 10 s Sample volume of 2 mL for analysis, measured in triplicate
Dritsakou et al,[35] 2015	To investigate the benefits of treating low birth weight infants predominantly with mother's own raw milk and early initiation of breastfeeding (raw human	The 2 groups show similar demographic and perinatal characteristics Predominantly raw milk-fed infants regained earlier their birth weight, suffered fewer	Human Milk Analyzer (MIRIS)	N/A	192 predominantly raw human milk-fed infants (70% of raw and 30% of	N/A

(continued on next page)

Table 4
(continued)

Author, Year	Purpose of Study (What Was Measured and for What Purpose?)	Results of Study/Conclusion	Model of Milk Analyzer Used and Setting	Calibration of Device	Sample Size and Characteristics (eg, Term, Preterm)	Sample Preparation/Handling and Storage (eg, Homogenized, Vortexed, Frozen, Thawed, How Much Volume in Analyzer?)
	milk/breastfed infants), in comparison with feeding only with donor banked milk (until the third week of life) and afterward a preterm formula until hospital discharge (donor banked/formula-fed infants)	episodes of feeding intolerance, and presented a higher body length and head circumference at discharge ($P<.001$) Those treated mainly with their mothers' milk were able to initiate breastfeeding almost 2 wk earlier compared with those fed with donor milk who achieved to be bottle fed later on postconceptual age Infants being breastfed until the 8th month of life conducted less visits for a viral infection to a pediatrician compared with those in the other group			donor milk) were matched to 192 donor/formula-fed ones	
Aceti et al,[63] 2009	To determine whether fat content, protein content, and osmolality of human milk before and after fortification may affect GER in symptomatic preterm infants	An inverse correlation was found between naive human milk protein content and acid reflux index Protein content of native human milk may influence acid GER in preterm infants A standard fortification of human milk may worsen nonacid GER indexes and, due to the extreme variability in human milk composition, may overcome both recommended	NIRA (cited papers who used MilkoScan)	Calibrated to human milk using covariation between instrumental readings and reference methods (Kjeldhal for nitrogen assay and Gerber for fat analysis)	GER was evaluated in 17 symptomatic preterm newborns fed native and fortified human milk	Requires 5 mL sample

	Aim	Findings	Device	Validation	Samples	Sample preparation
		protein intake and human milk osmolality Thus, an individualized fortification, based on the analysis of the composition of naïve human milk, could optimize both nutrient intake and feeding tolerance				
McLeod et al,[36] 2016	Randomized pragmatic study to test the hypothesis that growth and body composition of preterm infants more closely matches intrauterine growth if fortification based on measured milk composition is used to target consensus protein intakes according to PMA and energy intakes according to birth weight rather than using an assumed milk composition to target upper limits of consensus protein	At discharge (intervention vs routine practice) total protein and energy intakes from all nutrition sources, weight gain velocity and percentage fat mass did not significantly differ between groups A protein intake >3·4 g/kg/d reduced percentage fat mass by 2% Nutrition and growth was not improved by targeting milk fortification according to birth weight criteria and PMA using measured milk composition, compared with routine practice Targeting fortification on measured composition is labor intensive, requiring frequent milk sampling and precision measuring equipment, perhaps reasons for its limited practice Guidance around safe upper levels of milk fortification is needed	Human Milk Analyzer (MIRIS)	N/A	40 preterm infants recruited	Milk frozen at −20°C Before analysis, samples were defrosted, warmed in a water bath to 40°C, homogenized (1.5 s/mL of sample; Sonics Vibra-Cell, Model VCX-130; Sonics and Materials Inc.)
Rochow et al,[57] 2015	Model the impact of various frequencies of breast milk analysis measurements on	1. Fixed dose fortification of breast milk was not sufficient to provide macronutrients at	SpectraStar (Unity Scientific)	Previously validated	210 samples from pooled 24 h breast milk	Before analysis, samples were homogenized for

(continued on next page)

Table 4
(continued)

Author, Year	Purpose of Study (What Was Measured and for What Purpose)?	Results of Study/Conclusion	Model of Milk Analyzer Used and Setting	Calibration of Device	Sample Size and Characteristics (eg, Term, Preterm)	Sample Preparation/Handling and Storage (eg, Homogenized, Vortexed, Frozen, Thawed, How Much Volume in Analyzer?)
	the effective macronutrient intake of very low birth weight infants	the recommended level in all preterm infants 2. Target fortification with daily measurements precisely achieved recommended target intake 3. The reduction of measurement frequency increased the day-to-day variation 4. Measurements twice a week ensured that, on average, no infant received an intake that was below the recommended targets 5. The higher amount of carbohydrates and fat in some of the batches was owing to the composition of native breast and/or fixed dose fortifier, but not an effect of target fortification			batches Fresh milk was preferred	15 s using a sonicator 1 mL stored at −80°C
Rochow et al,[4] 2013	Establish the infrastructure to safely perform target fortification of breast milk in neonatal intensive care unit by measuring and adjusting fat, protein, and carbohydrate content on a daily basis	All 650 pooled breast milk samples required at least 1 macronutrient adjusted Biochemistry was normal in the 10 target fortified infants Matched pair analysis of infants indicated a higher milk intake but similar weight gain No adverse event was observed	SpectraStar (Unity Scientific)	Measurements are adjusted according to internal validation Precision and accuracy of the milk analyzer was evaluated by comparison with traditional methods	10 healthy preterm babies were enrolled in study	Before analysis, breast milk samples were homogenized using a sonicator for 3 × 10 s (VCX 130; Chemical Instruments AB) The osmolality was measured with a

Source	Objective	Main findings	Device	Reference method / calibration	Sample	Milk handling / comments
		Measurements of macronutrients by breast milk analyzer and traditional method correlated with a R^2 of 0.91 for carbohydrates, 0.95 for fat and 0.95 for protein		freezing point osmometer (sample volume of 20 μL, 3320 Micro-Osmometer; Advance Instruments)		
Morlacchi et al,[37] 2016	To assess the safety of targeted fortification of human milk in preterm infants compared with standard fortification, as well as the effects on infant growth	Weekly weight gain and daily growth rates were higher in infants receiving target fortification than in infants receiving standardized fortification	Human Milk Analyzer (MIRIS)	The instrument was calibrated for breast milk measurements using the Kjeldahl method for proteins, high-pressure liquid chromatography for lactose and the Rose-Gottlieb method for fat	A total of 10 preterm infants (birth weight 1223 ± 195 g; gestational age 29.1 ± 1.03 wk) were enrolled and 118 samples of pooled milk were analyzed	Nurses mixed a bottle containing the milk collected during the previous 24 h using a vortex shaker. Approximately 2 mL of breast milk from each bottle was aliquoted for the macronutrient analysis. Before composition analysis, samples of native breast milk were frozen. After 24 h, the thawed milk was homogenized using an ultrasonic homogenizer. The linear relationship between milk intake and weight gain observed in study babies but not seen in matched controls may be related to the variable composition of breast milk. Daily target fortification can be safely implemented in clinical routine and may improve growth
Simpson et al,[38] 2016	To study whether a system of DEBM energy content categorization and distribution would improve energy intake from DEBM	Cumulative energy intake from DEBM can be improved by categorizing and distributing milk according to energy content	Human Milk Analyzer (MIRIS)	N/A	85 samples, 20 babies	

Abbreviations: DEBM, donor expressed breast milk; GER, gastroesophageal reflux; H2FM, human milk-based human milk fortifier; HACCP, hazard analysis and critical control point; IR, infrared; N/A, not applicable; NIRA, near-infrared reflectance analysis; OMM, own mother's milk; PMA, postmenstrual age.

Findings of Included Studies

Evaluation of the device

To evaluate the accuracy of milk analyzers, study groups compared the measurements obtained from IR analysis with those obtained from reference chemical methods. To measure fat, the following chemical reference methods were used: a modified Folch method (n = 1),[8] a spectroscopic esterified fatty acid method (n = 1),[9] the Gerber method (n = 2),[10,61] the Roese-Gottlieb method (n = 2),[11,40] the Bligh and Dyer method (n = 1),[6] the Mojonnier method (n = 4),[51,59,60,65] and a modified Mojonnier method (n = 2).[5,52] One study did not specify their reference method for fat measurements.[41]

To measure protein, the following chemical reference methods were used: the Kjeldahl method (n = 9),[6,8,11,40,51,59–61,65] the Bradford method (n = 2)[6,10] a modified Bradford method using a commercial protein reagent (n = 1),[9] and elemental analysis (n = 2).[5,52] One study did not specify their reference method for protein measurements.[41] Multiple mentions are possible within each study.

To measure lactose content, the following chemical reference methods were used: high-performance liquid chromatography (n = 5),[8,51,59,60,65] an enzymatic spectroscopic method (n = 1),[9] the Chloramine-T method (n = 1),[10] the automated orcinol method (n = 1),[6] an enzymatic assay (n = 1),[40] high-pH anion exchange chromatography with pulsed amperometric detector (n = 1)[11] and the ultraperformance liquid chromatography tandem mass-spectrometry method (n = 2).[5,52] One study did not specify their reference method for lactose measurements.[41]

Among the 14 studies that aimed to evaluate the accuracy and precision of milk analyzers, the following results were found for fat IR measurements: fat IR measurements are accurate (n = 10)[5,6,8,40,41,51,52,59,61,65] and fat IR measurements are inaccurate (n = 5).[5,9–11,60] For protein IR measurements, the following results were found: protein IR measurements are accurate when compared with chemical reference methods (n = 10)[5,6,8,40,41,51,52,59,61,65] and protein IR measurements are inaccurate (n = 4).[5,9–11] For lactose measurements, the following results were found: lactose measurements are accurate (n = 4),[51,59] carbohydrate measurements are accurate (n = 1)[6], lactose measurements are only accurate when they are between 6 and 7 g/dL (n = 1),[8] lactose IR measurements correlated moderately to those obtained from reference methods (n = 1),[65] and carbohydrate/lactose IR measurements are inaccurate representations of true lactose values (n = 5).[5,9–11,40] Multiple mentions are possible within each study.

In terms of precision, nine studies found that the fat IR measurements are precise.[5,6,9,10,40,41,52,61,65] For protein IR measurements, nine studies reported precision.[5,6,9,10,40,41,52,61,65] For lactose IR measurements, five studies[6,9,10,40,65] found that they were precise, whereas 1 study[5] showed that they are not precise.

Among the 14 studies that evaluated their milk analyzers, ten studies[5,6,9,11,40,41,51,52,61,65] suggested new calibration curves for their devices, and four studies[41,51,52,61] validated their devices using an independent sample set, after recalibration.

Measurement of samples under various clinical conditions

Table 3 depicts the results of studies that used milk analyzers to measure samples under various clinical conditions. Among the studies that investigated the effect of fortification on macronutrient content, the following results were found: individual fortification significantly reduced the variability in nutritional intakes compared with standard fortification (n = 1),[42] human milk protein content after standard fortification fails to meet the recommended intake for preterm infants in approximately half of the cases (n = 1),[62] individualized fortification resulted in milks closer to target recommendations (n = 1),[3] even with fortification 39% of samples fail to meet the minimum protein requirements (n = 1)[13] and standard fortification result in only a small increase in protein and no significant change for lipid concentrations (n = 1).[71]

Among the studies that investigated the effect of freezing and thawing, the following results were reported: a decrease in the concentration of fat by freezing at −20°C (n = 4),[14,19,22,45] total nitrogen and lactose contents revealed a variable, low-magnitude, and not constant reduction with freezing time at −20°C (n = 1),[14] significant increases in protein and lactose concentrations after freezing at −20°C (n = 1),[43] freezing at −80°C significantly decreases the energy content of human milk, both from fat and carbohydrates compared with −20°C (n = 1),[20] freezing at −20°C significantly decreases lactose (n = 1),[22] and freezing at −20°C decreases protein concentration (n = 1).[45]

Among the studies that investigated the effect of lactation period on macronutrient content, the following results were reported: there were increases in lactose, lipid, calorie, and phosphate concentrations, and decreases in protein and secretory immunoglobulin A throughout the lactation period (n = 1);[16] the protein content decreased with lactation period (n = 7);[25,26,29,32,33,47,70] mean lipid levels varied among different lactational period groups but presented no significant difference (n = 2);[47,70] fat content decreases with lactation period (n = 2);[25,29] fat and energy were lower in colostrum, increased in transitional milk and decreased on the 30th day's mature milk (n = 1);[33] lactation period has no impact on lactose content in breast milk (n = 3);[29,47,70] and lactose increases with lactation period (n = 2).[25,33]

Clinical trials

Table 4 depicts the results of clinical trials that used milk analyzers. Overall, the following results were found: individualized fortification of human milk improves growth rate (n = 1), individual fortification reduces the variability in nutritional intakes (n = 1),[42] human milk-derived cream to fortified human milk had improved weight and length velocity (n = 1),[55] the addition of human milk-based human milk fortifier and cream to human milk provides both the benefits of bioactive elements from mother's milk and increased fat delivery (n = 1),[56] predominantly raw milk-fed infants regained earlier their birth weight, suffered less episodes of feeding intolerance, and presented a greater body length and head circumference at discharge compared with infants who were only fed donor banked milk (n = 1),[35] individualized fortification can optimize nutrient intake and feeding tolerance (n = 1),[63] nutrition and growth was not improved by targeting milk fortification (n = 1),[36] target fortification with daily measurements precisely achieved recommended target intake (n = 1),[57] target fortification can be implemented safely in clinical routine and may improve growth (n = 2),[4,37] and cumulative energy intake from donor expressed breast milk can be improved by categorizing and distributing milk according to energy content (n = 1).[38]

Preanalytical Sample Treatment of Included Studies

Among the 62 studies included in this review, six[11,17,43,45,51,71] measured fresh samples and the rest have stored their samples until analysis. The following sample storage temperatures were reported: 4°C (n = 9),[12,14,16,20,23,33,42,54,61] −5°C (n = 1),[36] −20°C (n = 23),[8,10,11,14,18,22,24,27,29,34,36,38,40,43,45,47,51–53,56,59,70] −25°C (n = 1),[44] −30°C (n = 1),[67] and −80°C (n = 9).[5,11,15,19,20,25,28,30,32] Twenty studies[3,4,9,13,21,26,31,35,37,41,46,48,49,55,57,60,62,63,65,69] did not report the storage temperature of the samples. Multiple mentions are possible within each study.

For storage period before analyses, the following were reported: 2–3 hours (n = 1),[71] 24 hours (n = 7),[14,16,20,37,43,45,54] 48 hours (n = 1),[19] 72 hours (n = 1),[42]

1 week (n = 1),[36] three months (n = 2),[53,67] between 8-83 days (n = 1),[20] between 30-180 days (n = 1),[22] 6 months (n = 1),[38] and no limit (n = 1). Fourty-five[3-6,8-10,12,13,15,18,21-35,40,41,44,46-49,52,55-57,59,60-63,65,69,70] studies did not report the storage period of samples prior to analyses. Six studies[11,17,43,45,51,71] measured fresh samples and hence did not store their samples. Multiple mentions are possible within each study.

For sample thawing temperature, the following were reported: 4°C (n = 2),[19,24] 25°C (n = 1),[53] 37°C (n = 7),[5,8,13,38,42,47,52] 38°C (n = 1),[65] 40°C (n = 24),[9-11,14,16,18,20-23,25,27-29,36,40,44,45,51,54,59,60,69,71] 45°C (n = 1),[34] and 50°C (n = 1).[6] Some studies reported a range of thawing temperatures: 20-40°C (n = 1)[26] and 25-33°C (n = 1).[56] Two studies[43,45] thawed their samples in a micro-wave and twenty-two studies[3,4,12,15,17,30-33,35,37,41,46,48,49,55,57,61-63,67,70] did not report the temperature used to thaw their samples. Multiple mentions are possible within each study.

For sample homogenization, the following techniques were reported: the Calais internal mechanism (n = 1),[59] a sonicator (n = 24),[4-6,9-14,16,18-20,22,24,27-29,34,36-38,56,57] a vortex (n = 2),[26,65] shaking the samples by hand (n = 3),[14,51,52] unspecified stirring method (n = 1),[8] manual homogenization (n = 1),[33] unspecified homogenization technique (n = 7),[21,23,24,40,47,53,69] and no homogenization (n = 1).[11] Twenty five studies[3,15,17,25,30-32,35,41-46,48,49,54,55,60-63,67,70,71] did not report homogenization.

For homogenization time and rate, the following were reported: shaking the samples ten times (n = 1),[14] 10s (n = 1),[56] 15s (n = 2),[52,57] 20s (n = 1),[65] 30s (n = 1),[11] 3 × 10s (n = 2)[4,5], and 1.5s/mL (n = 13).[9,10,13,14,16,18-20,22,24,27,36,38] A study[6] reported homogenization rates that were dependent on the volume of the sample: 30s/mL for 2.5mL samples and 5s/mL for 4-74mL samples. Forty-two studies[3,8,12,15,17,21,23-26,28-35,37,40-49,51,53-55,59-63,67,69-71] did not report their sample homogenization time/rate.

DISCUSSION

In this systematic review and critical evaluation of all studies that use IR milk analyzers for macronutrient (fat, protein, and lactose) measurement of human milk, the major finding is a significant lack of consistency among study groups using IR milk analyzers. Discrepancies arise in 2 areas: (1) the validation of IR milk analyzers for accurate detection of macronutrient content in breast milk and (2) preanalytical treatment and measurement procedure followed. It is important to note that in our current international multicentre trial on an identical set of quality control samples, results revealed significant differences in measurements among the participating 15 centres.[72]

Discrepancies in the Validation of Devices

Among the 14 studies that evaluated human milk analyzers, some have found IR measurements to be accurate and precise, whereas others have found the opposite. These differences likely result from 3 sources: (1) the choice of chemical reference methods for macronutrient measurement, (2) the size and characteristic of the sample set, and (3) sample preparation before measurement. Evaluation of accuracy is a critical step in the adaptation of IR milk analyzers for clinical and research purposes. A lack of uniformity in study design gives rise to these differences that subsequently lead to different results.

Carefully selected chemical reference methods provide the true macronutrient concentration against which the accuracy of the IR measurement values can be compared. Many of the published evaluations of IR analyzers for human milk apply chemical reference methods for macronutrient detection in dairy milk, because there are currently no standard methods to measure macronutrient content in human milk. These methods, however, require proper adjustment and validation for macronutrient measurement of human milk. This adjustment is necessary because the macronutrient composition of human milk differs greatly from that of cow milk. Notably, breast milk contains a different fatty acid profile, as well a significant amount of oligosaccharides, when compared with cow's milk. These matrix differences need to be taken into account when determining the true macronutrient content in a sample of human milk. Once properly established through a rigorous validation process, a chemical method provides the basis for a precise evaluation of IR milk analyzers.

Particular attention must be given to the measurement of lactose content with IR milk analyzers. Oligosaccharides present in significant numbers in human milk cannot be differentiated from lactose by IR technology. This produces an erroneous readout of the lactose concentration. Several studies[51,59] claim that IR milk analyzers are capable of measuring lactose. These studies, however, apply chemical reference methods that may be inappropriate for the chemical matrix of breast milk, especially when it comes to lactose measurement using high-pressure liquid chromatography (HPLC). Although HPLC is the method of choice to detect lactose in cow milk, there is no agreed HPLC method for lactose detection in human milk. The gold standard guidelines of dairy industry clearly emphasize that HPLC (like ISO 22662:2007; IDF 198:2007) is only applicable for lactose measurement of milk that does not contain oligosaccharides. The use of HPLC for detection of lactose in breast milk requires a setup and validation to account for differences in the chemical matrix between human and dairy milk. This step has yet to be demonstrated in previously published papers that validate milk analyzers for lactose measurement. Such difficulties may be overcome with the use of ultraperformance liquid chromatography tandem mass-spectrometry technology.[73]

Another crucial component in the evaluation process of IR milk analyzers is the selection of an appropriate sample set. Optimal evaluation of IR milk analyzers requires a sufficiently large sample size that is representative of breast milk encountered in the clinical setting. This includes milk that spans the full range of gestational ages and lactation periods. A sufficiently large sample size will ensure that the full range of macronutrient content seen in the clinical setting is also covered in the evaluation of the devices. Moreover, a larger sample size will ensure that the impact of random error from measurements with both chemical methods and IR milk analysis will be minimized.

The type of milk used in the evaluation process is also of great importance in determining whether or not the devices can be adopted for clinical practice. Human milk composition is highly variable. IR analysis of breast milk, in turn, is able to measure the concentration of a given macronutrient (fat, protein, and lactose) based on specific wavelength of light absorbed by functional groups present in the macromolecule. The functional group under IR analysis, however, may be shared with another macronutrient of interest. Thus, a change in the ratio of macronutrients in breast milk may affect measurement results. Breast milk that varies from term to preterm, and early to late lactation will cover the full range of macronutrient variation expected in breast milk and minimize the errors in measurement that are produced from matrix measurement. To produce a wider range of macronutrient concentration for the evaluation of milk analyzers, 3 procedures are commonly undertaken in the aforementioned studies: (1) the dilution of milk samples before measurement, (2) the addition of lactose, and (3) defatting of milk samples before IR analysis. However, these procedures will affect the matrix of breast milk and may lead to false measurement results, thus affecting the calibration and validation of the devices.

After testing, if a device is found to have a systematic offset in the measurement of certain macronutrients, a recalibration should be performed. This requires the plotting of measurement readouts generated by the IR milk analyzer against those generated through chemical reference methods. The inverse linear function of the resulting regression equation should be used as a correction algorithm to be applied to future readouts of the IR milk analyzer. Obviously, the accuracy and precision of the correction needs to be validated using an independent sample set. As with testing of the accuracy of the device as mentioned earlier, an appropriate sample set containing breast milk that is representative of the clinical setting should also be used in these sensitive processes. The appropriateness of this quality improvement approach has recently been confirmed by the results of our current international multi-centre trial.[72]

Discrepancies in Sample Preparation and Preanalytical Treatment

Another important factor that contributes to the diverging results in the reliability of IR milk analyzers is inappropriate sample preparation for measurement. Overall, among the studies examined in the current review, there is heterogeneity in sample preparation, handling, and storage. Samples are not always reported to be homogenized, and even if they are, there are inconsistencies with homogenization time. Homogenization of samples is important to avoid the loss of fat sticking to vials, and to ensure that the milk measured is representative of the sample.[5] A lack of, or insufficient, homogenization can lead to erroneous fat values measured.

Samples are also not always reported to be stirred, and when they are, there are different ways to do so; some groups vortex the samples at different rates, whereas others shake the samples in an arclike fashion. Again, these discrepancies can lead to the measurement of milk that is not representative of the sample, thus leading to erroneous measurements.

Furthermore, before measurement, samples are stored at various temperatures ($-20°C$, $-80°C$), and thawed at various temperatures ($4°C$, $25°C$, $37°C$, $40°C$), for different time periods. Although there are currently no conclusions on the impact of storage temperature and thawing temperature on the macronutrient content of breast milk, different temperatures may lead to different measurements of macronutrient.

Impact of Inappropriate Validation of Devices and Sample Preparation

Missing or inappropriate validation and standardization of IR milk analyzer handling may place doubt on the methodologic rigor of clinical studies using the devices. These clinical studies assess the effect of macronutrient variation in breast milk on the growth of preterm infants. This is of special importance when it comes to target fortification, whereby nutritionally deficient breast milk is supplemented with fat, protein, and lactose. Precise knowledge of macronutrient content is required to fortify human milk to the correct macronutrient levels. When macronutrient content is determined through IR milk analyzers before fortification, it must not be assumed that the devices measure properly with the manufacturer-provided calibration. Great care must be taken to ensure that the devices measure accurately. Failure to do so could lead to suboptimal macronutrient levels in breast milk after fortification, or even an overfortification, which can all affect growth patterns in infants.

In the present review, several studies examined the clinical viability of target fortification. De Halleux and colleagues[42] performed a validation of their milk analyzer that is used to determine macronutrient content before fortification. However, a small number of samples (n = 40) are used. Moreover, there is no description of the chemical reference methods or the characteristic of the milk used in the validation process. Similarly, Morlacchi and colleagues[37] aimed to assess the impact of target fortification on infant growth. Although this group mentioned the chemical reference methods used to validate their milk analyzer, the sample size was rather small (n = 10). McLeod and associates[36] do not perform or mention a prior validation of their IR milk analyzer. Other clinical studies in the present review are also affected by a lack of validation of their IR milk analyzer. Hair and coworkers[55] use IR milk analyzers to determine the effect of a human milk-derived cream supplement on premature weight gain. In this case, however, IR milk analysis is used to determine the caloric content of human milk before the addition of cream. Without proper validation, IR milk analyzers are unable to provide an accurate caloric content of the batch of interest. Another study by Dritsakou and associates[35] compares the feeding of preterm infants with raw human milk and banked human milk. Target fortification is attempted for both types of milk. However, without a properly validated IR milk analyzer, this will likely fail to lead to nutritionally appropriate breast milk being fed to premature infants. This aspect of methodologic study design could further explain the slower rate of growth in the donor milk group. Because donor milk is generally lower in protein content, macronutrient deficiencies arising from improper fortification are more likely to affect infants being fed donor milk. Because these various factors can affect the results of the studies, it is difficult to draw conclusions on the benefits of individual fortification and on the other results.

These discrepancies in validation of the milk analyzer and sample preparation may explain the different results obtained from the studies in group 2 (those aiming to assess the impact of various clinical processes on the macronutrient content of breast milk). Although some studies found that freezing can lower certain macronutrient content, others have found the opposite results. Similarly, different groups have found different impacts of lactation period on the macronutrient content of breast milk; however, most groups agree that protein content decreases with the lactation period. Most groups also agree that individualized fortification resulted in milks closer to target recommendations and can reduce the variability in macronutrient content.

It is, therefore, important for individuals using human milk analyzers to ensure that their devices are validated and calibrated appropriately, following good laboratory and clinical practice guidelines. To validate the device, it is important to choose reference chemical methods and to use a large sample size that covers a wide range of macronutrient levels, as Smilowitz and collegaues,[65] Rigourd,[41] Fusch and associates,[5] and Zhu and coworkers[11] have done. Research groups using milk analyzers should also describe their sample preparation to document its complex impact on macronutrient content. These groups should also ensure that different clinical conditions such as freezing and thawing are not affecting the macronutrient content of their milk samples. As per the good laboratory and clinical practice guidelines, it is also important for research groups to measure quality control samples using their milk analyzer before measuring any clinical samples, to check the status of their device.

SUMMARY

IR human milk analyzers have the potential for bedside use in the neonatal intensive care unit, because they allow for individual fortification of breast milk that can improve patient outcomes. However, research groups using these devices need an understanding of the impact of various clinical conditions on the macronutrient content in breast milk and should be cautious about their measurements until more is known about these devices. These devices must also be calibrated and validated following good laboratory and clinical practice, and appropriate sample preparation must be done.

REFERENCES

1. American Academy of Pediatrics Committee on Nutrition. Nutritional needs of low-birth-weight infants. Pediatrics 1985;75(5):976–86.
2. Maggio L, Costa S, Gallini F. Human milk fortifiers in very low birth weight infants. Early Hum Dev 2009;85(10 Suppl):S59–61.
3. Radmacher PG, Lewis SL, Adamkin DH. Individualizing fortification of human milk using real time human milk analysis. J Neonatal Perinatal Med 2013;6(4):319–23.
4. Rochow N, Fusch G, Choi A, et al. Target fortification of breast milk with fat, protein, and carbohydrates for preterm infants. J Pediatr 2013;163(4):1001–7.
5. Fusch G, Rochow N, Choi A, et al. Rapid measurement of macronutrients in breast milk: how reliable are infrared milk analyzers? Clin Nutr 2015;34(3):465–76.
6. Billard H, Simon L, Desnots E, et al. Calibration adjustment of the mid-infrared analyzer for an accurate determination of the macronutrient composition of human milk. J Hum Lact 2015;32(3):NP19–27.
7. MIRIS. Home Page. 2016. Available at: http://miris.se/. Accessed September 17, 2016.
8. Menjo A, Mizuno K, Murase M, et al. Bedside analysis of human milk for adjustable nutrition strategy. Acta Paediatr 2009;98(2):380–4.
9. Casadio YS, Williams TM, Lai CT, et al. Evaluation of a mid-infrared analyzer for the determination of the macronutrient composition of human milk. J Hum Lact 2010;26(4):376–83.
10. Silvestre D, Fraga M, Gormaz M, et al. Comparison of mid-infrared transmission spectroscopy with biochemical methods for the determination of macronutrients in human milk. Matern Child Nutr 2014;10(3):373–82.
11. Zhu M, Yang Z, Ren Y, et al. Comparison of macronutrient contents in human milk measured using mid-infrared human milk analyser in a field study vs. chemical reference methods. Matern Child Nutr 2016. [Epub ahead of print].
12. He BZ, Sun XJ, Quan MY, et al. Macronutrients and energy in milk from mothers of premature infants. Zhongguo Dang Dai Er Ke Za Zhi 2014;16(7):679–83.
13. Cooper AR, Barnett D, Gentles E, et al. Macronutrient content of donor human breast milk. Arch Dis Child Fetal Neonatal Ed 2013;98(6):F539–41.
14. Garcia-Lara NR, Escuder-Vieco D, Garcia-Algar O, et al. Effect of freezing time on macronutrients and energy content of breastmilk. Breastfeed Med 2012;7: 295–301.
15. Jans G, Matthys C, Lannoo M, et al. Breast milk macronutrient composition after bariatric surgery. Obes Surg 2015;25(5):938–41.
16. Hsu YC, Chen CH, Lin MC, et al. Changes in preterm breast milk nutrient content in the first month. Pediatr Neonatol 2014;55(6):449–54.
17. Dizdar EA, Sari FN, Degirmencioglu H, et al. Effect of mode of delivery on macronutrient content of breast milk. J Matern Fetal Neonatal Med 2014;27(11): 1099–102.
18. Khan S, Prime DK, Hepworth AR, et al. Investigation of short-term variations in term breast milk composition during repeated breast expression sessions. J Hum Lact 2013;29(2):196–204.
19. Chang YC, Chen CH, Lin MC. The macronutrients in human milk change after storage in various containers. Pediatr Neonatol 2012;53(3):205–9.
20. Lev HM, Ovental A, Mandel D, et al. Major losses of fat, carbohydrates and energy content of preterm human milk frozen at -80 degrees C. J Perinatol 2014; 34(5):396–8.

21. Zachariassen G, Fenger-Gron J, Hviid MV, et al. The content of macronutrients in milk from mothers of very preterm infants is highly variable. Dan Med J 2013; 60(6):A4631.

22. Garcia-Lara NR, Vieco DE, De la Cruz-Bertolo J, et al. Effect of Holder pasteurization and frozen storage on macronutrients and energy content of breast milk. J Pediatr Gastroenterol Nutr 2013;57(3):377–82.

23. Anderssen SH, Lovlund EE, Nygaard EA, et al. Expressing breast milk at home for 24-h periods provides viable samples for macronutrient analysis. Acta Paediatr 2015;104(1):43–6.

24. Garcia-Lara NR, Escuder-Vieco D, Alonso Diaz C, et al. Type of homogenization and fat loss during continuous infusion of human milk. J Hum Lact 2014;30(4): 436–41.

25. Yang T, Zhang Y, Ning Y, et al. Breast milk macronutrient composition and the associated factors in urban Chinese mothers. Chin Med J 2014;127(9):1721–5.

26. Kreissl A, Zwiauer V, Repa A, et al. Human MILK Analyser shows that the lactation period affects protein levels in preterm breastmilk. Acta Paediatr 2016;105(6): 635–40.

27. Pines N, Mandel D, Mimouni FB, et al. The effect of between-breast differences on human milk macronutrients content. J Perinatol 2016;36(7):549–51.

28. Lubetzky R, Sever O, Mimouni FB, et al. Human milk macronutrients content: effect of advanced maternal age. Breastfeed Med 2015;10(9):433–6.

29. Moran-Lev H, Mimouni FB, Ovental A, et al. Circadian macronutrients variations over the first 7 weeks of human milk feeding of preterm infants. Breastfeed Med 2015;10(7):366–70.

30. Mangel L, Ovental A, Batscha N, et al. Higher fat content in breastmilk expressed manually: a randomized trial. Breastfeed Med 2015;10(7):352–4.

31. Say B, Dizdar EA, Degirmencioglu H, et al. The effect of lactational mastitis on the macronutrient content of breast milk. Early Hum Dev 2016;98:7–9.

32. Thakkar SK, Giuffrida F, Bertschy E, et al. Protein evolution of human milk. Nestle Nutr Inst Workshop Ser 2016;86:77–85.

33. Dritsakou K, Liosis G, Valsami G, et al. The impact of maternal- and neonatal-associated factors on human milk's macronutrients and energy. J Matern Fetal Neonatal Med 2016;1–7 [Epub ahead of print].

34. Hahn WH, Song JH, Lee JE, et al. Do gender and birth height of infant affect calorie of human milk? An association study between human milk macronutrient and various birth factors. J Matern Fetal Neonatal Med 2016;1–14 [Epub ahead of print].

35. Dritsakou K, Liosis G, Valsami G, et al. Improved outcomes of feeding low birth weight infants with predominantly raw human milk versus donor banked milk and formula. J Matern Fetal Neonatal Med 2015;29(7):1131–8.

36. McLeod G, Sherriff J, Hartmann PE, et al. Comparing different methods of human breast milk fortification using measured v. assumed macronutrient composition to target reference growth: a randomised controlled trial. Br J Nutr 2016;115(3): 431–9.

37. Morlacchi L, Mallardi D, Gianni ML, et al. Is targeted fortification of human breast milk an optimal nutrition strategy for preterm infants? An interventional study. J Transl Med 2016;14(1):195.

38. Simpson JH, McKerracher L, Cooper A, et al. Optimal distribution and utilization of donated human breast milk: a novel approach. J Hum Lact 2016. [Epub ahead of print].

39. FOSS. MilkoScan™ FT1-Milk analysis using FTIR. 2016. Available at: http://www.foss.dk/industry-solution/products/milkoscan-ft1/. Accessed September 17, 2016.

40. Michaelsen KF, Pedersen SB, Skafte L, et al. Infrared analysis for determining macronutrients in human milk. J Pediatr Gastroenterol Nutr 1988;7(2):229–35.

41. Rigourd V. Mid-infrared spectrometric analysis to evaluate nutritional content of human milk bank. Arch Pediatr 2010;17(6):772–3 [in French].

42. de Halleux V, Rigo J. Variability in human milk composition: benefit of individualized fortification in very-low-birth-weight infants. Am J Clin Nutr 2013;98(2):529s–35s.

43. Abranches AD, Soares FV, Junior SC, et al. Freezing and thawing effects on fat, protein, and lactose levels of human natural milk administered by gavage and continuous infusion. J Pediatr (Rio J) 2014;90(4):384–8.

44. Michaelsen KF, Skafte L, Badsberg JH, et al. Variation in macronutrients in human bank milk: influencing factors and implications for human milk banking. J Pediatr Gastroenterol Nutr 1990;11(2):229–39.

45. Vieira AA, Soares FV, Pimenta HP, et al. Analysis of the influence of pasteurization, freezing/thawing, and offer processes on human milk's macronutrient concentrations. Early Hum Dev 2011;87(8):577–80.

46. Stoltz Sjostrom E, Ohlund I, Tornevi A, et al. Intake and macronutrient content of human milk given to extremely preterm infants. J Hum Lact 2014;30(4):442–9.

47. Chang N, Jung JA, Kim H, et al. Macronutrient composition of human milk from Korean mothers of full term infants born at 37-42 gestational weeks. Nutr Res Pract 2015;9(4):433–8.

48. Faerk J, Skafte L, Petersen S, et al. Macronutrients in milk from mothers delivering preterm. Adv Exp Med Biol 2001;501:409–13.

49. de Halleux V, Close A, Stalport S, et al. Advantages of individualized fortification of human milk for preterm infants. Arch Pediatr 2007;14(Suppl 1):S5–10 [in French].

50. Scientific U. Near infrared spectroscopy. 2016. Available at: http://www.unityscientific.com/products/near-infrared-spectroscopy. Accessed September 17, 2016.

51. Sauer CW, Kim JH. Human milk macronutrient analysis using point-of-care near-infrared spectrophotometry. J Perinatol 2011;31(5):339–43.

52. Kotrri G, Fusch G, Kwan C, et al. Validation of correction algorithms for near-IR analysis of human milk in an independent sample set—effect of pasteurization. Nutrients 2016;8(3):119.

53. Mokha JS, Davidovics ZH. Improved delivery of fat from human breast milk via continuous tube feeding. JPEN J Parenter Enteral Nutr 2016. [Epub ahead of print].

54. Stellwagen LM, Vaucher YE, Chan CS, et al. Pooling expressed breastmilk to provide a consistent feeding composition for premature infants. Breastfeed Med 2013;8:205–9.

55. Hair AB, Blanco CL, Moreira AG, et al. Randomized trial of human milk cream as a supplement to standard fortification of an exclusive human milk-based diet in infants 750-1250 g birth weight. J Pediatr 2014;165(5):915–20.

56. Tabata M, Abdelrahman K, Hair AB, et al. Fortifier and cream improve fat delivery in continuous enteral infant feeding of breast milk. Nutrients 2015;7(2):1174–83.

57. Rochow N, Fusch G, Zapanta B, et al. Target fortification of breast milk: how often should milk analysis be done? Nutrients 2015;7(4):2297–310.

58. Calais Human Milk Analyzer. 2016. Available at: http://www.calaisanalyzer.com/calais-human-milk-analyzer.html. Accessed September 28, 2016.

59. Groh-Wargo S, Valentic J, Khaira S, et al. Human milk analysis using mid-infrared spectroscopy. Nutr Clin Pract 2016;31(2):266–72.

60. O'Neill EF, Radmacher PG, Sparks B, et al. Creamatocrit analysis of human milk overestimates fat and energy content when compared to a human milk analyzer using mid-infrared spectroscopy. J Pediatr Gastroenterol Nutr 2013;56(5):569–72.

61. Corvaglia L, Battistini B, Paoletti V, et al. Near-infrared reflectance analysis to evaluate the nitrogen and fat content of human milk in neonatal intensive care units. Arch Dis Child Fetal Neonatal Ed 2008;93(5):F372–5.

62. Corvaglia L, Aceti A, Paoletti V, et al. Standard fortification of preterm human milk fails to meet recommended protein intake: bedside evaluation by Near-Infrared-Reflectance-Analysis. Early Hum Dev 2010;86(4):237–40.

63. Aceti A, Corvaglia L, Paoletti V, et al. Protein content and fortification of human milk influence gastroesophageal reflux in preterm infants. J Pediatr Gastroenterol Nutr 2009;49(5):613–8.

64. Instruments D. LactoScope FTIR Advanced. 2016. Available at: http://delta instruments.com/Products/Processors/LactoScopeFTIRAdvanced/tabid/246/Default.aspx. Accessed September 28, 2016.

65. Smilowitz JT, Gho DS, Mirmiran M, et al. Rapid measurement of human milk macronutrients in the neonatal intensive care unit: accuracy and precision of Fourier transform mid-infrared spectroscopy. J Hum Lact 2014;30(2):180–9.

66. Instruments A. The Acudairy. Available at: http://www.testmilk.com/acudairy.html. Accessed September 28, 2016.

67. Wojcik KY, Rechtman DJ, Lee ML, et al. Macronutrient analysis of a nationwide sample of donor breast milk. J Am Diet Assoc 2009;109(1):137–40.

68. Instruments M. York Dairy Analyzer. 2011. Available at: http://www.metron instruments.com/products/sample-page/. Accessed September 28, 2016.

69. Brooks C, Vickers AM, Aryal S. Comparison of lipid and calorie loss from donor human milk among 3 methods of simulated gavage feeding: one-hour, 2-hour, and intermittent gravity feedings. Adv Neonatal Care 2013;13(2):131–8.

70. Michaelsen KF, Larsen PS, Thomsen BL, et al. The Copenhagen Cohort Study on Infant Nutrition and Growth: breast-milk intake, human milk macronutrient content, and influencing factors. Am J Clin Nutr 1994;59(3):600–11.

71. Krcho P, Vojtova V, Benesova M. Analysis of human milk composition after preterm delivery with and without fortification. Matern Child Health J 2015;19(8):1657–61.

72. Fusch G, Kwan C, Rochow N, et al. Milk analysis using milk analyzers in a standardized setting (mamas) study: preliminary results. Abstracts der 112. Jahrestagung der Deutschen Gesellschaft für Kinder- und Jugendmedizin (DGKJ). Gemeinsam mit der 68. Jahrestagung der Deutschen Gesellschaft für Sozialpädiatrie (DGSPJ), 54. Herbsttagung der Deutschen Gesellschaft für Kinderchirurgie (DGKCH), 38. Jahrestagung des Berufsverbandes Kinderkrankenpflege Deutschland (BeKD) und 31. Jahrestagung der Gesellschaft für Pädiatrische Gastroenterologie und Ernährung (GPGE). Monatsschr Kinderheilkd 2016;164(3):276–7.

73. Choi A, Fusch G, Rochow N, et al. Establishment of micromethods for macronutrient contents analysis in breast milk. Matern Child Nutr 2015;11(4):761–72.

Index

Note: Page numbers of article titles are in **boldface** type.

A

AcuDairy Mid-Range Infrared instrument, 211–263
Adiponectin, 151–164
Advocacy, for lactation maintenance, 3
Alanine, 151–164
Albuminuria, 182–183, 186
Allergies, incidence of, 24, 28
Amino acids, 151–164
Antiadhesives, oligosaccharides as, 199
Antimicrobial proteins and peptides, 29–33
Antioxidants, 106–109
α_1-Antitrypsin, 184
Arachidonic acid supplements, **85–93**
Atopic diseases, incidence of, 24, 28

B

B cells, 27, 30, 33
Banked human milk, for preterm infants
    advantages of, 96–97, 109–110
    definition of, 131–132
    history of, 97–100
    labeling of, 110
    safety of, **131–149**
    treatment and quality of, **95–119**
"Bed side" milk analysis, **209–267**
Bile salt-stimulated lipase, 183, 186
Bioactive proteins, **179–191**
    assessment of, 181–182
    clinical trials of, 185–187
    digestion of, 179–181
    types of, 182–185
Body mass index, milk small molecules related to, 151–164
Body weight, measurement of, for milk consumption, 16–17
Bovine fortifiers, **173–178,** 185
Brain development. See Neurodevelopmental outcomes.
Breast milk. See Human milk.
Breast pumps, lactation maintenance and, 2–15
Bronchopulmonary dysplasia, 28, 124

Clin Perinatol 44 (2017) 269–274
http://dx.doi.org/10.1016/S0095-5108(16)30123-3
0095-5108/17

perinatology.theclinics.com

Moving?

Make sure your subscription moves with you!

To notify us of your new address, find your **Clinics Account Number** (located on your mailing label above your name), and contact customer service at:

Email: journalscustomerservice-usa@elsevier.com

800-654-2452 (subscribers in the U.S. & Canada)
314-447-8871 (subscribers outside of the U.S. & Canada)

Fax number: 314-447-8029

Elsevier Health Sciences Division
Subscription Customer Service
3251 Riverport Lane
Maryland Heights, MO 63043

*To ensure uninterrupted delivery of your subscription, please notify us at least 4 weeks in advance of move.

Printed and bound by CPI Group (UK) Ltd, Croydon, CR0 4YY

03/10/2024

01040391-0007